HORMONAL REGULATION OF SPERMATOGENESIS

CURRENT TOPICS IN MOLECULAR ENDOCRINOLOGY

Series Editors: Bert W. O'Malley and Anthony R. Means
Department of Cell Biology
Baylor College of Medicine
Houston, Texas

Volume 1:   *Hormone Binding and Target Cell Activation in the Testis*
Edited by Maria L. Dufau and Anthony R. Means

Volume 2:   *Hormonal Regulation of Spermatogenesis*
Edited by Frank S. French, Vidar Hansson,
E. Martin Ritzen, and Shihadeh N. Nayfeh

A Continuation Order Plan is available for this series. A continuation order will bring delivery of each new volume immediately upon publication. Volumes are billed only upon actual shipment. For further information please contact the publisher.

HORMONAL REGULATION OF SPERMATOGENESIS

Edited by

Frank S. French
University of North Carolina

Vidar Hansson
Rikshospitalet, Oslo, Norway

E. Martin Ritzen
Karolinska Sjukhuset, Stockholm, Sweden

and

Shihadeh N. Nayfeh
University of North Carolina

PLENUM PRESS·NEW YORK AND LONDON

Library of Congress Cataloging in Publication Data

Workshop on the Testis, 2d, Chapel Hill, N. C., 1975
   Hormonal regulation of spermatogenesis.

   (Current topics in molecular endocrinology; v. 2)
   Includes bibliographical references and index.
   1. Spermatogenesis in animals—Congresses. 2. Hormones, Sex—Congresses. I. French,
Frank S. II. Title. III. Series. [DNLM: 1. Spermatogenesis—Congresses. W1 CU82M v.
2/ WJ834 H812 1975]
QL966.W58 1975   599'.01'6   75-32541
ISBN 0-306-34002-X

Proceedings of the Second Annual Workshop on the Testis held
in Chapel Hill, North Carolina, April 2, 1975

© 1975 Plenum Press, New York
A Division of Plenum Publishing Corporation
227 West 17th Street, New York, N.Y. 10011

United Kingdom edition published by Plenum Press, London
A Division of Plenum Publishing Company, Ltd.
Davis House (4th Floor), 8 Scrubs Lane, Harlesden, London, NW10 6SE, England

Printed in the United States of America

Preface

The conference represented by this book was made possible
by support from NICHD and a planning committee headed by
Dr. Richard Sherins. Two general areas of research are included:
the first encompasses steroid hormone synthesis, metabolism and
transport in the testis; and the second relates to hormonal regulation of the seminiferous tubule with special emphasis on the control of Sertoli cell function. In addition, there are sections
on the purification of unique testicular proteins and morphological studies with particular emphasis on the Sertoli cell.

We would like to express our sincere thanks to Dr. Sherins
and his staff at NICHD and to all of the people at the
University of North Carolina who participated in the Conference
arrangements, to Dr. Judson J. Van Wyk, Chief of the Pediatric
Endocrinology Division, and Dr. H. Stanley Bennett, Director of
the Laboratories for Reproductive Biology. Our very special
thanks to Mrs. Carolyn Jaros for her help in handling the local
arrangements. Mrs. Martha Byrd and Mrs. Linda Rollins typed the
manuscripts. Miss Leslie Wells and Mr. Albert Smith kindly assisted
in proof reading, and Dr. Elizabeth Wilson gave much help with the
final editing process. To all of these people, we are most
grateful.

Frank S. French
Vidar Hansson
E. Martin Ritzen
Shihadeh N. Nayfeh

Contents

Purification of testicular proteins

Morphological studies on the seminiferous tubule

Steroid Synthesis and Metabolism: in Vitro Studies

DISTRIBUTION OF STEROIDS, STEROID PRODUCTION AND STEROID METABOLIZING ENZYMES IN RAT TESTIS

H.J. van der Molen, J.A. Grootegoed, M.J. de Greef-
Bijleveld, F.F.G. Rommerts and G.J. van der Vusse

Department of Biochemistry (Division of Chemical
Endocrinology)

Medical Faculty, Erasmus University Rotterdam,
Rotterdam, The Netherlands

INTRODUCTION

In the present paper some results are presented on:

1. the occurrence and age dependence of some enzyme activities
   in whole rat testis tissue as related to the development
   of spermatogenesis;
2. enzymes for steroid metabolism in isolated dissected rat
   testis tissue fractions with special emphasis on the age
   dependent variations of steroid 5α-reductase activity,
   and;
3. concentrations and production of steroids in isolated
   cellular and subcellular fractions of rat testis. These
   data are presented mainly to illustrate the limitation of
   results on enzyme activities, steroid concentrations and
   steroid production in total testis tissue and in isolated
   tissue fractions for the understanding of the regulation
   of specific processes in particular cell types, such as
   the regulation of spermatogenesis.

Nothing is known about the possible relationship between testicular steroids and the biochemical processes that are involved in
the development of spermatogenesis, although several studies in
the past 10-15 years have tried to correlate the presence and
activity of enzymes involved in steroid metabolism or the concentration of steroids in testis tissue with the known dependence of

3

spermatogenesis on testosterone (1-6). Part of the studies in the
developing testis have involved the relationship between the
appearance of spermatogenic cell types with age and the occurrence
of specific changes in testis parameters, such as enzyme activities
(7,8) or steroid concentrations (9). The observation of temporal
correlations between morphological and biochemical changes has
often been interpreted as the result of a mutually dependent development. We have compared in whole rat testis tissue the development of some enzyme activities which are not involved in steroid
metabolism with the activities of some steroid metabolizing enzymes
and the morphologic development of the testis and spermatogenesis.
For an organ consisting of several different cell types, as the
testis, such information for the whole organ, even if specific for
any individual cell type, does not permit conclusions about causal
relationships between different cell types. Therefore research
and discussion about biochemical changes in more defined cell
types of the developing testis was greatly stimulated when it was
found that relatively pure preparations of interstitial tissue and
seminiferous tubules could be isolated from whole testis tissue
(10). We have tried to study enzyme activities which can regulate
the levels of biologically active steroids in isolated dissected
testis tissue fractions. In addition to studies on 3β-hydroxy-
steroid dehydrogenase (11) and 20α-hydroxysteroid dehydrogenase
(12), we have been particularly interested in testicular steroid
5α-reductase activity. It has been known for a long time that rat
testis tissue can convert testosterone to 5α-reduced androstane
steroids (1-5), but the interest in these observations has in
recent years been stimulated by the observations that: 1. 5α-dihydro-
testosterone might be the biologically active steroid in androgen
dependent target tissues; 2. testosterone might have an effect on
certain steps in spermatogenesis (6): 3. testosterone can be converted by isolated spermatocyte fractions to 5α-dihydrotestosterone
(13-15). In light of the biological activity of 5α-dihydrotesto-
sterone and the ability of this steroid to interact with androgen
receptors in target tissues it was of interest to investigate whether
5α-dihydrotestosterone is an end-product of testosterone metabolism
or whether it only serves as an intermediate in a metabolic pathway
for conversion to other products, such as 5α-androstane-3, 17β-diols
(which in the prostate have a specific biological effect). Several
reports have now been published on the 5α-reductase activity in rat
testis, particularly on the cellular localization, the age of dependence and the possible control by LH (2-4, 18-22). We have
estimated and compared 5α-reductase activities in homogenates of
different testis tissue fractions of rats at different ages. The
in vivo significance of estimated enzyme activities in tissue
preparations in vitro depends greatly on the assay system used.
The finding of a specific enzyme activity, especially in tissue
homogenates, frequently reflects only the potential of the tissue
for a particular conversion.

Results from metabolic studies (incubation or superfusion) with intact tissues or cells using physiological substrate concentrations may more closely reflect the in vivo situation. Only estimation of endogenous steroid levels can reflect, however, the actual concentration of steroids. The presence of steroids in specific tissue compartments does not necessarily imply that these steroids are also produced in these tissue compartments. For the testis it has been demonstrated (16,17), that following administration of labeled testosterone, progesterone and pregnenolone these steroids will readily distribute between interstitial tissue and seminiferous tubules. In this respect we have studied not only the presence of steroids in cellular (and subcellular) fractions of the testis, but also the endogenous production of steroids by isolated testis tissue fractions (23,24), which might be a better parameter for the actual in vivo capacity of steroid production in different cell types. By correlating the development of spermatogenesis with the presence of steroids, the localization of steroid production and steroid metabolizing enzyme activities and other biochemical parameters in isolated cell types of the developing testis it is hoped. that more relevant information will be obtained, not only about the potential, but also about the actual relationships between steroid hormones and spermatogenesis.

METHODS

Male Wistar rats from the R-Amsterdam substrain were used for all experiments. Steroids and other chemicals were used as described previously (11,23-26). Testis tissue was dissected into interstitial tissue and seminiferous tubules using a wet dissection technique (25) essentially according to Christensen and Mason (10). Testosterone was estimated in tissue samples by radioimmunoassay (26) and pregnenolone was estimated using either gas-liquid chromatography or radioimmunoassay (24). The in vitro production of steroids from endogenous substrates in tissue homogenates (testosterone) or in isolated mitochondrial fractions (pregnenolone) was calculated from the difference in the amounts of steroid present in the incubation mixture after 1 h and at zero time (24). The following enzyme activities were estimated as described previously: 3β hydroxysteroid dehydrogenase (11), steroid sulfatase (11), 20α-hydroxysteroid dehydrogenase (12), carboxyl esterase (25), lactate dehydrogenase (24), monoamine oxidase (24) and cytochrome c oxidase (24). For the estimation of β-glucuronidase a modification of the method of Talalay et. al. (27) was used; this involved the measurement of the rate of phenolphtalein formation from phenolphtalein glucuronide. The activity of γ-glutamyl transpeptidase was measured according to Szasz (28).

The steroid 5α-reductase activity was estimated after incubation at 37°C for 15 min of ^{3}H-testosterone (25 nmol) with homogenized tissue fractions (2 mg protein) in the presence of an
NADPH-generating system (total incubation volume 1.0 ml). After
isolation and separation of the steroid products 5α--reductase
activity was expressed as the rate of formation (pmol/min/mg protein) of the sum of 5α-androstane-3, 17β-diols (DIOL), 5α-dihydro-
testosterone (DHT), 5α-androsterone and 5α-androstanedione. These
assay conditions were strictly standardized, because the estimated
enzyme activity appeared to depend on the amount of tissue and
substrate used, and the formation of the relative amounts of the
quantitatively most important metabolites, DIOL, varied with the
duration of incubation. The formation of DHT increased during the
first 15 min of incubation, but showed a significant decrease
thereafter, whereas the formation of DIOL increased almost linearly
during the first 30 min of incubation.

RESULTS AND DISCUSSION

Effect of Age on Some Enzyme Activities in Rat Testis

In a first attempt to correlate enzyme activities with specific cell types in testis tissue it was tried to correlate the age
dependence of non-steroidal enzyme activities (as markers for specific cell types during development of spermatogenesis) with 5α--re-
ductase activity using whole testis tissue. The decrease of β-
glucuronidase activity (Fig. 1) as described by Males et. al. (7),
was used as a potential marker for the development of spermatocytes and γ-glutamyltranspeptidase (Fig. 2) as a marker for
Sertoli cell development. It appears that the age-dependence of
5α-reductase activity in whole testis tissue (Fig. 3 and 4) does
not correspond with the pattern of either of these two enzymes.
The results for β-glucuronidase are in agreement with those of
Males et. al. (7), showing a high specific activity in the immature
rat which decreased during further development (Fig. 2) Males
et. al. (7) have suggested that the change in activity of this
lysosomal enzyme, having detectable activity only in Sertoli cells
and spermatogonia, reflects the increase of testis tissue through
the development of the spermatocytes. The specific activity of
γ-glutamyltranspeptidase (GTP) increased during the development of
the immature rat reaching a plateau on day 28. Hodgen et. al. (8)
made similar observations. In their experiments GTP activity increased between day 15 and 20 and there was no further increase
after day 20. The rapid increase in the specific activity of GTP
between day 15 and 20 coincides with the cessation of Sertoli cell
division and maturation and it has been suggested that GTP might be

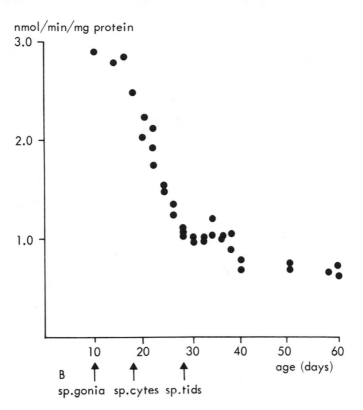

Figure 1. The development of β-glucuronidase activity in rat testis tissue.

used as a marker for Sertoli cell development. In our experiments GTP activity increased up to day 28. However, in the Holtzman rate used by Hodgen et al (0), Golgi phase spermatids were the most advanced germ cell type at day 25 and in the rats which were used for the present experiments stage I spermatids appeared around day 28. The specific activities of β-glucuronidase and GTP reached a maximum on day 28-30. During this time the first pachytene spermatocytes finish meiose I and II and give rise to the first spermatids. The increase in testis weight is almost linear during this period. Therefore the change in enzyme activities at day 28 can be related

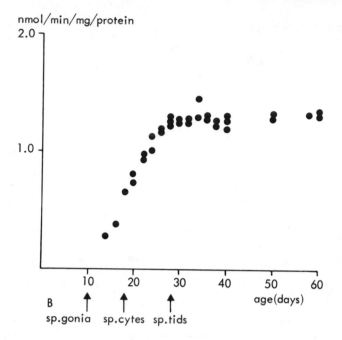

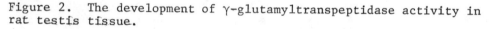

Figure 2.   The development of γ-glutamyltranspeptidase activity in rat testis tissue.

to a change in the enzyme profile of some cell types and/or it may result from a change in the number of different cell types in the germinal epithelium.

From Fig. 3 and 4 it appears that the amount of testosterone metabolized by whole testis tissue or by isolated interstitial tissue or seminiferous tubules depended on the age of the animals. In agreement with observations in the literature the most active conversion occurred in tissues from 30-40 day old animals.   The main metabolites were always androstanediol (s), DHT and andro-stenedione.   In the young animals androstanediols were produced in much larger amounts than any of the other metabolites.   The highest specific activities of the 5α-reductase were found in testis tissue of rats between 20 and 40 days of age.   The specific activities in testes of animals of 60-90 days were at least 10-20 times lower than the specific activities found in animals of 30-40

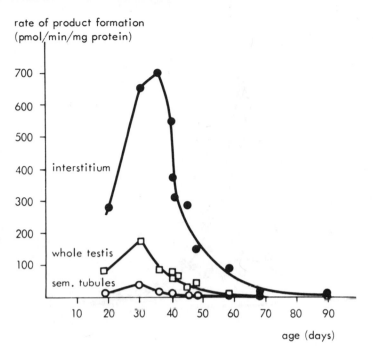

Figure 3. The effect of age on steroid 5α-reductase activity in whole testis tissue, interstitial tissue and seminiferous tubules of rat testis.

days. These results might reflect that the 5α-reductase is mainly present in cell types that do not further increase after day 30-40 (i.e. Leydig cells or Sertoli cells) and that the decrease in specific activity reflects the development of other testis cell types lacking 5α-reductase activity. Another explanation may be, that the change in 5α-reductase activity reflects a decrease in the enzyme activity of one specific cell type.

Localization and Activity of Enzymes in Isolated Testis Tissue Compartments

The localization and activities of steroid metabolizing enzymes in different testis tissue compartments may give an impression

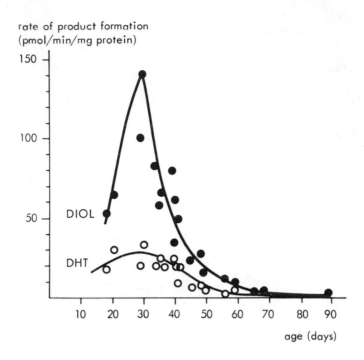

Figure 4.   The rate of formation of 5α-dihydrotestosterone (DHT) and 5α-androstane-3α, 17β-diol (DIOL) during incubation of whole rat testis tissue with testosterone.

about the potential of the different cell types for steroid meta-bolism.   It is important, however, to use well-defined tissue pre-parations and to prevent the possible destruction or artifactual cross-contamination of isolated tissue preparations.   In our initial attempts to study the metabolism of testosterone by isolated germ cell fractions we used the method described by Yamada et. al. (13) for the isolation of seminiferous tubules from immature rat testis. The testes after removal of the capsules were incubated for 30 min at 37°C in a buffer containing 0.1% collagenase.   Subsequently the unravelled seminiferous tubules were collected, washed with phosphate buffer and centrifuged, and the pellet was used as the seminiferous tubules fraction.   The supernatant obtained after removal of the un-ravelled tubules was centrifuged, and the pellet after washing with phosphate buffer was used as the interstitial tissue fraction.   From the results in Table 1 it appears, however, that metabolism of testo-sterone by such fractions isolated after collagenase treatment was

TABLE 1

Metabolism of Testosterone by Testis Tissue Prepara-
tions of a 34 Day Old Rat. Isolated Interstitial
Tissue and Seminiferous Tubules were Prepared Either
Following Collagenase Treatment (13) or Using a Wet
Dissection Technique (10,25)

	Rate of Product Formation (pmole/min. mg protein)			Carboxyl esterase pmole/min mg protein
	DHT	DIOL	$\Delta^{4\dagger}$	
WET DISSECTION				
Whole testis	20	65	5	0.15
Interstitial tissue	80	620	10	0.90
Seminiferous tubules	7	4	0	0.10
COLLAGENASE TREATMENT				
Whole testis	21	82	3	0.10
Interstitial tissue	20	11	31	0.08
Seminiferous tubules	35	120	24	0.15

$\dagger\Delta^4$ = 4-androstene – 3,17-dione

quite different from results obtained with dissected tissue
fractions. In "interstitial tissue" of 34 day old rats the 5α-
reductase activity, and the ensuing conversion to DHT and DIOL,
was much lower than in control experiments with dissected tissue
fractions (cf. Fig. 5 and 6). After collagenase treatment the 5α-
reductase activity was decreased, whereas much more 4-androstenedione
was produced. In contrast the conversion of testosterone by
"seminiferous tubules" resulted in much higher conversions than
expected. The distribution of the carboxyl esterase activity, which
has previously been used as a marker for interstitial tissue (25),
suggests that the "seminiferous tubules" were probably highly con
taminated with interstitial tissue.

Based on these results all further studies were done with
isolated interstitial tissue and seminiferous tubules obtained by
wet dissection (10,25). Using such dissected and washed testis
tissue fractions (25) we have studied in some detail the localization and distribution of 3β-hydroxysteroid dehydrogenase, 5α-re-
ductase (including 3α/β-hydroxysteroid dehydrogenase) and 20α-
hydroxysteroid dehydrogenase activities.

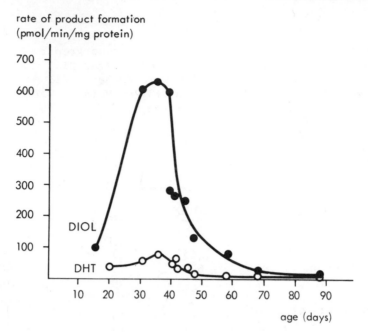

Figure 5. The rate of formation of 5α-dihydrotestosterone (DHT) and 5α-androstane-3α, 17β-diol (DIOL) during incubation of isolated rat testis interstitial tissue with testosterone.

3β-Hydroxysteroid Dehydrogenase

The results (see Table 2) of specific activities of 3β-hydroxy-steroid dehydrogenase in homogenates of different testis tissue preparations, clearly show that most of this enzyme activity is located in the interstitial tissue compartment. In further studies (11) concerning the subcellular distribution of this enzyme, it was found that most of the 3β-hydroxysteroid dehydrogenase activity in homogenates of total testis tissue could be isolated in microsomal fractions, whereas only 7-15% was isolated in mitochondrial fractions.

5α-Reductase

The specific activity of 5α-reductase in isolated interstitial tissue was much higher than the specific activities in total testis

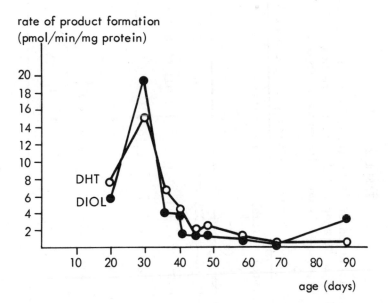

Figure 6. The rate of formation of 5α–dihydrotestosterone (DHT) and 5α–androstane–3α,17β–diol (DIOL) during incubation of isolated rat testis seminiferous tubules with testosterone.

TABLE 2

Intercellular Distribution of 3β-hydroxysteroid Dehydrogenae and Other
Enzymes in Rat Testis Tissues. All Results are Mean Values (±s.d.) of
at Least 4 Independent Experiments

Enzyme	Enzyme activity (mU/mg protein)			Ratio b/c
	Total testis tissue (a)	Interstitial tissue (b)	Seminiferous tubules (c)	
3β-SDH	0.140 ± 0.025	1.030 ± 0.140	0.008 ± 0.002	129
Steroid sulfatase	0.019 ± 0.003	0.056 ± 0.011	0.016 ± 0.003	3.1
Carboxyl esterase	280 ± 90	1250 ± 50	60 ± 9	20.8
Cytochrome c oxidase	155 ± 55	206 ± 71	182 ± 97	1.1
Lactate dehydrogenase	550 ± 110	170 ± 80	560 ± 100	0.3
Monoamine oxidase	0.84 ± 0.15	3.02 ± 1.15	0.82 ± 0.15	3.7

3β-SDH = 3β-hydroxysteroid dehydrogenase

or seminiferous tubules (Fig. 3). This is particularly clear for
testis tissue from the younger animals. For animals from 30-40 days
the ratio of specific activities in interstitial tissue to seminiferous tubules was in the order of 10-20. Assuming that whole
testis of young rats contains at least 10% interstitial tissue, this
would indicate that in 30-40 day old rats the interstitial tissue
would contribute in the order of 50-70% of the total 5α-reductase
activity in whole testis tissue. From these observations it is
also evident, that contamination of isolated seminiferous tubules
with a small amount of interstitial tissue, would significantly
increase the 5α-reductase activity. This may well explain the
close correlation between the age dependency of 5α-reductase activities in isolated interstitial tissue and seminiferous tubules.
It is not clear at the moment which factor(s) might cause the changes
of 5α-reductase activity in interstitial tissue with changes of age.
Under the conditions used for the present experiments the amount
of DIOL formed by homogenates of whole testis tissue (Fig. 4) and
of isolated interstitial tissue (Fig. 5) was for the younger animals
5-10 times higher than the amount of DHT formed. This difference
disappeared with increasing age of the animals. For isolated seminiferous tubules the accuracy of estimating the small conversion was
rather low, and the amounts of DHT and DIOL produced appeared to
be rather similar for animals of all ages (Fig. 6). The ratio of
DIOL/DHT formed in incubations with interstitial tissue, in the
order of 5-10, versus a ratio in the order of 1-1.5 for seminiferous tubules might reflect, that the specific activity of 3α-
hydroxysteroid dehydrogenase is higher in interstitial tissue than
in seminiferous tubules. Dorrington and Fritz in studies with
isolated intact cells have shown, that 5α-reductase activity is
present in Sertoli cells and spermatocytes but not in spermatids.
This might indicate that the higher specific activity in tubules
from immature rats reflects the higher proportion of Sertoli cells
and spermatocytes in these preparations, whereas the lower specific
activity in adult tubules might be caused by the high proportion
of inactive spermatids. The specific activity of 3α-hydroxysteroid
dehydrogenase for conversion of DHT to DIOL, according to Dorrington
and Fritz, is much higher in Sertoli cells than in spermatocytes.

20α-Hydroxysteroid Dehydrogenase

From the results in Table 3 it appears that 20α dehydrogenase
is mainly located in the seminiferous tubules. A calculation of
the enzyme activity per total testis on the basis of these results
would indicate that 97% of the 20α-hydroxysteroid dehydrogenase is
of tubular origin. These observations are in accordance with the
results reported by Lacy and Pettitt (30) and Bell et al. (31) who
also observed 20α-hydroxysteroid dehydrogenase activity in isolated
seminiferous tubules, although they did not quantitatively compare
the activity in tubules with the activity in interstitial tissue.

TABLE 3

Intercellular Distribution and Relative Specific
Activities of 20α-Hydroxysteroid Dehydrogenase
Between Rat Testis Tissues

	Carboxyl esterase (μmole/min. mg protein)	20α-SDH* pmole/min. mg prot.	nmole/min. testis
Seminiferous tubules	0.018	39	3.6
Interstitial tissue	0.86	8	0.2

*20α-SDH = 20α-hydroxysteroid dehydrogenase

Due to the lack of a specific marker for cells in seminiferous
tubules it was impossible to calculate the extent of contamination
of isolated interstitial tissue with cellular material from tubular
origin. Therefore it is not possible to conclude definitely from
the present results whether the small activity in isolated interstitial tissue reflects either true endogenous enzyme or is the
result of contamination with a small amount of tubular material.
If 20α-hydroxysteroid dehydrogenase activity would be quantitatively
significant under in vivo conditions, this enzyme could metabolize
C-21 steroids which would then be unavailable for conversion to C-19
steroids (including testosterone).

Endogenous Concentrations and Production of Steroids in
Cellular and Subcellular Fractions of Rat Testis

Concentrations and productions of endogenous steroids rather
than enzyme activities involved in steroid metabolism should give
a much better reflection of the actual in vivo presence of steroid.
The results in Table 4 reflect that concentrations of testosterone
in total homogenates and of pregnenolone in isolated mitochondrial
fractions are higher in interstitial tissue preparations than in
preparations from isolated seminiferous tubules. It is not certain
to which extent the low levels found in seminiferous tubules, which
are in agreement with previous observations (32), reflect contamination from interstitial tissue due to the dissection procedure.

The concentrations of testosterone in homogenates of whole
testis, interstitial tissue and seminiferous tubules were significantly increased with factors of 6.1, 3.7 and 3.2 respectively

TABLE 4

Concentrations of Testosterone in Testis Tissue Homogenates and of Pregnenolone
in Mitochondrial Fractions of Testis Tissue from Normal Adult Rats (Control) and
from Rats which had Received 100 I.U. (HCG) Subcutaneously Each Day for 5 Days (HCG)
Mean Values ± s.d.

	Testosterone (pmole/mg protein)		Pregnenolone (pmole/mg mitochondr. prot.)	
	control	HCG	control	HCG
Whole testis	6.2 ± 2.8	38.4 ± 14.5(4)*	29.3 ± 1.7	45.7 ± 11.0(6)
Interstitial tissue$^\phi$	18.8 ± 11.3	68.8 ± 17.3(5)	37.0 ± 15.1	115.0 ± 77.0 (6)
Seminiferous tubules$^\phi$	5.1 ± 2.9	16.4 ± 2.2(5)	1.3 ± 0.8	5.1 ± 2.5(6)

ϕ Values not corrected for losses of protein during dissection
* Number of determinations in parenthesis

(P < 0.05, P < 0.025 and P < 0.025) after HCG treatment. Pregnenolone concentrations in isolated mitochondrial fractions from whole
testis tissue, interstitial tissue and seminiferous tubules were
likewise increased with factors of 1.6, 3.1 and 3.9 respectively
(P < 0.05, P < 0.10 and P < 0.05).

The differences between steroid concentrations in isolated
seminiferous tubules and isolated interstitial tissue might reflect that steroids originate mainly from the interstitial tissue,
but it cannot be excluded that dissection of the whole testis
tissue causes a translocation of steroids between the different cell
types. Therefore endogenous production of steroids by the isolated
tissue compartments might give a better impression about the localization of steriod production. It appears from the results in
Tables 5 and 6 that the in vitro production of steroids in interstitial tissue preparations is much higher than the production in
preparations of seminiferous tubules.

Assuming that 10% of rat testis protein is present in the interstitial compartment, it can be concluded that for these in vitro
experiments the contribution of interstitial testosterone production
to the production in whole testis tissue is approximately 98%. With
respect to seminiferous tubules the testosterone production in homogenates and pregnenolone production in isolated mitochondrial
fractions was very small. It cannot be excluded that cell type(s) in
the spermatogenic compartment of the testis produce this small amount
of steroid, but on the other hand this apparent tubular production
may well reflect contamination with material from the interstitial
tissue.

Prolonged treatment of intact rats with HCG results in increased
testosterone production from endogenous substrates in homogenates
of whole testis tissue. Testosterone production in homogenates of
interstitial tissue, expressed either per mg interstitial tissue
or per amount of interstitial tissue obtained from two testes was
significantly increased with factors of 2.0 and 2.4 respectively
(P < 0.05 and P < 0.05), whereas no significant increase was observed in incubations with material from seminiferous tubules. No
corrections were made for losses of material during the dissection
procedure and therefore the sum of the testosterone production in
homogenates of interstitial tissue and seminiferous tubules is lower
than the production in preparation of whole, undissected tissue.
The in vitro results with isolated interstitial tissue preparations
indicate that the increased testicular steroid production is caused
by stimulation of the steroid production in the interstitial compartment. In that respect the present results are compatible with results
concerning in vitro stimulation by LH of testosterone biosynthesis
in isolated interstitial tissue and seminiferous tubules obtained from
hypophysectomized rats (3). HCG treatment resulted in a 2-3 times

TABLE 5

Production (pmole/mg protein h) of Testosterone and Pregnenolone in vitro by Testis Tissue Preparations Obtained from Normal Adult Rats (Control) and from Rats which had Received 100 I.U. HCG Subcutaneously Each Day for 5 Days (HCG) Mean Values ± s. d.

Tissue	Testosterone production by total homogenates (pmole/mg protein h)		Pregnenolone production by isolated mitochondria (pmole/mg protein h)	
	control	HCG	control	HCG
Whole testis	112 ± 47	267 ± 44(4)*	580 ± 165	1420 ± 390(5)
Interstitial tissue	1041 ± 228	2031 ± 628(5)	2665 ± 1000	7050 ± 2850(5)
Seminiferous tubules	2 ± 2	7 ± 5(5)	17 ± 15	37 ± 21(6)

* Number of determinations in parenthesis.

TABLE 6

Production of Testosterone and Pregnenolone In Vitro by Rat Testis Tissue Preparations (Expressed as nmol/2 Testes, h.). Testosterone Productions were Calculated From Experiments With Whole Tissue Homogenates. Pregnenolone Productions Were Calculated From Experiments With Isolated Mitochondrial Fractions. Values (Means ± S.D.) Were Not Corrected For Losses of Tissue During Dissection.

Tissue	Testosterone production		Pregnenolone production	
	control	HCG	control	HCG
Whole Testis	23.7 ± 9.6	60.2 ± 15.7(4)*	16.0 ± 4.5	38.3 ± 6.9(5)
Interstitial Tissue	13.6 ± 3.1	33.1 ± 3.8(5)	6.1 ± 3.5	20.7 ± 6.9(5)
Seminiferous Tubules	0.20 ± 0.18	0.57 ± 0.49(5)	0.16 ± 0.13	0.32 ± 0.12(6)

*Number of determinations in parenthesis.

higher pregnenolone production from endogenous precursors in testicular mitochondrial fractions in fractions, obtained from whole testis tissue as well as from isolated interstitial tissue. This observation strongly suggests that the enhanced androgen biosynthesis may be caused by stimulation of the mitochondrial pregnenolone production in the interstitial tissue.

CONCLUSIONS

Our results concerning the distribution of 5α-reductase activity and the distribution of DHT and DIOL formation between interstitial tissue and seminiferous tubules are in agreement with those of several other groups (13-15,18-21), with the exception of the results by Rivarola and Podesta (18) who reported a much larger conversion of T to DIOL and DHT in tubules than in interstitial tissue.

The present results of endogenous steroid levels and production are in agreement with the general accepted belief that most, if not all, of the testicular steroid production results from interstitial tissue production. It has been reported (16,17) that exogenous radioactive steroids are rapidly and equally distributed across all cell types of the rat testis. In light of these observations it would appear that the origin of endogenous testicular steroids is of little importance for the actual presence of endogenous steroids in different cell types. Nevertheless the results of endogenous concentrations reflect a much higher concentration of testosterone in interstitial tissue than in seminiferous tubules. It remains to be resolved, therefore, which processes or barriers might restrict the free diffusion of testosterone and other steroids across the testis. The presence of a specific androgen binding protein (ABP) (34,35) and a specific androgen receptor (36,37) in seminiferous tubules, but not in interstitial tissue, might even suggest a possibility for specific localization of androgens in seminiferous tubules. In this respect the recent results from Podesta and Rivarola (9) further indicate that in the developing rat, testis DIOL and DHT might be present only in seminiferous tubules, but not in interstitial tissue where they found only T. Such a distribution pattern of endogenous steroids is rather surprising, because on basis of the distribution of enzyme activities it would be expected that the interstitial tissue has the capacity to produce DHT and DIOL. Therefore these results could reflect a specific binding of DIOL and DHT by the seminiferous tubules. Future results of specific activity estimations in isolated tissue fractions after administration of radioactive steroids and measuring radioactive as well as endogenous steroids, might yield information on the metabolism as well as the production and possible intercellular transport of testicular steroids.

REFERENCES

1. Stylianou, M., Forchielli, E. and Dorfman, R.F., J. Biol. Chem. 236: 1318, 1961.

2. Nayfeh, S.N., Barefoot, S.E. Jr., and Baggett, B., Endocrinology 78: 1041, 1966.

3. Inano, H., and Tamaoki, B., Endocrinology 79: 579, 1966.

4. Inano, H., Hori, Y., and Tamaoki, B.F., CIBA Found. Colloq. Endocrinol. 16: 105, 1967.

5. Ficher, M., and Steinberger, E., Steroids 12: 491, 1968.

6. Steinberger, E., Physiol. Rev. 51: 1, 1971.

7. Males, J.L., and Turkington, R.W., Endocrinology 88: 579, 1971.

8. Hodgen, G.D., and Sherins, R.J., Endocrinology 93: 985, 1973.

9. Podesta, E.J. and Rivarola, M.A., Endocrinology 95: 455, 1974.

10. Christensen, A.S., and Mason, N.R., Endocrinology 76: 646, 1965.

11. Van der Vusse, G.J., Kalkman, M.L., and Van der Molen, H.J., Biochim. Biophys. Acta 348: 404, 1974.

12. De Bruijn, H.W.A. and Van der Molen, H.J., J. Endocr. 61: 401, 1974.

13. Yamada, M., Yasue, S., and Matsumoto, K., Acta Endocr. (Kbh) 71: 393, 1972.

14. Matsumoto, K., and Yamada, M., Endocrinology 93: 253, 1973.

15. Dorrington, J.H., and Fritz, I.B. Biochem, Biophys. Res. Comm. 54: 1425, 1973.

16. Parvinen, M., Hurme, P., and Niemi, P., Endocrinology 87: 1082, 1970.

17. Van Doorn, L.G., De Bruijn, H.W.A., Galjaard, H. and Van der Molen, H.J., Biol. Reprod. 10: 47, 1974.

18. Rivarola, M.A., and Podesta, E.J., Endocrinology 90: 618, 1972.

19. Folman, Y., Sowell, J.G., and Eik-Nes, K.B., Endocrinology 91: 702, 1972.

20. Folman, Y., Ahmad, N., Sowell, J.G., and Eik-Nes, K.B , Endocrinology 92: 41, 1973.

21. Moger, W.H., and Armstrong, D.T., Can. J. Biochem. 52: 744, 1974.

22. Lloret, A.P., and Weisz, J., Endocrinology 95: 1306, 1974.

23. Van der Vusse, G.J., Kalkman, M.L., and Van der Molen, H.J., Biochim. Biophys. Acta 297: 179, 1973.

24. Van der Vusse, G.J., Kalkman, M.L., and Van der Molen, H.J., Biochim. Biophys. Acta 000: 000, 1975.

25. Rommerts, F.F.G., Van Doorn, L.G., Galjaard, H., Cooke, B.A., and Van der Molen, H.J., J. Histochem. Cytochem. 21: 572, 1973.

26. Verjans, H.L., Cooke, B.A., De Jong, F.H., De Jong, C.C.M., and Van der Molen, H.J., J. Steroid Biochem. 4: 665, 1973.

27. Talalay, P., Fishman, W.H., and Huggins, C., J. Biol. Chem. 166: 757, 1946.

28. Szasz, G., Clin. Chem. 15: 124, 1969.

29. Wroblewski, F., and LaDue, J.S., Proc. Soc. Exp. Biol. Med. 90: 210, 1955.

30. Lacy, D., and Pettitt, A.J., Brit. Med. Bull. 26: 87, 1970.

31. Bell, J.G., Vinson, G.P., and Lacy D., Proc. Roy. Soc. London 176: 433, 1971.

32. Cooke, B.A., De Jong, F.H., Van der Molen, H.J., and Rommerts, F.F.G., Nature 237: 255, 1972.

33. Cooke, B.A., Rommerts, F.F.G., Van der Kemp, J.W.C.M., and Van der Molen, H.J., Mol. Cell Endocrin. 1: 99, 1974.

34. Hansson, V., Reusch, E., Trygstad, O., Torgersen, O., Ritzen, E.M. and French, F.S., Nature New Biol. 246: 56, 1973.

35. Vernon, R.G., Kopec, B. and Fritz, I.B., Mol. Cell. Endocrinol. 1: 167, 1974.

36. Hansson, V., McLean, W.S., Smith, A.A., Tindall, D.J., Weddington, S.C., Nayfeh, S.N., French, F.S. and Ritzen, E.M., Steroids 23: 823, 1974.

37. Mulder, E., Peters, M.J., De Vries, J., and Van der Molen, H.J., Mol. Cell. Endocrinol. 2: 171, 1975.

ANDROGEN METABOLISM IN THE SEMINIFEROUS TUBULE

M.A. Rivarola, E.J. Podesta, H.E. Chemes and
S. Cigorraga

Centro de Investigaciones Endocrinologicas,
Hospital de Ninos, Buenos Aires, Argentina

FSH, LH and androgens are involved in the hormonal control of spermatogenesis. While FSH acts directly on the seminiferous tubules, LH seems to exert its action by stimulating testosterone production by Leydig cells. This concept has been supported by the finding of specific binding of FSH in tubular cells (1) and of LH in the membranes of Leydig cells (2). Testosterone can cross the "blood testis barrier" and presumably enter the tubules through the Sertoli cells (3). It is also possible that precursors of testosterone produced by Leydig cells are transported into the tubules and converted to testosterone and its reduced derivatives, since it has been found that seminiferous tubules can convert pregnenolone into testosterone in vitro (4).

The germinal epithelium of the mature rat undergoes a continuing process of cellular differentiation and proliferation from spermatogonia to spermatozoa. It is not yet clear which steps of spermatogenesis are controlled by androgens. However, it has been postulated that androgens act on the formation of type A spermatogonia and also during the meiotic division (5). Androgens may act directly on proliferating germ cells or indirectly via Sertoli cells. The seminiferous tubules are localized in close proximity to the Leydig cells and are exposed to high concentrations of testosterone. It seems that the androgen-responsive cells of the seminiferous tubules need more androgen for their normal function than the cells of the prostate, seminal vesicles or other target organs (6), with the possible exception of the epididymis. In the present work, we have carried out studies on the metabolism of androgens in the seminiferous tubules with particular attention to the formation of the 5α-reduced derivatives of testosterone at different stages of sexual development.

25

TESTOSTERONE REDUCING ACTIVITY IN RAT SEMINIFEROUS TUBULES AT THE
TIME OF THE FIRST MEIOTIC DIVISION

Some years ago we became interested in studying whether or not
reduction of testosterone (T) to 5α–dihydrotestosterone (DHT) might
occur in the seminiferous tubules. For this purpose, we incubated
isolated seminiferous tubules and interstitial tissue of mature rats
with ³H–T as substrate (7). The time course of the accumulation of
radioactivity as T, DHT, 5α–androstane–3α, 17β–diol (3α–DIOL) and
androst–4–ene–3, 17–dione (androstenedione) was determined. In the
tubules, 3α–DIOL emerged as the main metabolite with only little
formation of DHT. On the contrary, in the interstitial tissue
fraction, no reduced products were observed and androstenedione was
the main metabolite formed. Since 3α–DIOL had been found by other
investigators (8) to be the main metabolite of T in preparations of
whole testis of maturing rats, we speculated that these authors could

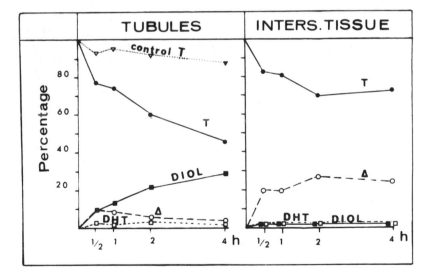

Figure 1.   Time–course of the percentage of total radioactivity in
T, DHT, 3α–DIOL and androstenedione (Δ) after incubation of 60–
day–old rat seminiferous tubules and interstitial tissue with T–¹⁴C.
Incubation were carried out at 31°C without addition of NADPH.

have been measuring at least in part, 5α-reductase of the seminiferous tubules. We then incubated isolated tubules and interstitial
tissue of 20-day-old rats (9). As illustrated in Fig. 2, both the
rate of T utilization and 3α-DIOL formation in the seminiferous
tubules of immature rats was much faster than that of mature animals.
Furthermore, the interstitial tissue fraction did not show any formation of androstenedione as previously shown in the mature rats.

We then proceeded to study the formation of 3α-DIOL by seminiferous tubules from birth to maturity. Since separation of tubules
from surrounding tissue is very difficult during the first two
weeks of life, studies were carried out in preparations of whole
testis in these very young rats. In rats 14 days or older, however,
studies were carried out in isolated seminiferous tubules. In
Fig. 3, we have plotted percentage of radioactivity in 3α-DIOL in
incubations of seminiferous tubules at different ages. 5α-reductase
activity became evident around the 12th day of life and increased
rapidly during the following week. In 2-hour-incubations, the
formation of 3α-DIOL was lower in 45-day-old animals and decreased
even further in the mature testis to remain low in 1-year-old rats.

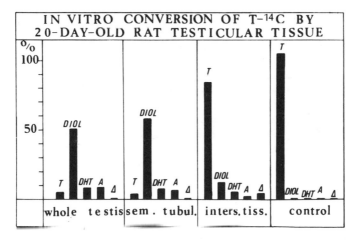

Figure 2. Percentage distribution of radioactivity in 20-day-old
rat whole testis, seminferous tubules and interstitial tissue after
3 hours of incubation with T-^{14}C at 31°C without addition of NADPH.
T: testosterone, DIOL: 5α-androstan 3α, 17β – diol, DHT: dihydrotestosterone, A: androsterone, Δ: androstenedione.

Histological studies were carried out in the testis of these developing rats. After the 10th day of life, seminiferous tubules
of maturing rats started showing a very active process of cellular
differentiation and multiplication. The first histological changes
in the nuclei of resting primary spermatocytes indicating the onset of meiosis were seen between the 10th and 12th day of life.
From days 14 to 20 there was a progressive development of meiosis.
First zygotene and pachytene spermatocytes were observed on day 16.
By day 20, meiosis was already well developed except for the absence of diplotene spermatocytes. Meiosis was completed in the
26-day-old rat. These changes coincided with a gradual and progressive increase in the formation of 3α-DIOL from T by the tubules
(Fig. 3). Full spermatogenesis was reached by day 60, at the time
when formation of 3α-DIOL had decreased. From these studies, we
proposed that 3α-DIOL might be involved in the stimulation of the
first meiotic division.

CONCENTRATION OF T, DHT AND 3α-DIOL IN RAT WHOLE TESTIS, SEMINIFEROUS
    TUBULES AND INTERSTITIAL TISSUE DURING SEXUAL DEVELOPMENT

     We have measured the content of T, DHT and 3α-DIOL in whole
testis, interstitial tissue and seminiferous tubules of rats at
different stages of sexual development in order to see if our in
vitro studies would correlate with this in vivo approach. Androgens
were determined by a competitive binding technique after purification
by thin layer chromatography (10). Values were confirmed in a selected group of samples by gas-liquid chromatography. In Fig. 4,
we have plotted the concentrations of T, DHT and 3α-DIOL in interstitial tissue and seminiferous tubules at different ages. Values
are expressed as ng per 100 mg proteins. In the interstitial tissue,
T reached values between 3000 and 4000 at sexual maturation, probably higher than any other tissue. DHT and 3α-DIOL could not be
detected in this tissue. In the seminiferous tubules, there was a
marked increment in the concentrations of T in 20-day-old rats that
decreased by day 26. Since then and up to sexual maturation there
was a marked increase in T with a decline of unknown significance
from 60 to 90 days. There was no early peak in DHT concentrations
in the seminiferous tubules, but after 50 days of age, at the time
of maturation of the first spermatozoa, DHT concentrations increased
markedly and were equal to T in the 90-day-old rats. 3α-DIOL concentrations in the seminiferous tubules increased at the same time
as T, from 10 to 20 days, but remained high also at 26 days of age
after which it decreased steadily and remained low after sexual
maturation. Therefore, at age 26 days, when meiosis is completed,
3α-DIOL was the androgen present in the highest amounts concentration in the seminiferous tubules. In tubules of sexually mature
rats, however, T and DHT were the major androgens.

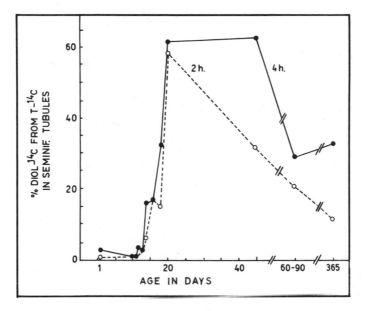

Figure 3. Percentage radioactivity in 3α-DIOL after incubating rat seminiferous tubules with T-^{14}C, from birth to maturity. Dotted line, 2 hours of incubation; full line, 4 hours.

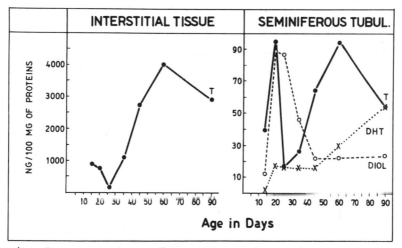

Figure 4. Concentrations of T, DHT and 3α-DIOL in rat interstitial tissue and seminiferous tubules during development and at maturation. DHT and 3α-DIOL were undetectable in the interstitial tissue.

Determination of T, DHT and 3α-DIOL by Gas-liquid Chromatography

The values for androgens obtained by the competitive binding technique were checked by gas-liquid chromatography. The purification of the androgens metabolites included one TLC on precoated silica-gel sheets, formation of pentafluorobenzoate derivatives (11) and a second TLC using the system of solvents benzene: actetone (140:7, v/v) for the monoderivatives of T and DHT and benzene: hexane (1:1, v/v) for the dipentafluorobenzoate of 3α-DIOL. Results obtained by gas chromatography were in good agreement with those measured by protein binding. A gas chromatography tracing of 3α-DIOL dipentafluorobenzoate obtained from seminiferous tubules of 20-day-old rats is shown in Fig. 5. A clear peak with a retention time corresponding to the 3α-DIOL derivative was present. This peak was absent in a similar sample obtained from interstitial tissue of the same rats, as well as in control blanks without tissue.

Ratios of 3α-DIOL/T in Interstitial Tissue and Seminiferous Tubules

3α-DIOL could not be detected in the interstitial tissue at any age while it was present in the corresponding tubular tissue in relatively greater amounts. Figure 6 shows the 3α-DIOL/T ratios in interstitial tissue and seminiferous tubules. In the interstitial tissue of the 20-day-old rat, as inferred by the sensitivity of the method, there was less than 0.1 ng per testis of 3α-DIOL. Using this value, the 3α-DIOL/T ratio was 35 times lower in the interstitial tissue than in the seminiferous tubules. The marked difference in these ratios confirm that, technically, the separation of seminiferous tubules from surrounding tissue was satisfactory.

Concentrations of T, DHT and 3α-DIOL in Testis of 26-Day-Old Rats Treated with a Combination of Estradiol Benzoate (E_2B) Plus Either T, DHT or 3α-DIOL

Rats were treated from the 5th to the 25th day of life with either vehicle, E_2B (5 µg/10 g body weight per day), E_2B plus T (1.5 mg/100 g body weight per day), E_2B plus DHT (same dose) or E_2B plus 3α-DIOL (same dose). All animals were sacrificed at 26 days of age. The contents of T, DHT and 3α-DIOL were measured in the testis (Table I). It can be seen that while E_2B administration resulted in a depletion of the androgen contents of the testis, the addition of a large dose of exogenous T reestablished both protein and androgen contents suggesting that 5α-reduction and 3α-oxido-reductase were active.

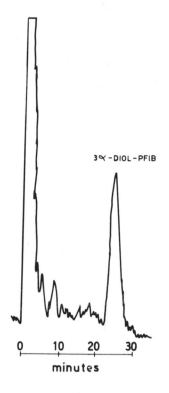

Figure 5. Gas chromatography tracing of 3α-DIOL dipentafluorobenzoate (3α-DIOL-PFlB) derived from 20-day-old rat seminiferous
tubules. After extraction and one TLC, samples were reacted with
pentafluorobenzoyl chloride and purified by a second TLC. Samples
were injected on a 130-cm-long, 4 mm internal diameter, coiled glass
column packed with 3% SE-30 on Chromosorb W (HP) (Pierce Chemical
Co.). Inlet, column and detector temperatures were set at 225°C.
A Packard 7424 Gas Chromatograph was used with Model 885 ^{3}H-electron
capture detector. 3α-DIOL/T ratios in seminiferous tubules and
interstitial tissue.

The addition of either DHT or 3α-DIOL had a similar effect, except
for the absence of T.

TESTOSTERONE REDUCING ACTIVITY IN SUBCELLULAR FRACTIONS OF RAT
SEMINIFEROUS TUBULES AT COMPLETION OF THE FIRST MEIOTIC DIVISION

The pattern of metabolism of ^{3}H-T and ^{3}H-DHT was investigated

TABLE I

Protein and Androgen Contents in Testes of 26-Day-Old Rats. Rats
Were Treated With Estradiol Benzoate (E_2B) Alone (50 µg/100 g Body
Weight) or in Combination With Different Androgens (1.5 mg/100 g
Body Weight) from the 5th to the 25th Day of Life.

	Testicular Proteins mg/testis	Testicular androgens ng/testis		
		T	DHT	3α-DIOL
Vehicle	4.08	0.98	0.31	2.35
E_2B for 20 days	1.11	ND	ND	ND
E_2B + T for 20 days	4.30	1.97	0.51	2.66
E_2B + DHT for 20 days	4.87	ND	0.90	4.95
E_2B + 3α-Diol	5.03	ND	2.12	4.61

in homogenates of seminiferous tubules of 26 day-old rats as well
as in subcellular fractions obtained by differential centrifugation. A 800 x g pellet was obtained, and this nuclear fraction
was purified as published by Moore and Wilson (12). The supernantant
was spun at 15000 x g for 30 min to obtain the mitochondrial pellet.
This supernatant was then spun at 105,000 x g for 60 min to yield
a microsomal pellet and a final supernatant containing the cell sap
(cytosol). Percentage distribution of radioactivity is shown in
Fig. 7. 3α-DIOL was the main metabolite of T in incubations of
tubular tissue homogenates, a finding similar to what we had previously found without homogenization. The cytosol had a pattern of
metabolism identical to the homogenate. In mitochondrial, microsomal and nuclear fractions, considerable conversion to DHT and 5α-
androstan-3β, 17β-diol (3β-DIOL) was also found. When DHT was used
as substrate, results were comparable. It is interesting that both
5α and 3α reductases were detected in the soluble fraction of this
tissue.

DISCUSSION

The finding that the 5α- and 3α-reductase activities described
by various investigators (8,13,14) in the immature testis were to
a great extent localized in the seminiferous tubules, prompted us

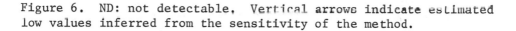

3α-DIOL / T RATIOS — NANOGRAMS PER TESTIS

	Interstitial Tissue	Seminiferous Tubules
14-day-old	$\frac{ND}{1.80} = \downarrow$	$\frac{0.66}{0.20} = 3.3$
20-day-old	$\frac{ND}{3.72} = \downarrow$	$\frac{3.12}{3.30} = 1.0$
26-day-old	$\frac{ND}{0.87} = \downarrow$	$\frac{3.47}{0.30} = 11.6$
45-day-old	$\frac{ND}{31.7} = \downarrow$	$\frac{1.80}{5.12} = 0.35$
60-day-old	$\frac{ND}{51.5} = \downarrow$	$\frac{1.95}{8.50} = 0.23$
90-day-old	$\frac{ND}{45.8} = \downarrow$	$\frac{2.55}{6.10} = 0.42$

Figure 6. ND: not detectable. Vertical arrows indicate estimated low values inferred from the sensitivity of the method.

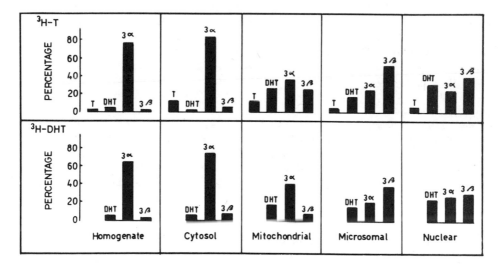

Figure 7. Percentage distribution of radioactivity in 26-day-old rat seminiferous tubules homogenates and in subcellular fractions incubated for 30 minutes in the presence of NADPH. ^{3}H-T (above) and ^{3}H-DHT (below) were used as substrates.

to postulate that activation of these enzymes was related to the
stimulation of the initiation of spermatogenesis. Even though
testes from 15- to 45-day-old rats are usually called "immature",
at this age the germinal epithelium is going through an extremely
active process of cellular growth and differentiation. "Maturing
testis" should be a proper denomination for these testes.
Steinberger and Duckett showed that exogenous T could stimulate
spermatogenesis in immature animals (15). The germinal epithelium,
particularly at the stage of the meiotic cellular division, could
then be considered a target organ for androgens. This concept
has been reinforced by the demonstration of the presence of androgen receptors in the testis (16,17). The close temporal relationship between the development of the first meiotic division and
the increased ability of the seminiferous tubules to convert T to
3α-DIOL led us to propose that the two events might be related.
By measuring the androgen contents in whole testis, interstitial
tissue and seminiferous tubules we could demonstrate that stimulation of 5α-reductase and 3α-oxido-reductase activities resulted, as
it might be expected, in an accumulation of 3α-DIOL in the seminiferous tubules at the time of the first meiotic division. The
different pattern in concentrations of androgen metabolites in
seminiferous tubules of immature and mature rats is very interesting.
DHT was the predominant reduced androgen present in tubules with complete spermatogenesis.

    Conversion of T to DHT and 3α-DIOL was also present in rats
receiving estradiol benzoate, suggesting that this conversion is
not completely dependent on gonadotropins. Formation of 5α and 3α
reduced androgens were found in all subcellular fractions of
seminiferous tubules at meiosis. However, the pattern of distribution of T metabolites showed differences. In total tissue homogenates and in the cytosol T was reduced to DHT and 3α-DIOL in
comparable amounts. In the particulate fractions much less 3α-
DIOL was formed, whereas these fractions still revealed a high
formation of DHT. The particulate fractions also converted T and
DHT into 3β-DIOL. These results suggest that the type of metabolism
found in incubations of teased tubules, as well as the high level
of 3α-DIOL at the time of the first meiotic division, is due to the
activities of these enzymes.

REFERENCES

1. Means, A.R. and Vaitukaitis, J., Endocrinology 90: 39, 1972.

2. Catt, K.J., Dufau, M.L. and Tsuruhara, T., J. Clin. Endocr.
    32: 860, 1971.

3. Van Doorn, L.G., De Bruijn, H.W.A., Galjaard, H. and Van der Molen, H.J., Biol. Reprod. 10:47, 1974.

4. Hall, P.F., Irby, D.C. and de Krester, D.M., Endocrinology 84: 488, 1969.

5. Steinberger, E., Physiol. Rev. 51: 1, 1971.

6. Neumann, F. and von Berswordt-Wallrabe, R., J. Endocr. 35: 363, 1966.

7. Rivarola, M.A. and Podesta, E.J., Endocrinology 90: 618, 1972.

8. Nayfeh, S.N. and Baggett, B., Endocrinolgoy 78: 460, 1966.

9. Rivarola, M.A., Podesta, E.J. and Chemes, H.E., Endocrinology 91: 537, 1972.

10. Podesta, E.J. and Rivarola, M.A. Endocrinology 95: 455, 1974.

11. Zmigrod, A., Landany, S. and Lindner, H.R., Steroids 15: 635, 1970.

12. Moore, R.J. and Wilson, J.D., Endocrinology 93: 581, 1973.

13. Inano, H., Hori, Y. and Tamaoki, B., CIBA Found. Collo. Endocrin. 16: 105, 1967.

14. Ficher, M. and Steinberger, E., Steroids 12: 491, 1968.

15. Steinberger, E. and Ducket, G.E., Endocrinology 76: 1184, 1965.

16. Hansson, V., Trygstad, O., French, F.S., McLean, W.S., Smith, A.A., Tindall, D.J., Weddington, S.C., Petrusz, P., Nayfeh, S.N. and Ritzen, E.M. Nature (Lond.) 250: 387, 1974.

17. Mulder, E., Peters, M.J. von Beurden, W.M.D. and van der Molen, H.J., FEBS Letters 47: 209, 1974.

ANDROGEN SYNTHESIS AND METABOLISM BY PREPARATIONS FROM THE SEMINIFEROUS TUBULE OF THE RAT TESTIS

Jennifer H. Dorrington and Irving B. Fritz

Banting and Best Department of Medical Research

University of Toronto, Toronto, Canada, M5G 1L6

INTRODUCTION

Sertoli cells maintain an intimate association with germ cells at all stages of differentiation. Based for the most part on ultra-structural studies, several important functions have been attri-buted to the Sertoli cell including the formation and maintenance of the blood-testis barrier, secretion of tubular fluid, nourish-ment and mechanical support of the germ cells, and steroidogenesis (1, 2). In addition, in vitro studies have shown that the Sertoli cell is the target for FSH action in the testes. FSH increased cyclic adenosine 3'5'-monophosphate (cyclic AMP) production in tubular preparations enriched in Sertoli cells but not in germ cells or interstitial cells (3). Sertoli cells have been implicated as the site of synthesis of androgen-binding protein (ABP) under the control of FSH (4-6).

The concept has therefore developed that the process of spermatogenesis is intimately associated with Sertoli cell functions. The effects of FSH on Sertoli cells may influence germ cell differ-entiation. We were motivated by these concepts to develop methods for the isolation of Sertoli cell-enriched preparations, and for the maintenance of those cells in culture. The method of isolation of Sertoli cells will be described, and this and the subsequent paper will deal with one aspect of Sertoli cell function, namely androgen synthesis and metabolism.

Preparation of Sertoli Cell-Enriched Aggregates

The method used for the preparation of Sertoli cell aggregates was based on that described in detail by Dorrington et. al. (7). A flow chart of the procedure is outlined in Fig. 1.   Scanning electron microscopy has been employed to demonstrate the effectiveness of the sequential enzyme digestion of the whole testes to isolate the cell aggregates (8).   The treatment with trypsin and DNase, followed by the washing procedure, dispersed the network of inter- stitial cells in the intertubular space, thereby releasing the tubule fragments.   Subsequent digestion of the tubule fraction with collagenase, followed by brief agitation, effectively removed the peritubular cells and layers of collagen.   Agitation with a Pasteur pipette disrupted the tubular structure and at the same time tended to dislodge germ cells remaining in the tubule fragments.   The final preparation consisted of groups of Sertoli cells (approximately 70%) in which were embedded germ cells.

Culture Conditions

The cell pellet was resuspended in standard culture medium and approximately 1.5 mg cell protein was plated in each culture flask containing 5 ml culture medium.   The standard culture medium con- sisted of Eagle's minimum essential medium, supplemented with anti- biotics, non-essential amino acids and additional glutamine (final concentration 4 mM).   Sertoli cell-enriched aggregates readily attached to the surface of the culture flask.   In contrast, most of the single germ cells remained floating in the medium.   The germ cells which were trapped in the aggregates tended to degenerate in the protein-free medium, or were released as the aggregates spread out on the surface of the culture flask.   Cultures were incubated at 32° in a water-saturated atmosphere of 95% air and 5% CO_2 for 48 hrs, the medium was then discarded and the attached cells were removed with trypsin.   Soy-bean trypsin inhibitor was added, and the cells were washed.   Degenerating cells were removed by this pro- cedure.   Electron microscopic examination of the resulting prepara- tion of cells revealed a relatively uniform population, having 90-95% of the same cell type.   Additional ultrastructural studies indicate that these cells have properties characteristic of Sertoli cells.   These properties, which have been described elsewhere (8), include indentated nucleus, prominent nucleoli, elongated mito- chondria, extensive Golgi apparatus, abundant smooth and rough endoplasmic reticulum, numerous microtubules and microfilaments, and evidence of characteristic tight junctions.

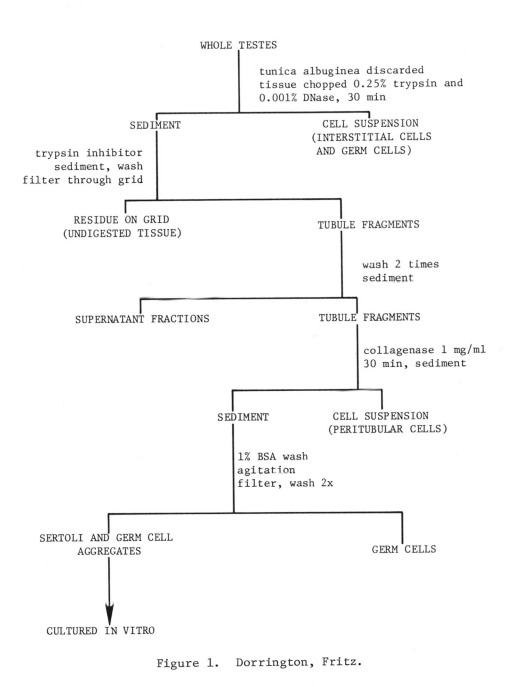

Figure 1.   Dorrington, Fritz.

The responsiveness of these cultured cells to FSH was mani-
fested by increased adenylate cyclase activity (7), an increase
in the incorporation of amino acids into protein (7), increased
synthesis of androgen-binding protein (9), increased conversion
of (^{14}C)-testosterone to (^{14}C)-estradiol-17β (10), and by altered
structural characteristics (8).

Incubation Conditions

Tubules (80 mg wet wt for the (^{14}C)-testosterone incubations,
40 mg for the (^{14}C)-pregnenolone incubations and 20 mg for the
(^{14}C)-DHT incubations and the various cell preparations were incubated at 32°C in an atmosphere of 95% O_2 and 5% CO_2 in 1 ml
Krebs-Ringer bicarbonate buffer pH 7.4 containing glucose, 1 mg/ml.
Labeled steroid (1 μg of (^{14}C)-testosterone, specific activity:
47.5 mCi/mmole, 1 μg of (^{14}C) DHT, specific activity 50.6 mCi/mmole
or 500 μg of (^{14}C)-pregnenolone, specific activity: 55.7 mCi/mmole)
was added in 20 μl dimethyl formamide. A blank incubation vessel
containing no tissue was included in every experiment.

Analytical Procedures

Following incubation with (^{14}C)-testosterone or (^{14}C)-DHT
(dihydrotestosterone) the steroids were extracted, purified and
identified as described previously (11). Following incubation
with (^{14}C)-pregnenolone the steroids were extracted as described
previously (11), and were separated by thin layer chromatography
in dichloromethane; diethyl ether, 5:2 at 4°C. The progesterone
and androstenedione were eluted and rechromatographed in benzene:
ethyl acetate 3:1, The pregnenolone, 17α-hydroxyprogesterone,
testosterone, androstanediol and androsterone areas were eluted
evaporated to dryness and acetylated overnight in 0.1 ml pyridine
and 0.1 ml acetic anhydride. The solution was evaporated to
dryness under N_2, and the residue was dissolved in chloroform:
methanol (1:1). The acetates were separated by thin layer chromatography in benzene:ethyl acetate (95:5), scraped from the silica
gel and counted.

RESULTS AND DISCUSSION

Synthesis of Androgens

Studies on the fine structure of Sertoli cells have revealed
the presence of certain inclusions typical of steroid-producing

cells (2). These include lipid droplets, abundant smooth endo-plasmic reticulum, granular endoplasmic reticulum, and numerous mitochondria. On the basis of these observations it has been suggested that the Sertoli cell is a source of steroid hormones which govern the differentiation of the germ cell. Androgen is essential for the completion of spermatogenesis within the semini-ferous tubule. Testosterone therapy alone will maintain spermato-zoa production if administered immediately after hypophysectomy. Therefore, it was of considerable interest to determine if the Sertoli cell had the potential to synthesise androgens.

The isolated tubule cannot convert exogenous (^{3}H)-cholesterol to (^{3}H)-androstenedione and (^{3}H)-testosterone (12). The use of exogenous cholesterol as a precursor for side-chain cleavage in short term in vitro incubations, however, has serious limitations as emphasised by the work of Armstrong (13) and Savard et. al. (14). These include the insolubility of cholesterol in the incubation medium, and the slow equilibration of exogenous cholesterol with the endogenous cholesterol pools.

Since exogenous pregnenolone enters the tubule readily (15) this steroid was used as a substrate for androgen synthesis. The ability to convert (^{14}C)-pregnenolone to androgens was assessed in isolated tubules from 35 day old rats, Sertoli cell-enriched aggregates prepared from isolated tubules and whole testes pre-parations from animals of the same age. Whole testes preparations converted pregnenolone to testosterone and also to 5α-androstane-diols and androsterone. Isolated tubules also converted pregnen-olone to androgens. However, the amounts converted were trivial compared to the capacity of the whole testis. Sertoli cell-enriched aggregates prepared from the isolated tubules by the pro-cedure described above and incubated immediately were unable to convert significant amounts of pregnenolone to androgens (Table 1).

Testosterone is synthesised by the interstitial cells of the testes, and this process is regulated by LH (16). The concentration of testosterone in the testicular lymph which bathes the seminiferous tubule is almost as high as that in the spermatic venous blood (1). The inability of the Sertoli cell to synthesise androgens from pregnenolone, together with the trivial ability of the isolated tubule, indicate that the tubule relies upon the interstitial cells for the testosterone required for the completion of spermatogenesis. There appears to be no barrier to the entry of testosterone into the tubule from the surrounding medium (15).

Conversion of Testosterone to 5α-Reduced Metabolites by Tubule and Cell Preparations

The prostate, seminal vesicles and certain other androgen-responsive tissues convert testosterone to DHT and other 5α-reduced

TABLE 1

Metabolism of (^{14}C)-Pregnenolone by Whole Testis Preparations,
Isolated Tubules and Sertoli Cell-Enriched Preparations
from 35 Day Old Rats

	Percentage of Total Radioactivity Recovered from		
	Whole Testis	Tubules	Sertoli Cells
Pregnenolone*	63.0 ± 4.0	96.1 ± 0.5	97.1 ± 1.0
Progesterone	7.9 ± 2.4	0.9 ± 0.1	0.4 ± 0.2
17αOH Progesterone	3.1 ± 0.6	0.7 ± 0.2	0.2 ± 0.1
Androstenedione	3.2 ± 0.5	0.3 ± 0.1	N.D.
Testosterone	1.3 ± 0.2	0.3 ± 0.1	N.D.
Androstanediol	5.5 ± 1.6	N.D.	N.D.
Androsterone	12.0 ± 2.2	N.D.	N.D.

*   Unmetabolised substrate

     Total testis tissue from 35 day old rats (40 mg wet wt),
isolated tubules (40mg wet wt) and freshly prepared Sertoli cell-
enriched aggregates (approximately 2mg protein) obtained from
the isolated tubules by the procedure described in the text, were
incubated in 1ml Krebs-Ringer bicarbonate buffer containing 1 mg
glucose and 500ng (^{14}C)-pregnenolone for 2 hr at 32° in an atmosphere
of 95%O_2 and 5% CO_2. The results were expressed as the mean ± SEM
of the percentage of the total radioactivity recovered after incubation of 2mg protein. Three separate experiments were performed
for each set of observations reported.

metabolites. It has been postulated that these metabolites may
be the active androgens in these tissues (17). The possibility
that the synthesis of 5α-reduced products from testosterone may
also play a role in the control of tubular function was raised
by the demonstration that DHT could effectively replace testosterone in maintaining spermatogenesis (18), and in permitting
spermatocytes to complete meiosis (19). The conversion of
testosterone to DHT is biologically irreversible, which suggests
that DHT or one of its metabolites can maintain spermatogenesis.

TABLE 2

Metabolism of (^{14}C)-Testosterone by Isolated Tubules from
Normal and Hypophysectomized Adult Rats

Metabolites	Percentage of Total Radioactivity Recovered*	
	Normal	Hypophysectomized** (1 week)
Androstanediol†	6.9 ± 0.7	8.9 ± 0.6
Dihydrotestosterone	1.5 ± 0.2	1.4 ± 0.2
Androsterone	1.1 ± 0.3	0.8 ± 0.2
Androstenedione	7.9 ± 0.7	4.9 ± 0.6

*Results are expressed as the percentage of products formed by
5.0 mg protein (80 mg wet wt approximately). Each value is the
mean ± SEM of 4 separate experiments. Tubules were incubated for
2 hr at 32°C in an atmosphere of 95%O_2 and 5%CO_2 in 1 ml Krebs
Ringer bicarbonate buffer containing 1 mg glucose and 1 μg (^{14}C)-
testosterone. Of the radioactivity not recovered in the above
metabolites, a low level (0.5%) was present at the origin and
in the solvent front area, and the remainder was recovered as
unmetabolized testosterone.

**Adult rats were hypophysectomized and allowed to regress for
one week.

†5α-androstan-3α,17β-diol and 5α-androstan-3β,17βdiol.

In the following study we have investigated the capacity of various
tubule and cell preparations to metabolise (^{14}C)-testosterone, in
order to determine which cell types in the tubule contribute to the
overall pattern of metabolites.

Tubules isolated from normal adult and immature rat testes
readily take up (^{14}C)-testosterone and convert it into (^{14}C)-
androstenedione and to the 5α-reduced products: (^{14}C)-DHT, (^{14}C)-
5α-androstane-3α-17β-diol and (^{14}C)-androsterone (Table 2, Fig. 2).
Tubules from immature rats converted a significantly higher proportion of (^{14}C)-testosterone to 5α-reduced metabolites than did
tubules from adult rats.

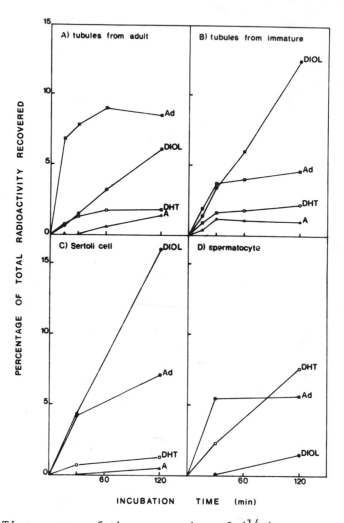

Fig. 2.   Time course of the conversion of (^{14}C) testosterone to
metabolites by: A) tubules from normal adult rats: B) tubules
from immature rats (26-28 days of age); C) Sertoli cell-enriched
preparations from 20 day old rats, and D) spermatocyte-enriched
preparations from 26-28 day old rats.   Tubule (80 mg wet wt) or
cell preparations (1-4 mg protein) were incubated with 1μg (^{14}C)-
testosterone.   All results are expressed as the mean ±SEM of the
percentage of total radioactivity recovered after incubation of
5.0 mg protein.   The metabolites formed were 5α-androstanediol
(DIOL), DHT, androstenedione (Ad), and androsterone (A).
* In each case, data shown are from a single experiment representative of results from 3 or 4 experiments (11).
* All but 0.5% of the radioactivity not accounted for by these
metabolites was unchanged ^{3}H-testosterone.

Sertoli cell-enriched aggregates were prepared from 20 day old rats and maintained in culture in standard culture medium for 48 hrs. The attached cells were removed from the surface of the flask by trypsinization, soy-bean trypsin inhibitor was added and the cells were washed in Krebs-Ringer bicarbonate buffer. These preparations of Sertoli cells contain 5α-reductase as well as 3α-hydroxysteroid dehydrogenase activity (Fig. 2,3).

Spermatocyte-enriched preparations were obtained from immature rats by procedures previously described (3). The preparations, which consisted of 85-90% spermatocytes at different stages of development, formed (^{14}C)-DHT as the major metabolite of (^{14}C)-testosterone (Fig. 2). A very low formation of 5α-androstane-3α-17β-diol was detected. However, it is possible that this was due to the contamination by Sertoli cells (approximately 2%).

Spermatids have little if any 5α-reductase activity or 3α-hydroxysteroid dehydrogenase activity (11). Consequently, the lower activities per unit weight of these enzymes in adult tubules compared to immature tubules may be a reflection of the higher proportion of spermatids, relative to the number of Sertoli cells and spermatocytes.

Of the cell types studied, Sertoli cells and spermatocytes contained 5α-reductase and metabolised (^{14}C)-testosterone to (^{14}C)-DHT. (^{14}C)-DHT was the major 5α-reduced metabolite produced by spermatocytes, whereas in the Sertoli cell further metabolism of the (^{14}C)-DHT to (^{14}C)-5α-androstane-3α,17β diol occurred. Qualitative and quantitative similarities between the steroids produced by the Sertoli cell preparation and the isolated tubule indicate that the Sertoli cell is mainly responsible for the overall spectrum of 5α-reduced metabolites formed from testosterone by the tubule.

Effect of Gonadotrophins on 5α-Reductase Activity

Several lines of evidence indicate that 5α-reductase activity in tubule cells is not directly dependent upon gonadotrophins. The 5α-reduction of (^{14}C)-testosterone by isolated seminiferous tubules from mature rats which had been hypophysectomized one week previously was quantitatively similar to that observed in tubules from intact adult rats (Table 2). The weight of the seminal vesicles was used as an index of the success of the hypophysectomy (mean seminal vesicle weight of the normal adults was 0.39g whereas in the group of hypophysectomized animals the weight was 0.10g). One week after hypophysectomy the cell population in the tubule is similar to that in the intact adult (20). These experiments suggested that the synthesis and activity of 5α-reductase in the tubule was independent of gonadotrophins. The possibility existed nevertheless that a change in the activity of 5α-reductase in the Sertoli cell, which comprised

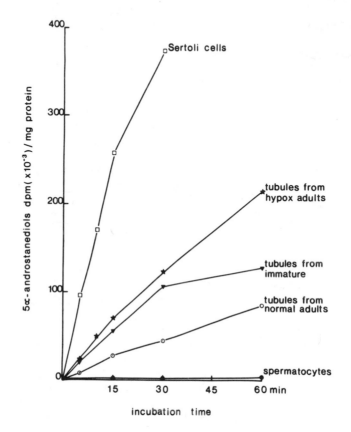

Fig. 3.   Time course of the conversion of (^{14}C)-dihydrotestosterone
to (^{14}C)-5α-androstanediols by various tubule and cell preparations
from the rat testis.   1 μg DHT was added to each incubation at zero
time.   Cell suspensions were prepared as described in the text.
Tubules (20 mg wet wt) were isolated from normal adult, from immature (26-28 days of age) and from hypophysectomized rats, killed
34-36 days postoperatively.   Results shown are from a single
experiment representative of results from two or more experiments
(11).

only a small proportion of the total cell population (4-5%) may not be detected. To obtain information on the possible gonadotrophic requirements of 5α-reductase activity in Sertoli cells, two series of experiments were performed. In the first series of experiments, adult rats were hypophysectomised and allowed to regress for 35 days. Saline, 25 µg NIH-FSH-S9 or 25 µg NIH-LH-S16 were injected subcutaneously twice daily for 3 days. One hour after the last injection the animals were killed, tubules were isolated and incubated with (^{14}C)-testosterone (1 µg) for 2 hrs. As shown in Table 3, 5α-reductase and also 3α-hydroxysteroid dehydrogenase activity was evident 35 days after hypophysectomy and the short term hormonal therapies employed did not significantly influence the formation of DHT and 5α-androstrane-3α,17β-diol.

TABLE 3

Metabolism of (^{14}C)-Testosterone by Isolated Tubules from Fully Regressed Hypophysectomized Rats* Treated for 3 Days with Saline, FSH or LH

Metabolite	Percentage of Total Radioactivity Recovered**					
	Treatment					
	Saline		FSH		LH	
Androstanediol	4.9	0.5	3.4	0.5	3.7	0.4
Dihydrotestosterone	0.8	0.2	0.9	0.2	0.8	0.3
Androsterone	0.4	0.1	0.6	0.2	0.3	0.1
Androstenedione	3.7	0.2	6.6	1.0	5.8	1.1

*Rats were allowed to regress for 35 days after hypophysectomy, Saline, 25 µg NIH-FSH-S9, or 25 µg NIH LH-S16 were injected subcutaneously twice daily for 3 days. There were three rats in each group.

** Data are expressed as described in legend to Table 2.

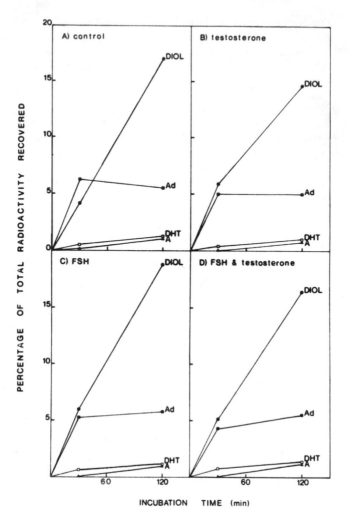

Figure 4. Time course of the conversion of (^{14}C)-testosterone to metabolites by Sertoli cell-enriched preparations. Cells were cultured in standard culture medium with A) no further additions, or containing B) testosterone 5×10^{-7}M, C) NIH-FSH, 5μg/ml, or, D) testosterone, 5×10^{-7}M, and FSH 5μg/ml. Medium and hormones were replaced after 24 hrs. After 48 hrs the cells were removed by trypsin treatment, trypsin inhibitor was added and the cells were washed. Cells were incubated in 1 ml Krebs-Ringer bicarbonate buffer containing 1 mg glucose and 1 μg (^{14}C)-testosterone. The metabolites formed were 5α-androstanediol (DIOL), DHT, androstenedione (Ad) and androsterone (A)
*Data are expressed as described in legend to Fig. 2.
*All but 0.5% of the radioactivity not accounted for by these metabolites was unchanged ^{3}H-testosterone.

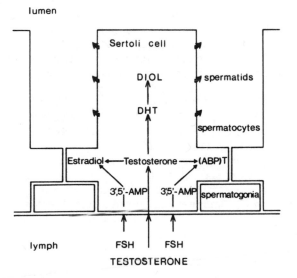

Figure 5. Schematic representation of the effects of FSH on testosterone metabolism in the Sertoli cell.

In the second series of experiments, Sertoli cells were prepared from 20 day old rats and were maintained in culture in
standard culture medium containing testosterone (5x10^{-7}M), FSH
(5 µg/ml), or testosterone (5x10^{-7}M) and FSH (5 µg/ml). After 48
hrs the cells were removed by brief trypsin treatment, soybean
trypsin inhibitor was added, the cells were washed and incubated
for either 30 min or 2 hr in the presence of (^{14}C)-testosterone
(1 µg). As shown in Fig. 4, the rate of conversion of testosterone
to 5α-reduced metabolites was not influenced by the pre-treatment
with hormones.

The data presented here reinforce the view that the Sertoli
cell cannot synthesise testosterone 'de novo' and is dependent
upon the interstitial cells for this hormone. Upon exposure to
testosterone the Sertoli cell has the ability to channel it along
one of at least three different routes and the choice clearly
depends upon the presence or absence of FSH (Fig. 5). ABP is
synthesised by the Sertoli cell and this process is controlled
by FSH (4-6). It follows therefore that the amount of high
affinity binding protein available to bind testosterone or DHT
and subsequently to secrete the complex into the adluminal space,
depends upon FSH. Another possible fate of testosterone in the
Sertoli cell involves its conversion to estradiol-17β. This process is also regulated by FSH. ABP has a high affinity for testosterone and DHT (K_d of approximately 10^{-9}M) and would be expected
to complete effectively with the 5α and 3α-reductases. In this
regard it is interesting to speculate that ABP may play an important
role in retaining and transporting sufficient testosterone (or DHT)
through the Sertoli cell layer, for sustaining spermatogenesis in
the adluminal compartments. In the absence of FSH, ABP production
and the aromatisation enzyme system would be non-functional and
the only known channel for testosterone or DHT metabolism remaining
available would permit accumulation of 5α-androstanediol. Some
support for this hypothesis comes from the work of Podesta and
Rivarola (21). The level of 5α-androstanediol is low in tubules
from normal adult rats, whereas the level of testosterone is high.
In view of the active 5α-reductase system present in tubules from
intact adults it is clear that the testosterone is being protected
in some manner from further metabolism. We suggest that ABP may
participate in this protection.

In conclusion, a central role of FSH in influencing androgen
metabolism by Sertoli cells has emerged. Stimulation of Sertoli
cells with FSH results in the regulation of the chemical form which
testosterone acquires on passing into the adluminal compartment
where androgen metabolites encounter the differentiating germ cells
(Fig. 5).

ACKNOWLEDGMENTS

This study was supported by grants from the Medical Research
Council of Canada and the Banting Research Foundation. The
authors gratefully acknowledge the technical assistance of
Heather McKeracher.

REFERENCES

1. Setchell, B.P., In Johnson, A.D., W.R. Gomes, and N.L. Vandemark
    (eds.) The Testis, vol 1, Academic Press, New York, 1970, p. 101.

2. Lacy, D., and Pettitt, A.J., Br. Med. Bull. 26: 87, 1970.

3. Dorrington, J.H., and Fritz, I.B., Endocrinology, 94: 395, 1974.

4. Vernon, R.G., Kopec, B., and Fritz, I.B., Molec. Cell.
    Endocrinol. 1: 167, 1974.

5. Hansson, V., Reusch, E., Trygstad, O., Torgersen, O., Ritzen,
    E.M., French, F.S., Nature New Biol. 246: 56, 1973.

6. Sanborn, B.M., Elkington, J.S.H., and Steinberger, E., In
    Dufau, M., and Means, A.R. (eds), Hormone Binding and Activation
    in the Testis, Plenum Press, 1974, p. 291.

7. Dorrington, J.H., Roller, N.F. and Fritz, I.B., Molec. Cell.
    Endocrinol. 1975 (in press).

8. Tung, P.S., Dorrington, J.H., and Fritz, I.B., Proc. Natl.
    Acad. Sci. U.S.A. 1975 (in press).

9. Fritz, I.B., Louis, B.G., Tung, P.S., Griswold, M., Rommerts,
    F.F.G., and Dorrington, J.H., this volume, p. 367.

10. Dorrington, J.H., and Armstrong, D.T., Proc. Natl. Acad. Sci.
    U.S.A. 1975 (in press).

11. Dorrington, J.H. and Fritz, I.B., Endocrinology 1975 (in press).

12. Hall, P.F., Irby, D.C., and de Kretser, D.M., Endocrinology 84:
    488, 1969.

13. Armstrong, D.T., J. Reprod. Fertil. Suppl 1: 101, 1966.

14. Savard, K., LeMaire, W., and Kumari, L. In The Gonads, McKerns, K.W. (ed) Appleton-Century-Crofts, New York, 1969, p. 119.

15. Parvinen, M., Hurme, P., and Niemi, M., Endocrinology 87: 1082, 1970.

16. Cooke, B.A., de Jong, F.H., van der Molen, H.J. and Rommerts, F.F.G., Nature New Biol. 237: 255, 1972.

17. Wilson, J.D., New England J. Med. 287: 1284, 1972.

18. Ahmad, N., Haltmeyer, G.C., and Eik-Nes. K.B., Biol. Reprod. 8: 411, 1973.

19. Lostroh, A.J., Endocrinology, 85 438, 1969.

20. Clermont, Y., and Morgentaler, H. Endocrinology 57: 369, 1955.

21. Podesta, E.J., and Rivarola, M.A., Endocrinology 95: 455, 1974.

GONADOTROPIC REGULATION OF 5α-REDUCTASE ACTIVITY IN THE INTERSTITIAL CELLS AND WHOLE TESTIS HOMOGENATE OF THE IMMATURE RAT

S.N. Nayfeh, J.C. Coffey, N.J. Kotite, and F.S. French

Departments of Biochemistry and Pediatrics, Dental
Research Center, and Laboratories for Reproductive
Biology, University of North Carolina, Chapel Hill,
North Carolina   27514   U.S.A.

INTRODUCTION

As early as 1965, it was first reported (1) that radioactive
progesterone is rapidly metabolized to testosterone (T) in homogenates of immature as well as mature rat testis, although T accumulation varies significantly with the age of the rat. It was observed
that testosterone is rapidly formed in vitro but accumulates in
inverse proportion to the rate of formation of 5α-androstane-3α,
17β-diol (3α-DIOL) (2,3). In the immature rat testis, the formation
of 3α-DIOL was extremely rapid and little testosterone accumulated
(3). At about the age of puberty, however, testosterone became the
major product and the formation of 3α-DIOL was greatly reduced (3).
Later studies in several laboratories confirmed these observations
and extended them to all ages of the rat, from birth to adulthood
(4-8). More recently, endogenous levels of 3α-DIOL were measured
in testicular extracts of seminiferous tubules and interstitial
cells from rats of various ages. 3α-DIOL concentrations in seminiferous tubules were found to be elevated between 25-35 days of
age, at which time testosterone levels were minimal (9). Following
the intravenous injection of ^{3}H-progesterone and ^{3}H-androstenedione
into immature rats, radioactive 3α-DIOL was also found to accumulate
as the major metabolite in testicular tissues (10).

5α-Dihydrotestosterone (DHT), which is an intermediate in the
conversion of T to 3α-DIOL (10,11), is an active androgen and is
thought to mediate T action in some androgen target organs. Since
the testis contains specific androgen receptors with high affinity
for T and DHT (12-14), it was presumed that both androgens may

play an important role in the initiation and maturation of
spermatogenesis and the onset of puberty in the rat. 5α–Reductase,
the enzyme that catalyzes the conversion of testosterone to DHT in
the rat testis, is present both in interstitial cells (10,15–17)
and seminiferous tubules (10,15–18); however, the mechanisms which
regulate its activity during various stages of development are not
yet known. Since 5α–reductase activity correlates closely with
maturational changes, the present experiments were designed to
study the effect of hypophysectomy and hormonal treatment on 5α–
reductase activity in immature rat testis. It is suggested that
gonadotropins regulate 5α–reductase activity, which, in turn, may
modulate the amounts of DHT and T accumulating during various
stages of testicular maturation.

MATERIALS AND METHODS

Hypophysectomized Sprague–Dawley rats were purchased from
Hormone Assay Laboratories, Chicago, Illinois. The interstitial
cells were obtained by teasing gently the decapsulated testis and
shaking in 0.15 M KCl solution for 2–3 minutes. The cell suspension
was filtered once over two layers followed by once over 4 layers
of nylon cloth. Cells were collected by centrifugation at 5000
rpm for 10 min. This preparation contained 60–75% Leydig cells,
25–40% tubular cells and other interstitial cells. Homogenates of
the interstitial cells and whole testis were prepared in a phosphate buffer containing saturating concentrations of NADPH–generating
system as described previously (2). 5α–Reductase was assayed by
incubating equal aliquots of each homogenate with saturating amounts
of [1,2-^{3}H]-testosterone and under conditions in which the reaction
rate was linear and proportional to enzyme concentration. The
products formed from the substrate were separated by thin–layer
chromatography on silica-gel plates in benzene:ethyl acetate (5:1)
after acetylation overnight at room temperature (10). The major
5α–reduced steroid metabolites were identified as described previously (7). Activity of 5α–reductase was determined as the sum
of DIOLS, DHT, and androsterone. 3α–DIOL and DHT accounted for
about 95% of radioactive 5α–reduced products.

RESULTS AND DISCUSSION

The Effect of Increasing Substrate Concentration on the
Accumulation of DHT and 3α–DIOL by Whole Testis
Homogenate of 30 Day–Old Rat

The effect of various concentrations of T in the incubation
medium on the amounts of DHT and 3α–DIOL formed is presented in
Figure 1. The amount of DHT accumulating rose from 0.02 at the

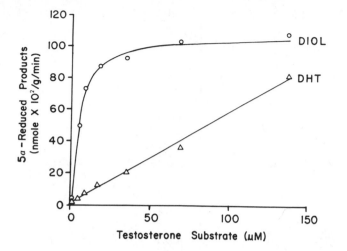

Figure 1. Effect of increasing concentrations of testosterone on its conversion to 5α-dihydrotestosterone (DHT) and androstanediol (DIOL) by testicular homogenates of immature rats. One hundred mg tissue was homogenized in 1.2 ml of phosphate buffer, pH = 7.4, containing NADPH-generating system and incubated for 1 hr at 37°. Non-radio-active testosterone was added to 6 mCi of ^{3}H-testosterone to obtain the appropriate specific activity.

lowest (^{3}H-T = 0.2 µM) to 0.81 nmole/g tissue/min at the highest concentration of ^{3}H-T (138.7 µM). At the same time, the amount of 3α-DIOL formed increased to almost maximal level (0.9 nmole/g tissue/min) at lower concentrations of ^{3}H-T (17.3 µM) and remained constant thereafter. As a consequence of the differential effect of increasing concentrations of ^{3}H-T on the accumulation of DHT and 3α-DIOL, the relative amounts of these products change so that DHT, the lesser metabolite at lower substrate concentrations, was formed in almost equal amounts as 3α-DIOL at higher concentrations. In a recent study, Lloret and Weisz (19) observed similar effects of increasing concentrations of T on the relative accumulation of DHT and 3α-DIOL in seminiferous tubules of adult rats. These in-vestigators suggested that the increase in DHT accumulation as compared with 3α-DIOL is possibly due to competition of T with DHT for 3α-oxidoreductase.

Unless otherwise stated, 5α-reductase activity was therefore quantitated as described under Methods following incubation with 17.3 x 10^{-6} M of ^{3}H-T and various tissue preparations. This sub-strate concentration was chosen to approach saturation of 5α-reductase (K_m = 7.6 x 10^{-6} M) without significant inhibition of 3α-oxidoreductase. Under these conditions, DHT should be rapidly

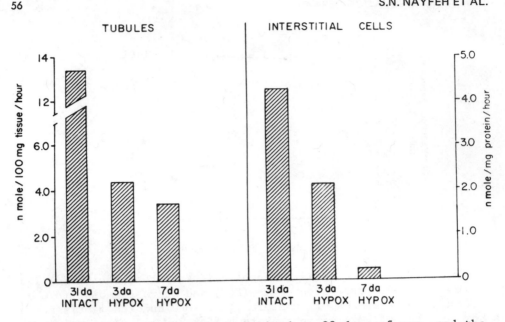

Figure 2.   Rats were hypophysectomized at 28 days of age, and the
5α-reductase activity was assayed at various intervals following
hypophysectomy.   Seminiferous tubules and interstitial cells from
each testis were prepared by teasing and washing with 0.154 M KCl.
The washed tubules and interstitial cells were homogenized in a
mixture of 0.154 M KCl and co-factors as described previously
(2).   1.2 ml of both homogenates were separately incubated with
20.8 nmol ^{3}H-T (S.A. 0.29 μCi/nmol) at 37° for 1 hr.   5α-Reductase
was quantitated by measuring the total radioactivity accumulating
in androstanediol, dihydrotestosterone and androsterone.   Protein
in interstitial cell preparation was determined by the Lowry method.
(Nayfeh et al., 1975 (10).)

converted to   3α-DIOL with only the 5α-reductase enzyme system being
rate-limiting.   To test this, ^{3}H-DHT, in amounts of 4 times those of
^{3}H-T, was incubated with immature rat testis homogenates for 1 hour,
and the DIOL formed was measured.   Even at this concentration,
very little DHT remained unmetabolized at the end of the incubation.

Effect of Hypophysectomy and Hormonal Treatment on 5α-Reductase in Immature Rat Testis

5α-Reductase was determined in interstitial cells and partially
purified seminiferous tubules of 28 day old rats at various intervals
following hypophysectomy.   The activity of 5α-reductase decreased

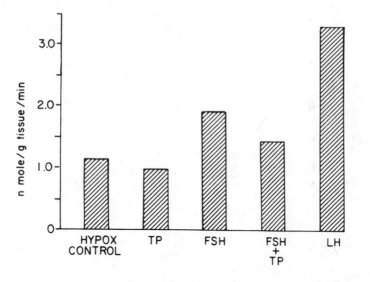

Figure 3.   Rats were hypophysectomized at 28 days of age, and
treatment was started 2 days later.   Rats in groups of 4 were injected daily either with 500 μg of NIH-FSH-S10 or 300 μg of NIH-LH-
S18 for 4 days.   Parallel groups were first treated for 3 days
with 2 mg of testosterone propionate (TP)/day followed by either
2 mg TP + 500 μg FSH or 2 mg TP alone daily for 4 additional days.
One testis from each rat was removed, and the four testes were
combined and homogenized as in Figure 1.   1.2 ml aliquots of the
homogenate (100 mg tissue) were incubated with ^{3}H-T and the 5α-
reductase activity determined.   (Nayfeh et al., 1975 (10).)

rapidly in both testicular compartments reaching low levels within
7 days (Figure 2).   The decline in the level of testicular 5α-
reductase during gonadal development and following hypophysectomy
prompted us to investigate the roles of gonadotropins and testosterone in regulation of 5α-reductase activity.

   Rats were hypophysectomized at 28 days of age, and two days
later groups of 4 were injected daily for 4 days with various hormonal preparations as described under the legend to Figure 3.   The
hypophysectomized control group was injected with the vehicle
only.   Twelve to 24 hours after the last injection the animals were
killed, and the testes removed into beakers containing ice-cold
0.154 M KCl solution.   Homogenates of whole testis and interstitial cells were prepared as described under Methods.   In these
studies, no attempt was made to measure 5α-reductase activity

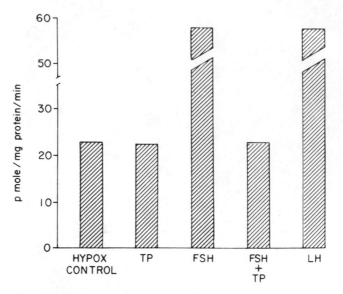

Figure 4. The remaining testes obtained from each group as described under Figure 3 were used for the preparation of the interstitial cell pellets (see Methods). Each pellet was homogenized
in 1.2 ml of incubation medium and incubated with ^{3}H–T for 1 hr
at 37°C. (Nayfeh et al., 1975 (10).)

in isolated seminiferous tubules, since the tubules obtained from
28 day old testis by microdissection were invariably contaminated
with interstitial cells. Aliquots of the homogenates were incubated
with ^{3}H–T for 1 hour at 37°C, and 5α–reductase activity was
quantitated. As shown in Figures 3 and 4, 5α–reductase activity
in homogenates of whole testis and isolated interstitial cells from
rats treated with LH was significantly higher than in those from
the hypophysectomized control rats. Although FSH injection was less
effective than LH in stimulating 5α–reductase activity in the whole
testis homogenate (Figure 3), it was equally as effective in
stimulating 5α–reductase activity of interstitial cells (Figure 4).

Testosterone propionate (1 mg/day) neither increased the
activity above the level of the hypophysectomized control group
nor augmented the response to FSH. Thus, gonadotropin stimulation
of 5α–reductase is not likely mediated through androgens. Endogenous
testosterone levels in testicular tissue from the testosterone-
treated rats were measured by competitive protein-binding after
purification of the tissue extracts on Sephadex LH-20 columns. The
concentration of testosterone was only 2% of the labeled testosterone

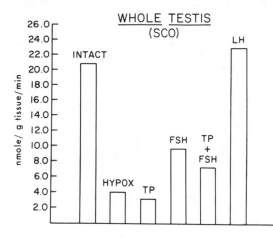

Figure 5.   Effect of hormonal treatment on 5α-reductase in
testicular homogenates from the Sertoli-cell only rats.   Rats
were hypophysectomized on the 24th day of age, and treatment
started 7 days later.   Hormonal treatment was similar to the
experiment described under Fig. 8, with the exception that the
LH dose was only 150 µg/day.   (Nayfeh et al., 1975 (10).)

substrate added, indicating that the lack of response could not
have resulted from substrate dilution.   In fact, testosterone inhibited the response to FSH.   Our results are in agreement with
previous studies of Gustafsson and Stenberger, Oshima et al.
and Frowein who have shown that androgen treatment in vivo
causes a decrease in 5α-reductase in rat liver (20) and in
5α-reductase (21) and 3α-oxidoreductase (22) in rat testis.
This is in contrast, however, to 5α-reductases in preputial
gland (19) and ventral prostate (23,24) which are dependent
on testicular androgens for full activity.

     The Sertoli cell is the primary target for FSH action in
the testis (25,26).   To augment the apparent increase in 5α-
reductase activity in whole testis homogenate following FSH
treatment, we next determined the effect of hormonal treatment of
5α-reductase in testis of the Sertoli-Cell-Only (SCO) rats.   SCO
rats were produced by irradiating (150 rads from Cobalt 60)
pregnant rats at 19-20 days of gestation.   This treatment has
been shown to produce male offspring with seminiferous tubules free
of germinal cells and containing only Sertoli cells (25).   SCO
rats were hypophysectomized on day 24 of age and treated with various
hormonal preparations 7 days following hypophysectomy.   Figures 5
and 6 show the effect of hypophysectomy and hormonal treatment on

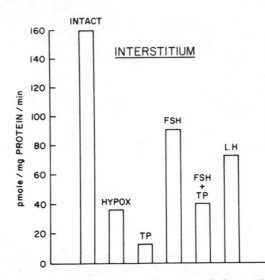

Figure 6.   Effect of hormonal treatment of 5α—reductase in interstitial cells from the Sertoli-cell only rats.   Interstitial cells
were obtained from the rats described under Figure 5 and 5α—
reductase activity was determined as described under Methods.
(Nayfeh et al., 1975 (10).)

5α—reductase activity in whole testis and isolated interstitial
cell homogenates. FSH stimulation of 5α—reductase activity
(Figures 5 and 6) was not significantly greater in the SCO testis
than in the non-irradiated testis (Figures 3 and 4). On the other
hand, LH stimulation of 5α—reductase activity in whole testis of
the SCO rat was greater than in the non-irradiated testis (Figure
3). These results, indicated that the 5α—reductase response to
either LH or FSH can occur in the absence of germ cells, and LH
target cells in the SCO testis are either more concentrated or
perhaps more sensitive to LH.

Since large doses of FSH (500 μg/day) were given in the above
experiments, it was important to determine whether the effect of
FSH on 5α—reductase activity might result from contamination with
LH. NIH—FSH—S9 preparation has been estimated to contain 1% of
LH activity when assayed by the ascorbic acid depletion method (27).
5α—Reductase activity was therefore measured in whole testis and
isolated interstitial cells following treatment with increasing doses
of LH and FSH in vivo, as described under the lgends to Figures 7
and 8. LH doses were chosen to be equivalent to or 4 times greater
than the amount of LH contamination present in the NIH—FSH—S9
preparation. Rats were hypophysectomized on day 28 of age, and 2
days later were injected with hormones. The hypophysectomized control was injected with the vehicle only. At the end of the treatment

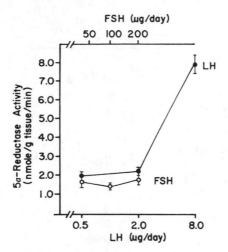

Figure 7. Log-dose response of 5α-reductase activity in whole
testis homogenate to injection of increasing doses of LH and FSH.
Rats were hypophysectomized on 28 days of age, and two days later
groups of 5-6 rats were injected subcutaneously with various doses
of hormones. 5α-reductase activity was assayed as described under
Methods. Each point represents the mean ± SEM of 5-6 whole testis
homogenates.

period, the rats were killed and one testis was saved for preparation
of interstitial cells as described under Methods. In doses up to
8 µg/day, LH resulted in an almost 5 fold increase (from 1.69 ± 0.12
in the control to 7.93 ± 0.57 nmole/g/min at the highest LH concentration) in 5α-reductase activity of whole testis homogenate
(Figure 7), while in much larger doses (50-200 µg/day), FSH was in-
effective in stimulating 5α-reductase activity (Figure 7). Since
a response was seen at a dose of LH above 2 µg/day, it is possible
that the 5α-reductase response in whole testis homogenates to
higher doses of FSH (500 µg/day, Figure 3) might have resulted
from LH contamination of the FSH preparation.

     In contrast, when 5α-reductase activity was measured in inter-
stitial cells isolated from the opposite testis, these same doses
of FSH resulted in a 6-fold increase (from 2.4 in the control to
12.8 pmole/mg protein/min at the highest FSH concentration) in 5α-
reductase activity, while LH, in doses up to 8 µg/day, resulted in
a much smaller increase in enzyme activity above the vehicle control
(Figure 8). The percent stimulation of 5α-reductase activity in
isolated interstitial cells following LH treatment was much less
than it was in whole testis homogenates, suggesting that LH may be
acting on cell type(s) not included in this interstitial cell
preparation.

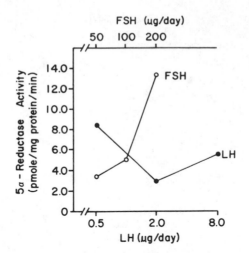

Figure 8.   Log-dose response of 5α-reductase activity in interstitial cells to increasing doses of LH and FSH.   Hormonal treatment similar to Figure 7.   Each point on the curve represents the
mean of duplicate incubation of pooled interstitial cells from
5-6 testis each obtained from individual rats.

These results demonstrated that 5α-reductase activity of the
immature testis, as assayed in vitro under linear kinetic conditions, decreases following hypophysectomy and is increased by
treatment with FSH or LH in vivo.   The results from the dose
response studies establish the ability of FSH treatment in vivo
to increase 5α-reductase activity in a preparation consisting
mainly of interstitial cells.   Unless the amount of LH present in
the NIH-FSH-S9 preparation is much greater than 4%, the FSH
stimulation of 5α-reductase activity in the interstitial cells
cannot be accounted for by LH contamination of the FSH preparation.   Kamiyoshi et al. (28) have recently shown that the
contamination of the NIH-FSH-S9 preparation with LH may be
estimated to be greater than 1% when bioassayed by a method other
than the ascorbic acid depletion test.   A second possibility for
the action of FSH is suggested by the reports that FSH may act
synergistically to potentiate the action of LH on the interstitial
cells (29,30).   Odell et al. (30) have postulated that FSH has a
role in the initiation of LH action by inducing responsiveness of
the interstitial cells to LH.   Since the rats in the present study
were treated with FSH alone and not with FSH + LH, FSH action
could be mediated through a similar mechanism only if FSH potentiates
the action of LH present as contaminant in the FSH preparation.

A second interesting aspect of the present studies is the demonstration that 5α-reductase in the whole testis is increased following in vivo treatment with relatively small doses of LH. This effect of LH appears to be specific to certain cell types that are not easily released into the interstitial cell preparation by shaking. These could be interstitial cells that are more tightly attached to connective tissue of the interstitial compartment or tubular wall and respond to LH treatment differently than cells released by preparative procedure. On the other hand, LH may directly or indirectly cause the stimulation of 5α-reductase activity in another cell type, such as peritubular or Sertoli cells. It appears unlikely that LH stimulates 5α-reductase in germ cells, since in the absence of germ cells (SCO testis), the response to LH was greater than in the non-irradiated testis.

Thus, these results demonstrate that 5α-reductase of the immature rat testis is present at least in two compartments and is stimulated either by FSH and/or LH. However, in these studies neither the site(s) of action of gonadotropins nor the temporal sequence of biochemical events leading to this stimulation has been established.

ACKNOWLEDGEMENTS

Financial support was provided by USPHS Grants HD-04466, DE-02668 and RR-05333, and University of North Carolina Research Council. Ovine FSH-S9 and S10 and LH-S-18 were generously supplied by NIAMDD.

REFERENCES

1. Baggett, B., and Nayfeh, S.N., Fed. Proc. 24: 638, 1965.
2. Nayfeh, S.N., and Baggett, B., Endocrinology 78: 460-470, 1966.
3. Nayfeh, S.N., Barefoot, S.W., and Baggett, B., Endocrinology 78: 1041-1048, 1966.
4. Inano, H., Hori, Y., and Tamaoki, B., Ciba Foundation Colloquia on Endocrinol. 16: 105, 1967.
5. Ficher, M., and Steinberger, E., Steroids 12. 491-506, 1968.
6. Strickland, A.L., Nayfeh, S.N., and Rrench, F.S., Steroids 15: 373-387, 1970.
7. Coffey, J.C., French, F.S., and Nayfeh, S.N., Endocrinology 89: 865-872, 1971.
8. Steinberger, E., and Ficher, M., Endocrinology 89: 679-684, 1971.
9. Podesta, E.J., and Rivarola, M.A., Endocrinology 95: 455, 1974.

10. Nayfeh, S.N., Coffey, J.C., Hansson, V., and French, F.S., J. Steroid Biochem. 6: 1975.

11. Lee, T.P., and Baggett, B. Presented at the Third Annual Meeting of the Society for the Study of Reproduction, abstract, 1970.

12. Hansson, V., McLean, W.S., Smith, A.A., Tindall, D.J., Weddington, S.C., Nayfeh, S.N., French, F.S., and Ritzen, E.M., Steroids 23: 823-832, 1974.

13. Mulder, E., Peters, M.J., DeVries, J., and van der Molen, H.J., Mol. Cell Endocrinol. 2: 171, 1975.

14. Smith, A.A., McLean, M.S., Hansson, V., Nayfeh, S.N., and French, F.S., Steroids 25: 569, 1975.

15. Folman, Y., Sowell, J.G., Eik-Nes, K.B., Endocrinology 91: 702, 1972.

16. Folman, Y., Ahmad, N., Sowell, J.G., Eik-Nes, K.B., Endocrinology 92: 41, 1973.

17. van der Molen, H.J., Grootegoed, J.A., de Greefbijleveld, M.J., Rommerts, F.F.G., and Vander Vusse, G.J., this volume.

18. Rivarola, M.A., and Podesta, E.J., Endocrinology 90: 618, 1972.

19. Lloret, A.P., and Weisz, J., Endocrinology 95: 1306, 1974.

20. Gustafsson, J.A., and Stenberger, A., J. Biol. Chem. 249: 711, 1974.

21. Oshima, H., Sarada, T., Ochiai, K., and Tamaoki, B.I., Endocrinology 86: 1215, 1970.

22. Frowein, J., J. Endocrinol. 57: 437, 1973.

23. Fencl, M., DeM and Villee, C.A., Steroids 21: 537, 1973.

24. Shimazaki, J., Matsushita, I., Furuya, N., Yamanaka, H., and Shida, K., Endocrinology (Jap.) 16: 453, 1969.

25. Means, A.R., and Huckins, C. In Hormone Binding and Target Activation in the Testis, Dufau, M., and Means, A. (Eds.), Plenum Press, N.Y., p. 145, 1974.

26. Dorrington, J.H., and Fritz, I.B., Endocrinology 94: 395-403, 1974.

27. Reichert, L.E., Jr., and Wilhelmi, A.E., Endocrinology 92: 1301, 1973.

28. Kamiyoshi, M., Tanaka, K., and Tanabe, Y., Endocrinology 91: 385, 1972.

29. Purvis, J.L., and Menard, R.H., this volume.

30. Odell, W.D., Swerdloff, H.S., Jacobs, H.S., and Hescox, M.A., Endocrinology 92: 160, 1973.

COMPARTMENTATION OF MICROSOMAL CYTOCHROME P-450 AND 17α-HYDROXYLASE ACTIVITY IN THE RAT TESTIS

J.L. Purvis and R.H. Menard

Department of Biochemistry, University of Rhode Island,
Kingston, Rhode Island 02881; The Rhode Island Hospital
and the Division of Biological & Medical Sciences,
Brown University, Providence, Rhode Island 02906

The adult testis consists of two functionally different tissue compartments: the interstitial tissue which serves in a hormonal role and the seminiferous tubules which function in a reproductive role. In addition to having dissimilar roles in the testis, the two tissues are also characterized by different functional cell types. The interstitial tissue, which is found interspersed between the seminiferous tubules, contains the steroid-producing Leydig cells; whereas the seminiferous tubules are composed of two cell types, the germinal and Sertoli cells. In recent years, an interest has increased as to whether the latter compartment in the testis, i.e., the seminiferous tubules, can also function in a hormonal or steroidogenic role. Such interest has been fostered particularly by the studies of Lacy and associates (1) who have implicated the Sertoli cells of the seminiferous tubules in an androgen synthetic pathway similar to that found in the Leydig cells. Their evidence is based on studies in which seminiferous tubules separated from interstitial tissue of the rat testis were capable of in vitro synthesis of testosterone from steroid precursors such as pregnenolone and progesterone. Other investigators (2-6) undertaking similar experiments have reported that the seminiferous tubules of the rat testis may account for 10 to 30% of the total testosterone biosynthesis from progesterone.

In the testis, the formation of androgens from pregnenolone or progesterone occurs by a microsomal enzyme system (7) which has been suggested to be located predominantly in the Leydig cells of the interstitial tissue. If a similar microsomal pathway does exist in the seminiferous tubules, then the individual enzymes must be present in the tubular compartment. One of these enzymes, the 17α-hydroxylase, which catalyzes the conversion of progesterone to

65

17α-hydroxy-progesterone, has been reported by us and by others
(8,9) to have for its active site the microsomal carbon monoxide
(CO) binding hemoprotein, cytochrome P-450. The detection of 17α-
hydroxylase activity in the seminiferous tubules would be of interest
since steroid 17α-hydroxylation has been reported to occur in only
one other tissue, namely the adrenal gland; whereas the activity
of other microsomal enzymes associated with testicular steroidogenesis, such as the 3β- and the 17β-hydroxysteroid dehydrogenases
are present in various tissues such as liver and, therefore, could
also exist in the seminiferous tubules without taking part in a
microsomal pathway from pregnenolone to testosterone.

Since the active site for microsomal steroid hydroxylation in
the testis is associated with its CO-binding hemoprotein, cytochrome P-450, and since our research has been related to the
functional role and regulation of cytochrome P-450 in endocrine
tissues (10-15), the question as to whether cytochrome P-450 and,
therefore, microsomal 17α-hydroxylation is present in the seminiferous tubules was studied by the following approaches: (1) By
tissue separation experiments in which the concentration of cytochrome P-450 and the activity of the 17α-hydroxylase were examined
in the microsomal fraction of rat interstitial and tubular cells,
(2) By following the rate of appearance of cytochrome P-450 and
microsomal protein during testicular development, and (3) By the
effect of the tissue-specific hormones LH and FSH on the synthesis
of 17α-hydroxylase and cytochrome P-450. During the course of
this investigation we have also attempted to localize intra-
testicularly the activities of other microsomal cytochrome P-450
enzymes, such as the C_{17}-C_{20} lyase in the rat testis.

INTRATESTICULAR LOCALIZATION OF CYTOCHROME P-450 AND

17α-HYDROXYLASE ACTIVITY IN THE RAT TESTIS

Testis Preparation

Rat testis tubules were gently teased apart with forceps from
the interstitial tissue according to the method of Christensen and
Mason (6). In each experiment testes were combined into two
groups: one for separation; the other served as controls. Control
testis were either decapsulated or teased and spread, and were suspended either in 0.15M KCl or in 0.25M sucrose for the duration of
the separation. At the completion of the dissection, the tubular
and interstitial tissue were individually combined for the preparation of the microsomes (8).

The method for measuring the amount of microsomal cytochrome
P-450 and the specific activity of the 17α-hydroxylase has been

described in detail elsewhere (8,10,15). Briefly, the reaction
mixture in a total volume of 0.20 ml contained: 50 μM (4-^{14}C) progesterone (SA 105,000 dpm/nmole in 1% propylene glycol), 50 mM Tris-
buffer pH 7.4, 150 mM KCl, 500 μM NADPH, 10 mM glucose-6-phosphate,
1 U/ml of glucose-6-phosphate dehydrogenase and 5 mM $MgCl_2$. The
reaction was started by the addition of microsomal protein in
amounts varying from 20 to 200 μg for whole testis, 10 to 60 μg for
interstitial, and 250 to 900 μg for tubules. The mixture was incubated at 37 C in air for 10 to 30 min. Rates of hydroxylation were
constant during this time period and were proportional to the amount
of microsomal protein added (8).

After termination of the reaction mixture, steroids were separated by TLC. Two major radioactive bands, corresponding to the
mobility of authentic progesterone and 17α-hydroxyprogesterone, were
detected by radioscanning. The 17α-hydroxyprogesterone band as
detected under ultraviolet light, was scraped from the plate into
scintillation vial and the radioactivity was measured quantitatively
by liquid scintillation spectrometry. The radioactive product 17α-
hydroxyprogesterone, was identified by recrystallization to constant
specific activity and more recently by mass spectrometry following
isolation by high pressure liquid chromatography (Dupont Instrument
Model 830) on a Zorbax SIL column.

In the above microsomal assay system, labeled 17α-hydroxy-
progesterone accumulates and is not further converted to androstenedione or testosterone. Since cytochrome P-450 is the active
site for both the 17α-hydroxylase and the $C_{17}C_{20}$ lyase enzymes
(8,11,16,17), saturation of the binding sites of cytochrome P-450
in vitro with high amount of progesterone will prevent the binding
of 17α-hydroxyprogesterone to cytochrome P-450, thereby, inhibiting
the conversion of 17α-hydroxyprogesterone to androstenedione. In
other assays such as the C_{17}-C_{20} lyase the enzyme level is adjusted
so that the product of this assay, androstenedione, never reaches
the Km value for a succeeding reaction.

The amount of cytochrome P-450 was determined from its carbon
monoxide absorption spectrum (18). Difference spectra of turbid
suspension were recorded at room temperature either in an Aminco
DW-2 or in a Cary recording spectrophotometer equipped with a high-
intensity light source Microsomes were suspended in 20 or 50 mM
Tris-buffer, pH 7.4, and were equally divided between two cuvettes
having an optical path of 1 cm. Microsomal protein concentrations
were: whole, 3 to 5 mg/ml; interstitial, 2 to 3 mg/ml; and tubular
4 to 6 mg/ml. The concentrations of cytochrome P-450 and its breakdown product, cytochrome P-420, were determined from the CO-
difference spectra using an extinction coefficient of 91 $mM^{-1}cm^{-1}$
for the absorption between 450 nm relative to 490 nm and an extinction coefficient of 110 $mM^{-1}cm^{-1}$ for the change between 420 and
490 nm (19).

Table 1

Concentration of Cytochrome P-450 and Activities of 17α-Hydroxylase and $C_{17}-C_{20}$ Lyase in Rat Interstitial Cell and Tubular Microsomes

Preparation	Cytochrome P-450		17α-Hydroxylase		$C_{17}-C_{20}$ Lyase	
	nmoles/mg protein	nmoles/testis	nmoles/min/mg protein	nmoles/min/testis	nmoles/min/mg protein	nmoles/min/testis
1. Whole:[a]	0.057	0.226	0.089	0.320	----	----
Interstitial	0.115	0.164(74)[c]	0.281	0.269 (84)	----	----
Tubular	<0.004	<0.014 (7)	<0.001	<0.003 (1)	----	----
2. Whole:[a]	0.040	0.167	0.093	0.331	----	----
Interstitial	0.053	0.143 (86)	0.169	0.274 (83)	----	----
Tubular	n.d.[d]	n.d.	0.012	0.034 (10)	----	----
3. Whole:[a]	0.048	0.197	----	----	----	----
Interstitial	0.086	0.162 (82)	----	----	----	----
Tubular	<0.003	<0.012 (6)	----	----	----	----
4. Whole:[b]	0.029	0.701	0.134	1.648	0.037	0.455
Interstitial	0.159	0.580 (83)	0.570	1.140 (69)	0.162	0.324 (71)
Tubular	0.010	0.072 (10)	0.047	0.118 (7)	0.013	0.052 (11)
5. Whole:[b]	0.030	0.708	0.118	1.493	0.056	0.708
Interstitial	0.100	0.552 (78)	0.310	0.651 (44)	0.110	0.231 (33)
Tubular	<0.003	<0.027 (4)	0.010	0.045 (3)	<0.003	<0.014 (2)

[a]Whole testis, decapsulated; [b]Whole testis, decapsulated, teased and spread; [c]Numbers in brackets indicate the percent of control; [d]Cytochrome P-450 and/or P-420, measured at a microsomal concentration of 5.5 mg/ml, was not detectable (n.d.) in this experiment.

Compartmentation of Cytochrome P-450 and 17α-Hydroxylase

Activity in the Rat Testis

The levels of cytochrome P-450 and the cytochrome P-450 dependent enzymes, the 17α-hydroxylase and the C_{17}-C_{20} lyase, were determined in the microsomal fraction of the separated interstitial and tubular cells (Table 1). When calculated either on the basis of per mg of microsomal protein or per testis, the concentration of microsomal cytochrome P-450 and the activities of the two cytochrome P-450 dependent enzymes were found to be 10 to 30-folds higher in the interstitial cells than in the seminiferous tubules. Measurements of the CO-hemoproteins in tubular microsomal suspensions of 4 to 6 mg protein per ml, revealed little, if any, cytochrome P-450 or its breakdown product, cytochrome P-420. A very low tubular 17α-hydroxylase activity was detected when the amount of microsomal protein added to the reaction mixture ranged from 20 to 160 µg (Table 1, experiment 1). The amount of 17α-hydroxylase activity was less than 0.4% of the interstitial cell concentration and less than 1% of the whole testis when calculated on the basis of per mg of microsomal protein. However, in other experiments, the cytochrome P-450 hydroxylating activity in the seminiferous tubules could only be detected accurately when the amount of microsomal protein varied from 250 to 900 µg (Table 1, experiment 2, 4, and 5); in this case the activity in the tubular microsomes was 10 to 30 times less than the activity in the interstitial microsomes. On the other hand, hydroxylating activity in the interstitial cell microsomes could be detected with the addition of only 10 µg of protein. Thus, the detection of cytochrome P-450 hydroxylase activity in the seminiferous tubules in the presence of only high microsomal protein concentration added to the reaction mixture may indeed indicate that the activity represents interstitial cell hydroxylase activity resulting from a contamination of the seminiferous tubules by interstitial tissue during the physical separation of the testicular cells. Although a 5 to 10% contamination of the seminiferous tubules by the interstitial cells would be difficult to observe histologically, gradient centrifugation techniques for the isolation of seminiferous tubules following the separation of the testicular cells by the method of Christensen and Mason (6) have revealed that, at least, 5 to 10% of the tubular cells are contaminated with interstitial cells (Lee, I.P., personal communication). This low amount of contamination would, therefore, account for the 6 to 7% detection of the activities of the cytochrome P-450 dependent enzymes in the seminiferous tubules.

The amount of cytochrome P-450 recovered in the microsomal fraction of the interstitial cells ranged from 74 to 86% of the whole testis. On the other hand, less than 10% (average 7%) of cytochrome P-450 and/or cytochrome P-420 was found in the tubular microsomes on a per testis basis. Differences in the values of

Table 2

Loss of the Microsomal Activities of Cytochrome P-450,
17α-Hydroxylase, and C_{17}-C_{20} Lyase in Teased, Spread Testes

Preparation	Time Spread hr	Cytochrome P-450 nmoles/mg protein	17α-Hydroxylase nmoles/min/mg protein	C_{17}-C_{20} Lyase nmoles/min/mg protein
Whole: teased and spread[a]	0	0.054	0.180	0.050
	1/2	0.050 (7)[b]	0.220	-----
	3-4	0.030 (44)	0.126 (30)	0.029 (42)
Tubules[c]		<0.002	0.007	-----

[a]Rat testes were decapsulated, teased and spread in 0.25M sucrose on petri dishes which were kept on ice. After different times periods, the testes were homogenized in 0.25M sucrose and the microsomes were prepared as described elsewhere (11). The activities of cytochrome P-450, 17α-hydroxylase, and C_{17}-C_{20} lyase were determined as described in Methods. Resulting values are averages of two experiments.

[b]Numbers in brackets indicate the percent decrease in the activities with respect to controls.

[c]Testis tubules were separated from interstitial cells for 30 minutes in a cold room set at 5 C. Whole testis which were teased and spread served as the control.

cytochrome P-450 either per mg of microsomal protein or per testis
in experiments 1-3 and 4-5 are due to the higher yield of microsomal protein recovered when the homogenate is fractionated in 0.25M
sucrose (experiments 4 and 5) compared to 0.15M KCl (experiments 1-
3). As noted in experiment 5 of Table 1, the activites of the 17α-
hydroxylase and the $C_{17}-C_{20}$ lyase recovered in the interstitial
fraction were only 44 and 33%, respectively, of the whole testis.
The low activities of the two hydroxylases in this experiment were
attributed to a 45% breakdown of cytochrome P-450 to its inactive
form, cytochrome P-420. This breakdown of cytochrome P-450, which
was detected in various amounts in most experiments, can take place
during the separation of the seminiferous tubules from the interstitial cells (Table 2). In the two experiments illustrated in
Table 2, a 30 to 45% loss occurred in the concentration of cytochrome P-450 and in the activites of the two cytochrome P-450
hydroxylases in microsomes prepared from testes which were teased
and spread for 3 to 4 hours; no significant loss, however, was
found when the activities were measured within a half-hour or when
the testes were only decapsulated and placed in cold KCl or sucrose
solution (Table 1, experiments 1, 2, and 3). Moreover, when the
concentration of cytochrome P-450 and the activity of the 17α-
hydroxylase were measured in tubular microsomes prepared from seminiferous tubules which were dissected within 30 minutes from the
interstitial tissue, less than 4% of the amount of the testicular
cytochrome P-450 and approximately 3% of the testicular 17α-
hydroxylase activity were recovered in the tubular fraction
(Table 2).

The possibility that the concentration of cytochrome P-450 in
the seminiferous tubules is too low to be detected by present
techniques cannot be excluded. If the activities of the microsomal
cytochrome P-450 hydroxylases are present in the seminiferous tubules, the action of these tubular enzymes during steroidogenesis
would probably play a small role in the microsomal androgen formation of such steroids as 17α-hydroxyprogesterone and androstenedione because of their low specific activities as compared to
the specific activities of the interstitial cell hydroxylases. The
latter conclusion is supported by the data shown in Table 1 in which
the specific activities of the microsomal cytochrome P-450 hydroxylases differ by 10 to 30 times between the interstitial tissue and
the seminiferous tubules. Thus, our biochemical studies support
the current view that the microsomal androgen pathway for the formation of testosterone from either pregnenolone or progesterone via
microsomal hydroxylation and side-chain cleavage is located mainly,
if not exclusively, in the Leydig cells of the interstitial tissue.
If synthesis of testosterone occurs in the seminiferous tubules of
the testis, then either a novel mechanism may exist for the formation of testosterone from precursors such as cholesterol or pregnenolone or that the last enzyme in the microsomal pathway of
testosterone biosynthesis, the 17β-hydroxysteroid dehydrogenase,

is active at a high rate in the seminiferous tubules and utilizes
as substrates steroid precursors which are first formed in the
Leydig cells.

LEVELS OF MICROSOMAL CYTOCHROME P-450 DURING TESTICULAR DEVELOPMENT

As indicated in Figure 1, the level of microsomal cytochrome
P-450 as a function of age during testicular development has a lag
period from day 15 to 25, then increases linearly to day 37, and
reaches a steady-state level at day 55 where the rate of synthesis
of testicular cytochrome P-450 equals the rate of degradation. In
contrast to the rate of synthesis of microsomal cytochrome P-450,
the rate of microsomal protein synthesis is linear between day 20
and 65 and attains a constant level only at 85 days of age. Moreover, at 44 days of age where the level of cytochrome P-450 per mg
protein reaches its maximum, the amount of cytochrome P-450 per
testis is 88% of its maximal while the level of microsomal protein
is only 53%. Because of the dissimilar rates of synthesis of testicular cytochrome P-450 and testicular microsomal protein, the level
of cytochrome P-450 per mg protein declines slowly after day 44 and
reaches a constant level at the time the microsomal protein becomes
constant. Thus, during the maturation of the rat testis, the fall
in the level of cytochrome P-450 per mg protein from 44 to 125 days
of age is caused by an increased synthesis of tubular microsomal
protein which does not contain cytochrome P-450, and which is
probably of germinal origin.

In Tables 3 and 4, the relation of microsomal cytochrome P-450
to the interstitial and tubular volumes of the testis of a seasonal
breeding animal was studied. In the adult Ring-necked Pheasant
(Phasianus colchinus) gonadal development either during the reproductive cycle or during photoperiodicity response may be characterized, according to testicular weight, into five stages (Table 3).
In each stage the interstitial and tubular volume is used as an
index to follow the development of either the interstitial or tubular compartment of the testis. As shown in Table 3, the two
testicular compartments increased markedly in size between stages
1 and 2 after which the development of the interstitial tissue
gradually plateaus to adult levels, whereas the size of the tubular
compartment continues to double. When the amount of microsomal
protein synthesized at each stage is compared to the development
of the two testicular compartments, the increase in microsomal protein formation correlated only with the increase in the tubular
compartment. A one to three fold increase in the amount of microsomal protein synthesized is in agreement with a similar increase
in the size of the seminiferous tubules. As noted during the
development of the rat testis, the testicular content of microsomal
cytochrome P-450 in the adult pheasant also increases 10 folds
during gonadal growth. This increase in the concentration of

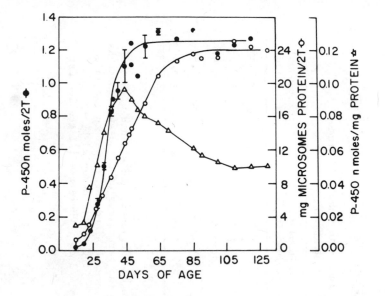

Fig 1.   Levels of Microsomal Cytochrome P-450 and Microsomal
Protein as a Function of Age

Microsomes of rates of different ages were prepared by method
of Purvis (11) in 0.25M sucrose after removing the mitochondrial
fraction, and cytochrome P-450 and mg microsomal protein determined:
●———● cytochrome P-450/2 testis, 0———0, mg microsomal protein/2
testis, △———△ cytochrome P-450/mg microsomal protein.   From
Jimenez, U. and Purvis, J.L. (unpublished).

cytochrome P-450 in the whole testis was found to be associated
with the increase in the development of the interstitial tissue
(Table 4).   This latter observation was assessed by determining
at each stage of gonadal growth the ratio of the testicular content of cytochrome P-450 to the size of either the interstitial or
tubular tissues.   As shown in Table 4, the rise in the level of
cytochrome P-450 during testicular growth corresponded to a similar
increase in the ratio of cytochrome P-450 to interstitial volume,
but not to that of the tubular volume.

Table 3

Level of Microsomal Protein, Interstitial Volume, and Tubular Volume
in Pheasant Testis During Sexual Maturation

Stage	Testis weight grams	N^a	Interstitial volume $(mm^3)^b$	Tubular volume $(mm^3)^b$	mg microsomal protein/bird
I	0.10–0.50	12	52 $\pm$ 1.8	76 $\pm$ 6	1.75 $\pm$ 0.19
II	0.50–1.00	8	105 $\pm$ 5	306 $\pm$ 37	6.77 $\pm$ 0.97
III	1.00–2.00	7	117 $\pm$ 4	706 $\pm$ 38	11.94 $\pm$ 0.97
IV	2.00–4.00	5	134 $\pm$ 6	1634 $\pm$ 54	26.16 $\pm$ 3.96
V	4.00–8.00	12	152 $\pm$ 4	3591 $\pm$ 24	49.12 $\pm$ 5.38

[a] N represents the number of experiments. Values are expressed as $\pm$ S.E.

[b] Pheasant testes were fixed in Bouin's fixative, paraffin embedded, sectioned, and stained with eosin and hematoxylin. Histological sections were photographed and the percentage of cross-section areas occupied by the interstitial tissue and seminiferous tubules were obtained. This percentage value was then used to calculate the percentage of the total volume of the testis occupied by these tissues. The total volume of the testis was computed from $V = 4/3$ ab^2, where $a = 1/2$ the longest and $b = 1/2$ the widest diameter of the testis.

Table 4

Correlation Between Cytochrome P-450, Interstitial Volume, and
Tubular Volume During the Development of the Adult Pheasant Testis

Testis weight grams	Cytochrome P-450 nmoles/bird	Cytochrome P-450 Interstitial volume	Cytochrome P-450 Tubular volume
0.25	$0.075 \pm .01^a$	1.44×10^{-3}	1.00×10^{-3}
0.75	$0.250 \pm .02$	2.38×10^{-3}	0.80×10^{-3}
1.50	$0.410 \pm .03$	3.50×10^{-3}	0.58×10^{-3}
3.00	$0.760 \pm .03$	5.65×10^{-3}	0.47×10^{-3}
6.00	$0.876 \pm .05$	5.75×10^{-3}	0.24×10^{-3}

[a]Values are the mean of five experiments $\pm$ S.E.

Thus, the decline in the level of microsomal cytochrome P-450
in the testis either during the gonadal development of the rat or
during the seasonal-development of the adult pheasant may result
from a proliferation in the endoplasmic reticulum of the seminiferous
tubules which, in turn, would cause a decrease in the concentration
of cytochrome P-450 in the interstitial tissue when calculated on a
basis of per milligram of microsomal protein. The latter supposition
is based on the evidence that microsomal cytochrome P-450 is localized only in the interstitial tissue of the testis and that the
greater amount of microsomal protein synthesized in the testis is
predominantly of tubular origin.

HORMONAL CONTROL OF CYTOCHROME P-450 AND CYTOCHROME

P-450 DEPENDENT ENZYMES IN THE TESTIS

Recently, Purvis et al. (11,12) have shown that testicular
mitochondrial and microsomal cytochrome P-450 may be altered by
hypophysectomy, which causes a decay of the microsomal cytochrome
P-450 level to 1% of the intact animal, or by treatment of intact
or hypophysectomized animals with HCG which causes an elevation in
the levels of testicular cytochrome P-450. Such hormonal alteration
in the rat may affect three enzyme systems in the testis which require cytochrome P-450: the mitochondrial cholesterol side-chain
cleavage enzyme which hydroxylates cholesterol at the C-20 and
C-22 position and cleaves the 20,22-dihydroxycholesterol to
pregnenolone and isocaproic aldehyde, the microsomal 17α-hydroxylase
which catalyzes the hydroxylation of progesterone to 17α-hydroxy-
progesterone, and the microsomal C_{17}-C_{20} lyase which catalyzes the
cleavage of 17α-hydroxyprogesterone to androstenedione.

The relationship of the concentration of microsomal cytochrome P-450 to the activities of the 17α-hydroxylase and the C_{17}-C_{20} lyase can be seen in Figure 2. If the level of microsomal cytochrome in the testis is varied over a 100-fold ranged by treating either hypophysectomized or intact rats with various amounts of either LH alone or LH in combination with other pituitary hormones, measurement of the activities of the 17α-hydroxylase and the C_{17}-C_{20} lyase at each cytochrome P-450 level clearly suggests that the enzymatic rates of the latter enzymes are dependent on the concentration of cytochrome P-450. The results in Figure 2 demonstrate that the increased activities of the 17α-hydroxylase and the C_{17}-C_{20} lyase are closely coupled to the increased levels of cytochrome P-450 so that increases in the concentration of cytochrome P-450 results in proportional increases in 17α-hydroxylase and C_{17}-C_{20} lyase activities, thereby, resulting in a constant ratio of either 17α-hydroxylase or C_{17}-C_{20} lyase to cytochrome P-450. The activities of the 17α-hydroxylase and the C_{17}-C_{20} lyase were 4.20 and 1.86 nmoles/min/ nmoles of cytochrome P-450, respectively. The ratio of the 17α-hydroxylase to the C_{17}-C_{20} lyase is 2.2 to 1 and indicates that the rate of synthesis of the 17α-hydroxylase is higher than the rate of synthesis of the C_{17}-C_{20} lyase.

The specificity of the pituitary hormones on the synthesis of microsomal protein and cytochrome P-450 was studied by injecting LH, FSH, and LH and FSH into hypophysectomized rats. The effect of the gonadotrophic hormones LH and FSH on the synthesis of microsomal cytochrome P-450 and of microsomal protein in the hypophysectomized rat is illustrated in Figure 3. Although FSH increases microsomal protein to a much greater extent than LH, LH has a much greater effect on the synthesis of cytochrome P-450. Expressed either as nmoles/2 testis or nmoles/mg protein, the concentration of cytochrome P-450 is 7 times higher after treatment with LH than with FSH. On the other hand, treatment of animals with both LH and FSH causes a 16 to 30 times increase in the level of microsomal cytochrome P-450. This effect of LH and FSH compared to LH alone is additive when the results are expressed as nmoles/mg protein (Figure 3B) but greater than additive when expressed as nmoles/2 testis (Figure 3A). This differential effect on microsomal cytochrome P-450 may be explained by different effects of FSH on the rat testis: a) an FSH-increase in microsomal protein synthesis which occurs in the seminiferous tubules and b) a synergistic effect of FSH on the LH-stimulation of cytochrome P-450 synthesis. Thus, in the rat testis a dual effect of FSH on microsomal protein synthesis in the seminiferous tubules and on the action of LH in the interstitial cells could result in changes in the levels of cytochrome P-450/2 testis without changing the levels of cytochrome P-450/mg protein.

Although a synergistic action of FSH on LH controlled cytochrome P-450 synthesis is postulated in the hypophysectomized rat,

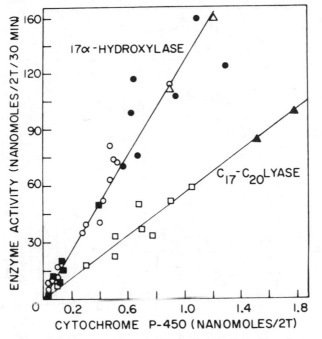

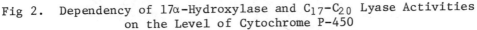

Fig 2.   Dependency of 17α-Hydroxylase and $C_{17}-C_{20}$ Lyase Activities
on the Level of Cytochrome P-450

Male rats (200 gms) were hypophysectomized and injected subcutaneously every 12 hours for seven days with different dosage of
GH, TSH, LH, and FSH alone or in various combinations. In a few
cases, rats with intact pituitaries were treated only with LH.
After seven days, animals were killed and testis microsomes were
prepared. The following equations and correlation coefficients
obtained were: 17α-hydroxylase, y = 2.34 + 124.1 x , r = 0.94;
$C_{17}-C_{20}$ lyase y = 0.95 + 55.3 x, r = 0.97. The different symbols
indicate the different hormonal combinations: Hx FSH ■; Hx LH o,
□ ; Hx LH+FSH ●; intact LH Δ,▲. From Latif, S.A. and Purvis, J.L.
(unpublished).

no synergistic effect is seen in one-day old chicks treated with
LH + FSH. The chick data, as illustrated in Table 5, shows that
LH stimulates cytochrome P-450 synthesis and that the effect of
FSH + LH on cytochrome P-450 is additive. Furthermore, if FSH is
contaminated with 3% LH then the effect of FSH on microsomal

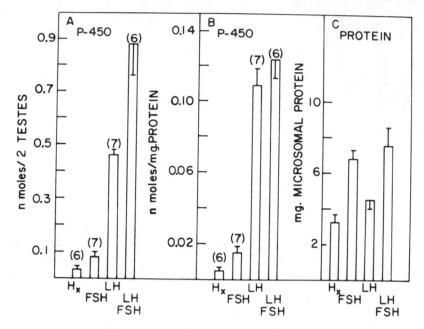

Fig 3.   The Effect of LH, FSH and LH + FSH on Microsomal Protein
         and Cytochrome P-450 in the Hypophysectomized Rat

        Rats, hypophysectomized for 30-60 days, were injected s.c.
every 12 hr with either LH 100 µg/day, or LH + FSH 100 µg/day.
Animals were killed 7 days later and testis microsomes were pre-
pared.   Numbers in parentheses indicate number of experiments.
Each determination shows the mean ± S.E.   From Latif, S.W. and
Purvis, J.L. (unpublished).

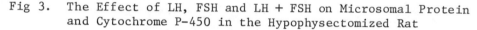

cytochrome P-450 in the chick testis can be completely accounted
for.

        The control of testicular cytochrome P-450 synthesis by the
pituitary gonadotropic hormone LH can be clearly seen by the log-
dose relationship of injected LH to the levels of microsomal and
mitochondrial cytochrome P-450.   The administration of 3 to 100 µg
of LH/day to hypophysectomized rats resulted in a linear increase
in the levels of mitochondrial and microsomal cytochrome P-450, expressed either as nmoles/mg protein or as nmoles/2 testis, (Figure
4).   Stimulation of the microsomal cytochrome P-450 levels by LH
was detected to be sensitive to the dose administered, requiring a
minimum dose of 5.6 µg/day to produce a 4-5 fold increase, whereas

Table 5

Effect of LH and FSH Administration on the Concentration
of Microsomal Cytocrome P-450 in the Chick Testis[c]

Treatment[a] (dose/chick)	Cytochrome P-450	
	nmoles/mg protein	nmoles/chick
Saline 0.10 ml	0.066	0.0038
LH 3.1 µg	0.085 (29)[b]	0.0060 (58)
LH 10 µg	0.133 (100)	0.0110 (189)
LH 31 µg	0.150 (127)	0.0154 (305)
LH 100 µg	0.183 (200)	0.0210 (453)
FSH 100 µg	0.048 (-27)	0.0071 (87)
FSH 100 µg + LH 31 µg	0.111 (68)	0.0195 (413)

[a]Testis from 50 chicks were pooled for each determination of cytochrome P-450. One day-old chicks were administered s.c. a single dose of hormone every 24 hr for a period of 2 days. Testis were removed 24 hr after the last administration. Chicks were 3 days old at the time of death. The mean relative potency of the ovine FSH (NIH-FSH-S9), as reported by the Endocrine Study Section, was 1.13 U/mg and the LH contamination was estimated to be less than 0.010 NIH-LH-S1 U/mg.

[b]Numbers in brackets indicate the percent increase with respect to controls.

[c]Data taken from Menard, R.H. and J.L. Purvis, Endocrinology 91, 1506 (1972).

mitochondrial cytochrome P-450 level is less sensitive requiring an amount of LH 3 times higher to produce a measurable effect. The results in Figure 4 also show that the rate of cytochrome P-450 synthesis induced by LH treatment is different for microsomal and mitochondrial cytochrome P-450. If calculated on a per testis basis, microsomal cytochrome P-450 synthesis is about 4 times faster than mitochondrial synthesis; whereas on a per mg protein basis, it is 2 times faster than mitochondrial synthesis.

In a few experiments, a 100 µg FSH/day was injected to hypophysectomized rats for 4 days prior to the administration of LH. The effect of FSH priming in such a manner resulted in increased levels of cytochrome P-450/2 testis, but was without any change on a per mg protein basis, (Figure 4). This effect of FSH could be caused by both an FSH-stimulation of tubular protein synthesis and

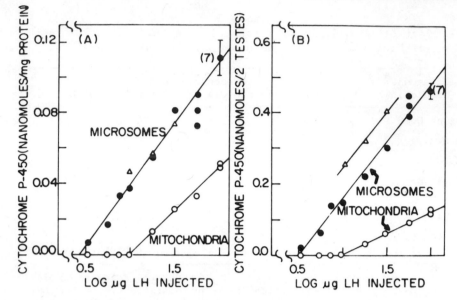

Fig 4.   Relationship Between Testis Microsomal and Mitochondrial
Cytochrome P-450 and the Log-Dose of LH Injected
After Hypophysectomy

Male rats, hypophysectomized for 40 to 55 days, were treated
with LH at a dosage of 3.3 to 100 µg/day (s.c. every 12 hr for 7
days). In some cases the animals were pre-treated for 4 days with
FSH (100 µg/day) before LH treatment. The following equations and
correlation coefficients were obtained: Microsomal P-450/mg protein: N = 18, y = −0.03 + 0.07x, r = 0.87; Mitochondrial P-450/mg
protein: N = 9, y = −0.047 + 0.048x, r = .986; Microsomal P-450/2T,
N = 15, y = −0.155 + .316x, r = .96; Mitochondrial P-450/2T, N = 9,
y = −.121 + .121x, r = .997. ● Microsomal P-450, O Mitochondria
P-450, and Δ microsomal P-450 after 4 day pre-treatment with FSH.
From Latif, S.A. and Purvis, J.L. (unpublished).

by a synergistic effect of FSH on the LH-stimulated synthesis of
cytochrome P-450 as described in Figure 3, or may be caused by a
contamination of FSH with LH. If the effect of FSH on cytochrome
P-450 synthesis is caused by LH contamination, then a 12-13% contamination of FSH with LH would be required to superimpose the two
curves.

An effect of FSH on the activity of the 17α-hydroxylase is
seen in Figure 5 in which the log-dose effects of LH and FSH on the

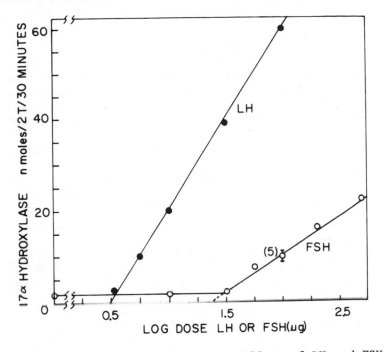

Fig 5.   The Comparison of Log-Dose Effect of LH and FSH on
17α-Hydroxylase Activity

    Different dose levels of LH and of FSH were injected for seven
days into 200 gm rats which had previously been hypophysectomized
for 54 days.   LH and FSH treatment was s.c. every 12 hours.   The
equations and correlation coefficients are as follows: LH stimulated 17α-hydroxylase, $y = -18.64 + 38.96\ x$, $r = 1.0$; FSH stimulated
17α-hydroxylase, $y = -19.3 + 15.16\ x$, $r = 0.96$.   From Latif, S.A.
and Purvis, J.L. (unpublished).

17α-hydroxylase activity are compared.   FSH administration to hypophysectomized rats has no effect on the 17α-hydroxylase activity
until the dosage injected per day reaches 56 µg (as compared to
5.6 µg for LH).   However, when FSH is administered at an amount
greater than 56 µg/day, the effect of FSH treatment on the activity
of the microsomal 17α-hydroxylase is linearly related to the dose
given.

DISCUSSION

It is apparent from the measurements of microsomal cytochrome
P-450 and the cytochrome P-450 dependent enzymes in the tubular and
interstitial compartments of the rat testis that the small amount
(6-7%) of the testicular 17α-hydroxylase activity found in the seminiferous tubules can be explained by interstitial cell contamination
which may occur during the physical dissection of the testicular
cells. This interpretation that cytochrome P-450 is an interstitial cell enzyme is consistent with the measurements of microsomal cytochrome P-450 and microsomal protein during testicular
development. These results show that a large amount of testicular
microsomal protein is synthesized by testicular elements which are
not forming cytochrome P-450. These elements are more likely the
germinal cells of the seminiferous tubules.

Since the action of the pituitary hormone, LH, is specific for
its target tissue, the Leydig cell (20) and since the administration
of LH to hypophysectomized animals regulates the levels of testicular
cytochrome P-450 and the cytochrome P-450 dependent enzymes (Figures
2, 3, and 4), the placing of microsomal cytochrome P-450 and the
microsomal enzymes, the 17α-hydroxylase and the $C_{17}-C_{20}$ lyase, in
the interstitial compartment of the testis naturally follows. However, in the rat the specificity of the hormonal effect of LH on
testicular cytochrome P-450 is not absolute. FSH treatment, although
requiring the administration of larger doses than LH, may cause a
stimulation in the synthesis of microsomal cytochrome P-450 and the
cytochrome P-450 dependent enzymes in the hypophysectomized rat.
However, the effect of FSH on microsomal cytochrome P-450 synthesis
may be explained by an FSH synergistic effect on the low level of
contaminating LH. Such a synergistic effect of FSH on the LH-
stimulation of cytochrome P-450 would explain the greater than
additive effect of the combined LH and FSH treatment compared to
the LH treatment alone on the level of testicular cytochrome P-450
(Figure 3). Moreover, the absence of any effect of FSH on the level
of the 17α-hydroxylase activity at a dosage below 56 μg/day (Figure
5) is consistent with the interpretation of a synergistic effect.
The reason for this possible synergistic effect of FSH on the LH-
induced 17α-hydroxylase activity in the rat testis is unclear. With
one-day old chicks as a model system, the stimulation in the level
of microsomal cytochrome P-450 detected after FSH administration
(100 μg/chick) can be accounted for by a 3% LH contamination. Although the FSH preparations used in this study (NIH-FSH-S1, S8, and
S9) were estimated to contain less than 1% LH when assayed by the
ascorbic acid depletion method (21), the possibility exists that
the contamination of FSH by LH may be greater when bioassayed by
a different method such as the ^{32}P uptake by chick testes (22,23)
or by the in vitro formation of testosterone using intact decapsulated rat testis (M.L. Dufau, personal communication).

Thus, in this study we have used three approaches--physical localization of cytochrome P-450 and the cytochrome P-450 dependent enzymes, the 17α-hydroxylase and the $C_{17}-C_{20}$ lyase, in the testis. From these studies, we have concluded that this prosthetic group, i.e., cytochrome P-450, and these steroidogenic enzymes are interstitial cell enzymes and are not present in the seminiferous tubules of the testis.

REFERENCES

1. Lacy, D., in The Endocrine Function of the Human Testis (eds., James V.H.T., Serio, M. and Martini, L.), vol. 1, Academic Press, New York, 1973, p. 493.
2. Van der Molen, H.J., de Bruijn, H.W.A., Cooke, B.A., de Jong, F.H. and Rommerts, F.F.G., in The Endocrine Function of the Human Testis (eds., James, V.H.T., Serio, M. and Martini, L.) vol. 1, Academic Press, New York, 1973, p. 459.
3. Dufau, M.L., de Kretser, D.M. and Hudson, B., Endocrinology 88: 825, 1971.
4. Inano, H., J. Steroid Biochem. 5: 145, 1974.
5. Hall, P.F., Irby, D.C. and de Krester, D.M., Endocrinology 84: 488, 1969.
6. Christensen, A.K. and Mason, N.R., Endocrinology 76: 646, 1965.
7. Shikita, M. and Tamaoki, B., Endocrinology 76: 563, 1965.
8. Menard, R.H. and Purvis, J.L., Arch. Biochem. Biophys. 154: 8, 1973.
9. Machino, A., Inano, H. and Tamaoki, B., J. Steroid Biochem. 1: 9, 1969.
10. Menard, R.H. and Purvis, J.L., Endocrinology 91: 1506, 1972.
11. Purvis, J.L., Canick, J.A., Latif, S.A., Rosenbaum, J.H., Hologgitas, J. and Menard, R.H., Arch. Biochem. Biophys. 159: 39, 1973.
12. Purvis, J.L., Canick, J.A., Mason, J.I., Estabrook, R.W. and McCarthy, J.L., Annals N.Y. Acad. Sciences 212: 319, 1973.
13. Purvis, J.L., Canick, J.A., Rosenbaum, J.H., Hologgitas, J. and Latif, S.A., Arch. Biochem. Biophys. 159: 32, 1973.
14. Mason, J.I., Estabrook, R.W. and Purvis, J.L., Annals N.Y. Acad. Sciences 212: 406, 1973.
15. Menard, R.H., Stripp, B. and Gillette, J.R., Endocrinology 94: 1628, 1974.
16. McMurty, R.J. and Hagerman, D.D., Steroids Lipids Res. 3: 8, 1972.
17. Betz, G., Roper, M. and Tsai, P., Arch. Biochem. Biophys. 163: 318, 1974.
18. Estabrook, R.W., Peterson, J., Baron, J. and Hildebrandt, A., in Methods in Pharmacology (ed., Chignell, C.F.)., vol. 11, Appleton-Century-Crofts, 1972, p. 303.
19. Omura, T., and Sato, R., J. Biol. Chem. 237: 2652, 1962.

20.   Catt, K.J. and Dufau, M.L., in Receptors for Reproductive
      Hormones (eds., O'Malley, B.W. and Means, A.R.) Plenum
      Publishing Corp., New York, 1973, p. 379.
21.   Reichert, L.E., Jr. and Wilhelmi, A.E., Endocrinology 92:
      1301, 1973.
22.   Burns, J.M., Comp. Biochem. Physiol. 34:   727, 1970.
23.   Kamiyoshi, M., Tanaka, K. and Tanabe, Y., Endocrinology 91:
      385, 1972.

SYNTHESIS OF ESTRADIOL -17β BY SERTOLI CELLS IN CULTURE:

STIMULATION BY FSH AND DIBUTYRYL CYCLIC AMP

David T. Armstrong[1], Young S. Moon, Irving B. Fritz
and Jennifer H. Dorrington

Departments of Physiology and Obstetrics & Gynecology

University of Western Ontario, London, Canada, and
Banting & Best Department of Medical Research
University of Toronto, Toronto, Canada

INTRODUCTION

The ability of the mammalian testis to secrete estrogens is
well established, although the testicular cell type(s) responsible
for secretion of this class of steroids has been somewhat contro-
versial. The Sertoli cell was initially implicated on the basis of
early observations of feminization of dogs with Sertoli cell tumours
(1); this was subsequently substantiated by the isolation of biologically active estrogenic material from Sertoli cell tumours (2,3).
On the other hand, Hunt and Budd (4) concluded that the Leydig cell
was the cell responsible for estrogen secretion, on the basis of
evidence of feminization in men with tumours believed to be of interstitial cell origin. Support for this conclusion came from the observations of Maddock and Nelson (5) that prolonged administration
of human chorionic gonadotropin (HCG) to normal and hypogonadal men
resulted in increased urinary estrogen secretion. This was associated
with histologic evidence of marked stimulation of the Leydig cells,
interference with normal spermatogenesis, and appearance of "degen-
erative" changes in the Sertoli cells.

More recent experiments have not resolved this controversy
unequivocally. De Jong et al. (6) reported concentrations of estradiol 17β to be 9 to 15 times greater in interstitial tissue than in

[1] Associate of the Medical Research Council of Canada.

seminiferous tubules dissected from the testes of adult rats. On the other hand, when these separated tissue preparations were incubated in vitro for 3 hours, no increase in the content of estradiol-17β occurred in the interstitial tissue, whereas the content in the seminiferous tubules was approximately doubled.

The roles of the pituitary gonadotropins in regulation of testicular estrogen secretion have not been established. The importance of luteinizing hormone (LH) has been inferred from the above cited observations of Maddock and Nelson (5) that HCG increased urinary estrogen excretion in men. However, the massive dosages which were used in these studies do not preclude the possibility of the responses being due to follicle-stimulating activity in the HCG preparations. In a more recent study, De Jong et al. (7) observed increased concentrations of estradiol-17β in the testicular venous plasma of intact male rats following acute i.v. injection of a large dose of HCG (100 I.U.) but not of a small dose of NIH-FSH (5 μg). These authors (6) also reported increased testicular tissue concentrations of estradiol-17β following chronic treatment of intact adult rats with HCG (100 I.U./day for 5 days), but not following acute administration of FSH (5-10 μg i.v.) to intact rats, or acute and/or chronic administration of FSH to hypophysectomized rats.

The recent development of methods for isolation and maintenance of Sertoli cells in primary culture (8,9) provided us with a more direct means of determining whether or not the Sertoli cells are capable of estrogen biosynthesis, as well as of investigating the roles of the two pituitary gonadotropins in regulating this biosynthesis.

MATERIALS AND METHODS

Sertoli cell aggregates were prepared from testes of 18- to 20-day-old rats, and cultured in Falcon plastic culture flasks, using methods described previously (9,10). The cells were maintained for 24 hours in the standard culture medium without steroid substrates or hormones, in an atmosphere of 95% air and 5% of CO_2. At the end of this pre-incubation period, the media were discarded and replaced with fresh media containing the substrate, hormones, or other substances under investigation. Incubations were continued for varying periods, media being harvested after appropriate intervals as described under Results. At the end of incubations, steroids were extracted from the cells with ethanol, and the cells were then scraped from the surfaces of the culture flasks, 1 M sodium hydroxide added, and aliquots taken for protein determination (11).

TABLE I

Effect of FSH on Estradiol-17β Synthesis by Rat Sertoli Cells
Cultured for 48 Hours in Medium Containing Various Steroid
Substrates

Hormone Treatment	Number of Flasks	Estradiol-17β Synthesis (pg/mg protein ± S.E.) in Medium Containing:		
		No Steroid Substrate	Testosterone 5×10^{-7} M	Pregnenolone 5×10^{-7} M
None	3	<10	187 ± 35	<10
NIH-FSH-S10 (5 µg/ml)	3	17 ± 4	1900 ± 47	19 ± 10

Hormone and substrates were added at the beginning of incubation, and again after
24 hours. From Dorrington & Armstrong (10).

Aliquots of culture media were extracted with 2 x 5 volumes of diethyl ether and the ether extracts evaporated to dryness in 12 x 75 mm disposable culture tubues. Aliquots of the ethanolic extracts of cells were evaporated to dryness in similar culture tubes. The estradiol-17β contents of these extracts were measured by specific radioimmunoassay, as described previously (10), utilizing an antiserum raised against estradiol-17β-6-BSA, kindly provided by Dr. Gordon Niswender.

RESULTS AND DISCUSSION

Synthesis of estradiol by Sertoli cells during 48 hours of culture in medium containing various substrates is shown in Table 1. In Medium containing no exogenous steroid substrate, estradiol synthesis was negligible either in the absence or presence of FSH. Addition of testosterone (5×10^{-7}M) to the medium resulted in significant synthesis of estradiol in the absence of FSH. Addition of FSH (5 μg NIH-FSH-S10/ml) to medium containing testosterone increased estradiol synthesis 10-fold. Exogenous pregnenolone (5×10^{-7}M) was not an effective substrate for estradiol synthesis, either in the absence or presence of FSH.

In order to determine the specificity of the stimulatory action of FSH, the abilities of a more highly purified FSH preparation (P-FSH, lot #G4-105C, kindly supplied by Dr. Harold Papkoff), and of NIH-LH-S18 to stimulate estradiol synthesis in the presence of testosterone, were compared to that of the NIH-FSH preparation. The results summarized in Table 2, indicate the relative ineffectiveness of NIH-LH (5 μg/ml), and the relatively greater effectiveness of the P-FSH (0.25 μg/ml) in stimulating estradiol synthesis. At these concentrations, the amount of LH activity present in the P-FSH is less than 0.1% of that present in the NIH-LH.

Since FSH stimulates cyclic-3',5'-AMP (cAMP) synthesis by Sertoli cells when cultured under similar conditions (12), dibutyryl cAMP was added to media to determine whether this cyclic nucleotide could mimic the action of FSH on estradiol synthesis. As summarized in Table 2, dibutyryl cAMP (10^{-4}M) was highly effective in stimulating estradiol production by Sertoli cells cultured in medium containing testosterone.

The kinetics of the stimulatory action of FSH was investigated in an experiment in which the culture medium was harvested after varying periods of incubation of Sertoli cells in the presence of testosterone. As illustrated in Figure 1, a lag period of at least two hours occurred before any stimulation of estradiol synthesis was seen.

TABLE II

Effects of Various FSH and LH Preparations, and
Dibutyryl Cyclic-3', 5' -AMP on Synthesis
of Estradiol-17β by Rat Sertoli Cells in Culture

Culture Conditions	Number of Flasks	Estradiol-17β Synthesis (pg/mg protein ± S.E.)
Control	3	18 ± 2
NIH-FSH-S10 (5 µg/ml)	3	687 ± 97
P-FSH-G4-105C (0.25 µg/ml)	3	930 ± 39
NIH-LH-S18 (5 µg/ml)	3	37 ± 3
Dibutyryl cAMP (10^{-4}M)	3	568 ± 18

Cells were cultured for 48 hours in medium containing testosterone
(5 x 10^{-7}M). Testosterone and stimulating agents were added at
the beginning of incubation, and again after 24 hours. From
Dorrington & Armstrong (10).

    In order to determine whether FSH by itself was able to induce
the ability to synthesize estradiol, or whether concomitant exposure
of cells to both FSH and testosterone was necessary, Sertoli cells
were pre-incubated for 24 hours in medium containing either FSH alone
(5 µg/ml) or FSH + testosterone (5 x 10^{-7}M). The media were harvested
for estradiol assay, and the cells were washed three times to remove
traces of hormone, substrate and product. Some cells were extracted
without further incubation, to determine their estradiol content;
others were incubated for 2, 6 or 10 hours further, in fresh medium
containing testosterone (5 x 10^{-7}M) but no FSH. The data presented
in Table 3 confirmed that FSH had been effective in stimulating
estradiol synthesis during the 24-hour pre-incubation in the presence
of testosterone. The amounts of estradiol contained in the cells
at the end of the pre-incubation period (i.e., at the beginning of
the succeeding incubation) are presented in Table 3. Accumulation
of estradiol in the media after 2, 6 and 10 hours incubation in the
presence of testosterone is illustrated in Figure 2. It is evident
that cells which have been exposed for 24 hours to FSH are able to
begin synthesizing estradiol immediately when they are placed in
medium containing testosterone, without a significant lag period.

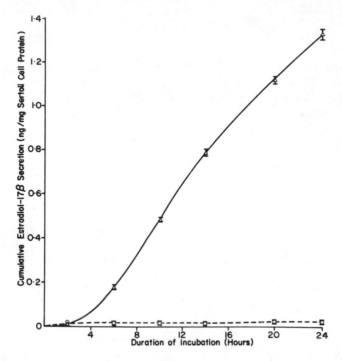

Figure 1.   Effects of FSH on cumulative secretion of estradiol-17β
throughout 24-hour culture in medium containing testosterone.
Medium added at a zero time, and replaced after 2, 6, 10, 14, and
20 hours, contained testosterone (5 x 10^{-7}M) and either no FSH
(0) or NIH-FSH-S10 (5 µg/ml) (Δ).

Thus, the two-hour lag seen in Figure 1 would appear to represent
the time necessary for induction of the response by FSH, rather than
the time necessary for the enzymatic reactions themselves to occur,
once initiated by FSH.

      There is no indication from these results that testosterone
participates in this induction process; cells exposed only to FSH
during the 24-hour pre-incubation period synthesized estradiol as
soon after being placed in fresh medium containing testosterone
as did cells which had been exposed to FSH plus testosterone.
Thus, it would appear that the role of testosterone is purely to
provide substrate for aromatization.

      In contrast to the nearly linear rate of estradiol synthesis
seen in the experiment summarized in Figure 1, a considerable decline in the initial rate of synthesis was evident after 2 hours
in the experiment summarized in Figure 2, especially in cells which

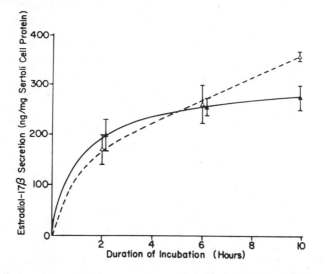

Figure 2. Effect of 24-hour pre-incubation of Sertoli cells in medium containing NIH-FSH-S10 (5 μg/ml) in the absence vs presence of testosterone (5 x 10⁻⁷M), as outlined in Table 3, on subsequent secretion of estradiol-17β- during incubation for varying periods in medium containing testosterone (5 x 10⁻⁷M) but no FSH. At the end of pre-incubation, cells were washed three times with medium containing no FSH or testosterone, then placed in fresh medium containing testosterone only.

had been pre-incubated with FSH plus testosterone. Possible reasons for this difference include: (a) Cells may require the continued presence of FSH for maintenance of estradiol synthesis (in the experiment of Figure 2, no FSH was present during the 10-hour experimental period, whereas it was present throughout the experiment of Figure 1); (b) Substrate may have become limiting and/or accumulated metabolites may have become inhibitory in the experiment of Figure 2 (in this experiment, medium containing testosterone was added at zero time, and not replaced, whereas in the experiment of Figure 1, fresh medium containing 5 x 10⁻⁷M testosterone was added at 2- or 4-hour intervals for the first 14 hours of culture).

In order to distinguish between these two alternatives, another experiment was performed in which cells were pre-incubated for 24 hours with FSH. After discarding the pre-incubation medium, the cells were rinsed and two sets of flasks were incubated for a further 10 hours in medium containing either testosterone alone, or testosterone + FSH; the media were harvested and replaced every

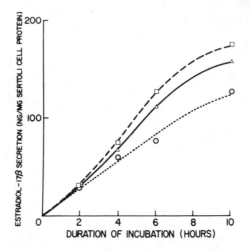

Figure 3.   Estradiol-17β secretion during 10-hour culture of
Sertoli cells under varying conditions following 24-hour pre-incubation with NIH-FSH-S10 (5 μg/ml). (a) ☐ Medium containing testosterone (5 x 10^{-7}M) and NIH-FSH-S10 (5 μg/ml) added at zero time
(i.e., at end of 24-hour pre-incubation), and replaced after 2, 4,
and 6 hours of incubation.   (b) Δ Medium containing testosterone
added at zero time and replaced after 2, 4, and 6 hours of incubation.   (c) O Medium containing testosteone added at zero time
only. Replicate flasks were then incubated for 2, 4, 6 or 10 hours
without replacing media. Analysis of variance indicated that the
slopes, over the linear portions of the time-courses (2 to 6 hours),
of curves (a) and (b) did not differ significantly, and that the
combined slope of (a) and (b) was significantly greater (p < 0.05)
than that of curve (c).

2 hours for the first 6 hours of incubation. To a third group of.
flasks, medium containing testosterone alone was added only at zero
time.   Incubations were carried out for 2, 4, 6 or 10 hours without
replacing media.   The results of this experiment are presented in
Figure 3.   Regression analyses of these curves indicated that the
slightly greater rate of estradiol synthesis observed during the
linear portion of the time-course (the first 6 hours) as a result of
continued presence of FSH was not statistically significant, whereas
the decreased rate due to addition of testosterone at zero time only
was significant (p < 0.05).   It cannot be concluded whether this

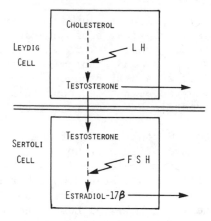

Figure 4.   The cell, two gonadotropin hypothesis for regulation
of estradiol-17β synthesis in the testis.

decrease was caused by insufficient testosterone as a result of
consumption via alternate metabolic pathways, or by inhibitory influences of accumulated metabolites.   The previous reports of extensive conversion of testosterone to ring A-reduced metabolites by
Sertoli cells (9) may be consistent with either interpretation.

     The results of our experiments unequivocally establish the
ability of the Sertoli cells to convert testosterone to estradiol-
17β.   Since the cells did not produce significant amounts of
estradiol in the absence of exogenous steroid substrate, or in
the presence of pregnenolone, it seems likely that the androgen
utilized for estrogen synthesis by the Sertoli cell in vivo is
produced elsewhere in the testis.   This interpretation is consistent with previous observations on the steroidogenic capabilities
of isolated seminiferous tubules and interstitial tissue.   Isolated
tubules were unable to synthesize testosterone from endogenous precursors (13) or from exogenous cholesterol-17α-^{3}H (14), whereas
interstitial tissue incubated under similar conditions synthesized
androgen 13,14).   The concentration of testosterone in testicular
lymph is almost as high as that in spermatic venous blood (15), and
there appears to be no barrier to the entry of testosterone to the
tubule (16,17).

     The ability of FSH, but not LH, to increase the rate of synthe-
sis of estradiol in the Sertoli cell in the presence of testosterone,

offers the first convincing evidence, in either sex, of a steroidogenic action of FSH at a biochemical site separate from that at
which LH stimulates steroidogenesis. This effect, which can be
mimicked by dibutyryl cAMP, is consistent with previous reports
that FSH, but not LH, increases cAMP production in isolated Sertoli
cells (12) and that seminiferous tubules containing Sertoli cells
but lacking germ cells contain FSH receptors (18).

The parallels between Sertoli cells of the testes and granulosa cells of the ovary have often been noted, since they are
believed to have similar embryological origins (19). Estrogen synthesis in the ovarian follicle has been demonstrated to involve
cooperation between two different cell types, the granulosa cells
and the theca interna cells (20,21), although the biochemical basis
for this cooperation has not been established. Our observations
pose the intriguing possibility that testicular estrogen synthesis
may also be the result of interactions between two cell types, as
well as offering an explanation of the separate roles of the two
gonadotropins in regulating this synthesis (Figure 4). In this
model, testosterone formed by the interstitial cells under the
influence of LH is transported to the Sertoli cells, where it is
converted to estradiol-17β under the influence of FSH.

In the absence of FSH, aromatization would be the rate-limiting
step in estradiol biosynthesis, whereas in the presence of FSH, the
rate-limiting factor would then be availability of substrate for
aromatization. Thus, this model could explain the previously reported
(7) ineffectiveness of LH-containing preparations in causing increases
in estradiol production in animals with intact pituitary glands.

The physiological significance of estrogen synthesis in the
testis is not known. Possible functions include systemic hormonal
roles, e.g., in feedback regulation of FSH secretion, or local roles
in maintaining the appropriate milieu within the seminiferous tubule
necessary for spermatogenesis. A third possibility is suggested by
the reports that interstitial cell cytoplasm and nuclei contain
specific estradiol-binding proteins with characteristics of receptors,
(22,23) and that interstitial cell nuclei concentrate radioactivity
following injection of ^{3}H-estradiol in immature rats (24). It is
conceivable that the estradiol produced by the Sertoli cells exert
a local regulatory effect on the metabolism of the interstitial
cells; thus the testosterone-estradiol system may constitute an
interstitial cell-Sertoli cell messenger system.

SUMMARY

Sertoli cells isolated from the testes of 18 to 20-day old rats
synthesize estradiol-17β when grown in primary culture in the

presence of testosterone (5×10^{-7}M). After an initial lag phase of
about 2 hours, follicle-stimulating hormone (FSH) stimulates synthesis of estradiol up to 50-fold, synthesis being approximately
linear for 24 hours when medium is changed every 2-6 hours.
Luteinizing hormone (LH) causes only a marginal stimulation, at concentrations consistent with contamination with FSH. Dibutyryl cyclic
3',5'-adenosine monophosphate (dbcAMP) (10^{-4}M) mimicks the effect
of FSH. No significant synthesis occurs in the absence of steroid
substrate or in the presence of pregnenolone (5×10^{-7}M). When
cells are pre-incubated for 24 hours with FSH in the absence of
testosterone, addition of testosterone results in an immediate
increase in estradiol synthesis without a lag phase, suggesting
that FSH or dbcAMP are capable of inducing the conditions necessary
for stimulation in the absence of testosterone. These observations
provide the first direct evidence of estradiol-17β synthesis by
Sertoli cells from normal animals, and offer evidence that synthesis
of this steroid is regulated at the level of the aromatizing enzyme
system by FSH and cyclic AMP.

ACKNOWLEDGEMENTS

Supported by grants from the Medical Research Council of
Canada (MT 3392 and MT 3292) and the Banting Research Foundation.

REFERENCES

1. Zuckerman, S., and McKeown, T., J. Path. & Bact. 46: 19, 1938.
2. Huggins, C., and Moulder, P.V., Cancer Res. 5: 510, 1945.
3. Berthrong, M., Goodwin, W.E., and Scott, W.W., J. Clin.
    Endocr. and Metab. 9: 579, 1949.
4. Hunt, V.C., and Budd, J.W., J. Urol. 42: 1242, 1939.
5. Maddock, W.O., and Nelson, W.O., J. Clin. Endocr. & Metab.
    12: 985, 1952.
6. DeJong, F.H., Hey, A.H., and van der Molen, H.J., J. Endocr.
    60: 409, 1974.
7. DeJong, F.H., Key, A.H., and van der Molen, H.J., J. Endocr.
    57: 277, 1973.
8. Welsh, M.J., and Wiebe, J.P., Proc. Can. Fed. Biol. Soc. 17:
    44, 1974.
9. Dorrington, J.H., and Fritz, I.B., Endocrinology (in press),
    1975.
10. Dorrington, J.H., and Armstrong, D.T., Proc. Nat. Acad.
    Sci. (in press), 1975.
11. Lowry, O.H., Rosebrough, N.J., Farr, A.L., and Randall, R.J.,
    J. Biol. Chem. 193: 265, 1951.
12. Dorrington, J.H., Roller, N., and Fritz, I.B., Hormone Binding
    and Target Cell Activation of the Testis, Vol. I, Dufau, M.,
    and Means, A.R. (Eds.), Plenum Press, N.Y., p. 237, 1974.

13. Cooke, B.A., DeJong, F.H., van der Molen, H.J., and Rommerts, F.F.G., Nature (New Biol.), 237: 255, 1972.
14. Hall, P.F., Irby, D.C., and de Kretser, D.M., Endocrinology 84: 488, 1969.
15. Setchell, B.P., The Testis, Vol. I, Johnson, A.D., Gomes, W.R., and Vandemark, N.L. (Eds.), Academic Press, N.Y., p. 101, 1970.
16. Parvinem, M., Hume, P., and Niemi, M., Endocrinology 87: 1082, 1970.
17. Podesta, E.J., and Rivarola, M.A., Endocrinology 95: 455, 1974.
18. Means, A.R., Life Sciences 15: 371, 1974.
19. Franchi, L.L., Mandl, A.M., and Zuckerman, S., The Ovary, Vol. 1, Zuckerman, S. (Ed.), Academic Press, N.Y., p. 1, 1962.
20. Falck, B., Acta Physiol. Scand. Suppl. 163: 1, 1959.
21. Short, R.V., Rec. Progr. Horm. Res. 20: 303, 1964.
22. Brinkmann, A.O., Mulder, E., Lamers-Stahlhofen, G.J.M., Mechielsen, M.J., and van der Molen, H.J., FEBS Letters 26: 301, 1972.
23. Mulder, E., Brinkmann, A.O., Lamers-Stahlhofen, G.J.M., and van der Molen, H.J., FEBS Letters 31: 131, 1973.
24. Stumpf, W.E., Endocrinology 85: 31, 1969.

COMPARISON OF STEROID METABOLISM IN TESTICULAR COMPARTMENTS OF HUMAN AND RAT TESTES

Anita H. Payne and Robert P. Kelch

Departments of Obstetrics and Gynecology,
Biological Chemistry and Pediatrics
The University of Michigan
Ann Arbor, Michigan 48104

Great interest has developed in recent years on the intratesticular site of enzymes necessary for steroid hormone synthesis
in mammalian testes. We have been interested in the intratesticular localization of steroid sulfatase. Steroid sulfates have been
observed to be present in high concentrations in human testicular
tissue. Ruokonen et al. (1) determined the amount of various free
steroids and steroid sulfates in testes obtained at the time of
orchiectomy for prostatic carcinoma. In their study the major
steroids isolated from human testes were testosterone, pregnenolone
sulfate and dehydroepiandrosterone sulfate; the concentration of each
expressed as μg free steroid/ 100 g of tissue was 55, 51 and 41
respectively. In earlier studies from our laboratory (2), we demonstrated that pregnenolone sulfate, dehydroepiandrosterone sulfate
and androstenediol-3-sulfate are cleaved by the same testicular
steroid sulfatase with pregnenolone sulfate exhibiting the lowest
K_m. Further studies on the steroid sulfatase activity of homogenates
or minces of testicular tissues from patients indicated that sulfatase activity was greater in isolated seminiferous tubules than in
intact testicular tissue (3). As part of the same study, when
pregnenolone was used as the substrate intact testicular tissue
metabolized more than twice as much pregnenolone as did tubules.
Intact testicular tissue produced approximately twice as much 17-
hydroxypregnenolone, four times as much androstenediol and four
times as much testosterone as did seminiferous tubules. However,
tubules yielded more than twice as much 5-pregene-3β,20α-diol than
did intact testicular tissue. These data suggest that the major
concentration of 20α-reductase is in tubules rather than interstitial tissue, while 17-hydroxylase and C_{17}-C_{20} lyase are concentrated
mainly in interstitial tissue. The concentration of 3β-hydroxy-

97

steroid-dehydrogenase-isomerase and 17β-hydroxysteroid reductase
activities were determined by incubating dehydroepiandrosterone with
isolated tubules and intact testicular tissue from the same testes.
The enzyme activities were found to be similar in both compartments.
This is in contrast to reports on the 3β-hydroxysteroid dehydrogenase-isomerase activity in isolated tubules and intact testicular
tissue from rat testes. Van der Vusse et al. (4) observed a 17 to 1
ratio of this enzyme activity in rat testes for intact tissue to
tubules.

        Additional studies from this laboratory (5) and by Rivarola
et al. (6) have demonstrated that the major site for 5α-reduction
in the adult human testis is in the seminiferous tubules. We reported
on the metabolism of ^{3}H androstenedione in seminiferous tubules and
interstitial cells from the testis of a 17 year old kidney donor
patient. The separation of the testicular compartments was accomplished by treatment of portions of testicular tissue with buffer
containing collagenase. Cells obtained in this manner consisted of
clusters of interstitial cells interspersed with some sperm and
germ cells, while the tubular preparation was essentially free of
interstitial cells. The following observations were made. Conversion to testosterone was approximately the same in both tissue compartments. However, the conversion to 5α reduced metabolites was
much greater in seminiferous tubules than in the interstitial cell
suspension. A difference in the type of 5α-reduced metabolites
in the two testicular tissue compartments was observed. Dihydrotestosterone was identified only in tubules, while androsterone, a
5α-C$_{19}$ steroid without androgenic properties was identified as a
product of androstenedione only in the interstitial cell suspension.
Both 5α-androstane-3α, 17β-diol and 5α-androstane-3β, 17β-diol in
addition to dihydrotestosterone were found as metabolites of andro-
stenedione·or testosterone in seminiferous tubules. Only a minute
amount of these androstanediols was identified in the incubation
of the interstitial cell suspension.

    The above studies on pregnenolone sulfate cleavage and dihydro-
testosterone formation in seminiferous tubules of the human testis
could not distinguish which cell types in the seminiferous tubules
brought about these enzyme reactions. The present investigation
describes studies on testosterone metabolism and steroid sulfate
cleavage in human seminiferous tubules containing only Sertoli cells,
the intratesticular localization of steroid sulfatase in rat testes,
as well as the intratesticular site of estrogen synthesis in the
rat and human testis.

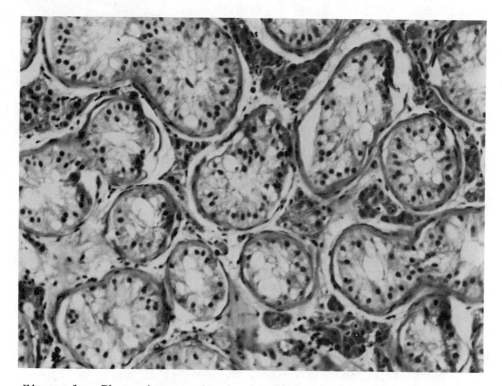

Figure 1. Photomicrograph of a section of the testis from patient
G.M. (H and E,x162). Testis consists of sharply defined seminiferous tubules lined by Sertoli cells. No germ cells could be
identified. Leydig cells are prominent and at least relatively
increased in number. Pathological diagnosis: cryptorchidism with
complete absence of spermatogenesis.

STEROID SULFATASE ACTIVITY AND TESTOSTERONE METABOLISM
IN HUMAN TESTICULAR TISSUE

Testicular tissue was obtained at the time of orchiectomy.
Patient G.M. was a 22 yr old healthy male with unilateral cypotor-
chidism; patient C.D.V. was a 61 yr old male with prostatic carcinoma and diffuse osteoblastic metastases. Tissue from patient
G.M. was divided into 2 portions, one was used for the separation

of seminiferous tubules from interstitial tissue and the remainder
was used for the incubation of intact testicular tissue. The testicular tissue of patient C.D.V. was used for obtaining isolated
seminiferous tubules; no intact tissue was used from this patient.
Portions of seminiferous tubules or intact testicular tissue from
patient G.M. were incubated for 2 hr in air with constant shaking
at 34° in 1ml of 2.5mM Hepes buffer, pH 7.4 containing Krebs Ringer
salts, 1mM NADPH, 1mg/ml glucose and 1.64μM ^{3}H-testosterone (1.95 x
10^7 dpm) or 3.8μM ^{3}H-pregnenolone sulfate (1.84 x 10^7 dpm). The
isolated tubules from patient C.D.V. were incubated for 1 hr with
1.64μM ^{3}H-testosterone under identical conditions are for G.M. All
incubations were carried out in duplicate. At the end of incubation
with ^{3}H-testosterone, ^{14}C-dihydrotestosterone was added for quantitation. Extraction and purification were carried out as previously
described (3,5).

     Histological studies on sections of testicular tissue from
patient G.M. revealed sharply defined tubules lined by Sertoli cells
(Fig.1). Sections of testicular tissue from patient C.D.V. (Fig 2)
revealed a normal testis with active spermatogenesis.

     The metabolism of testosterone by human seminiferous tubules
is shown in Table 1. Although the tubules from the cryptorchid
testis were incubated for 2 hr, only a small amount of dihydrotestosterone was produced and no 5α-androstane-3α, 17β-diol could be detected. The yield of androstenedione was greater in the 2 hr incubation of tubules from the cryptorchid testis than was observed for
the 1 hr incubation of the histologically normal testis.

     Pregnenolone sulfate cleavage by seminiferous tubules and in-
tact testicular tissue from patient G.M. after 2 hr incubation with
^{3}H-pregnenolone sulfate is presented in Table 2. These results are
compared to similar studies reported previously on patients J.W.R.
and P.H. (3). Steroid sulfatase activity is expressed as picomoles
free steroid produced per mg of protein. The amount of pregnenolone
sulfate cleaved is greater in seminiferous tubules than in intact
testicular tissue in the three patients. When the steroid sulfatase
activities of seminiferous tubules and intact testicular tissue
from the same patient are compared the greatest ratio is found in the
cryptorchid testis.

     The very small amount of 5α reduction seen in the seminiferous
tubules which contain Sertoli cells only, suggests that the major
site of 5α reduction in the human tubule is not the Sertoli cell.
This is in agreement with a study reported by Dorrington and Fritz
(7) in which they showed that dihydrotestosterone formation in
rat tubules occurs mostly in spermatocytes. In contrast to 5α
reduction, the cleavage of pregenolone sulfate was considerably
greater in the Sertoli cell only tubules than in normal seminiferous
tubules. This finding suggests that steroid sulfatase in the human
testis is located in Sertoli cells.

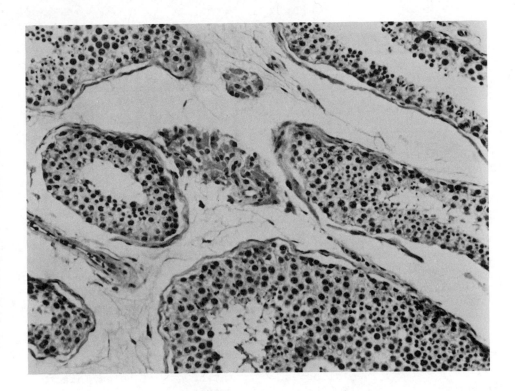

Figure 2. Photomicrograph of a section of the testis from patient
C.D.V. (H and E,x162). Seminiferous tubules are sharply defined
and contain germ cells at various stages of maturation. Interstitial cells are clearly defined and normal in appearance.
Pathological diagnosis: normal testis with active spermatogenesis.

STEROID SULFATASE ACTIVITY IN INTERSTITIAL TISSUE AND SEMINIFEROUS TUBULES OF ADULT RAT TESTES

Rats, approximately 90 days old, were killed by decapitation;
the testes were removed and placed in ice-cold buffer. Separation
of tubules from interstitial tissue was accomplished by the wet
dissection method first described by Christensen and Mason (8).
Interstitial tissue webs and tubules were washed separately several
times with fresh buffer to remove free cells. Intact testicular
tissue, isolated seminiferous tubules and interstitial tissue webs
were homogenized using 0.05M phosphate buffered saline, pH 7.4 or
Krebs Ringer Bicarbonate buffer, pH 7.4. Duplicate aliquots of
each homogenate were incubated at 34° with 3.6μM ^{3}H-pregnenolone
sulfate. Aliquots were removed at the indicated time and assayed

TABLE 1

Metabolites of Testosterone in Isolated Seminiferous
Tubules of Human Testes Expressed in Picomoles/Mg Protein

Metabolite	Patients	
	C.D.V.*	G.M.**
Dihydrotestosterone	3.82	1.47
5α-Androstane-3α, 17β-diol	2.43	N.D.
Total 5α Reduced Metabolites	6.25	1.47
Androstenedione	22.3	32.8

TABLE 2

Pregnenolone Sulfate Cleavage by Seminiferous Tubules
and Intact Testicular Tissue of Human Testes
Expressed as Picomoles/Mg Protein

Patient	Seminiferous Tubules	Intact Testis	Ratio Tubules/Intact Testis
G.M.	772	206	3.8
J.W.R.*	480	180	2.7
P.H.*	330	200	1.7

*Previously reported data (3).

for steroid sulfatase activity as described earlier (2). Steroid
sulfatase activity is expressed as picomoles of free steroid per
mg protein.

Fig. 3 illustrates the rate of pregnenolone sulfate cleavage
in seminiferous tubules, intact testicular tissue and interstitial
tissue. As can be seen steroid sulfatase activity is considerably
higher in interstitial tissue than in seminiferous tubules. Intact
testicular tissue exhibits steroid sulfatase activity slightly higher
than that observed in tubules. The same observation was recently
reported by Van der Vusse et al. (4) using dehydroepiandrosterone
sulfate as substrate. The finding that steroid sulfatase activity

TABLE 3

Effect of Hypophysectomy on Steroid Sulfatase Activity
(Picomoles Free Steroid/mg Protein) in Intact Tissue,
Isolated Interstitial Tissue and
Seminiferous Tubules of Adult Rat Testes

Treatment	Intact Tissue	Interstitial Tissue	Seminiferous Tubules
None	$108 \pm 5.3(3)*$	$358 \pm 10.8(4)$	$103 \pm 2.5(3)$
Hypophysectomy	$107 \pm 7.5(4)$	$209 \pm 15.8(4)**$	$106 \pm 8.0(4)$

*Each value is the mean $\pm$S.E. Number of rats in parenthesis.
**Significantly different from control p< 0.01.

is higher in interstitial tissue than in tubules is in contrast to
our observations in human testes, and may indicate that steroid
sulfates serve different functions in rat and human testes. A
marked difference in the concentration of steroids and steroid sulfates in the two species has been reported (9).

Additional evidence that the steroid sulfatase located in tubules
and interstitial tissue of rat testes might serve different functions
was obtained by studying the steroid sulfatase activity in the
respective testicular compartments in testes from hypophysectomized
rats. These studies were performed in adult rats 14 days post-
hypophysectomy. As illustrated in Table 3 hypophysectomy had no
effect on steroid sulfatase activity in seminiferous tubules while
significantly decreasing the activity in interstitial tissue. Since
interstitial tissue in rat testes comprises such a small percentage
of total testicular tissue, no effect of hypophysectomy could be discerned when examining the steroid sulfatase activity in intact
testicular tissue.

ESTRADIOL BIOSYNTHESIS IN INTERSTITIAL TISSUE AND
SEMINIFEROUS TUBULES OF RAT AND HUMAN TESTES

Rat Testes: Dissection of testicular compartments were performed as described above. Each testicular tissue was homogenized
in 0.1M phosphate buffered saline, pH 7.0 and subjected to centrifugation at 500xg for 10 min. One ml aliquots of the 500xg super-
nate were incubated for 2 hr at 34° with 20μCi $(1,2,6,7(n)-{}^{3}H)-$
androstenedione (252 picomoles) and an NADPH generating system. At
the end of incubation ${}^{14}D$-estrone and ${}^{14}C$-estradiol were added for
quantitation.

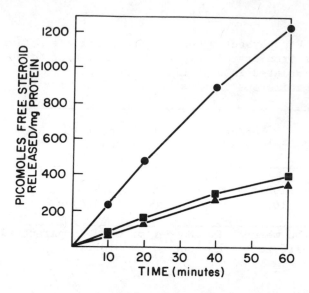

Figure 3. Rate of cleavage of 3.6μM ³H pregnenolone sulfate by homogenates of seminiferous tubules, ▲—▲, intact tissue, ■—■, and interstitial tissue, ●—●, of adult rat testes during 1 hr incubation.

Extraction of phenolic steroids was carried out as previously described (5). The phenolic fraction was subjected to paper chromatography, thin layer chromatography (ITLC-SA Gelman) for estrone fraction and recrystallization to constant specific activity with authentic crystalline estrogens. During aromatization of (1,2,6,7(n)-³H) androstenedione, approximately 67% of the ³H at carbon atoms 1 and 2 is lost as ³H₂0 (10). All results were corrected for these losses.

The amount of ³H 17β-estradiol formed from ³H androstenedione was small. As listed in Table 4, 22 times more estradiol per mg of protein incubated was synthesized by interstitial tissue than seminiferous tubules. The amount of estradiol synthesized by the tubular preparation may reflect contamination of the tubules with Leydig cells. When making the comparison between interstitial tissue and intact testicular tissue, interstitial tissue synthesized 13 times as much 17β-estradiol as the intact testicular

tissues .   Since interstitial tissue in rat testes comprises
approximately 10% of total testicular weight, the present results
would indicate that all or by far the vast majority of estradiol
in rat testes is synthesized in the interstitial tissue. No estrone
was detected in any of the tissue fractions.

Human Testes : A similar study was performed with homogenates of
isolated seminiferous tubules and intact testicular tissue from a
24 yr old patient who died of gunshot wounds to the head; testes
were obtained at autopsy.   In this experiment 1 ml aliquots of
homogenates were incubated with $10\mu Ci$ $(7\alpha-^3H)$ androstenedione
(877 picomoles).   The amount of estradiol formed per mg of protein
was 2.32 picomoles for intact testicular tissue compared to 0.86
picomoles for seminiferous tubules.   Although estradiol was synthesized by the seminiferous tubules, the much greater formation
in intact testicular tissue suggests that the major site of estradiol synthesis in the human testis is in interstitial tissue.   The
amount of estradiol synthesized by human testicular tissue per mg of
protein is more than 100 times the amount formed by rat testicular
tissue. This is consistent with differences observed in estradiol
concentrations in spermatic vein blood from human beings and rats.
No estrone was detected.

TABLE 4

Estradiol Synthesis (Femtomoles Estradiol/mg
Protein) in Isolated Interstitial Tissue,
Seminiferous Tubules and Intact Tissue of
Adult Rat Testes*

Interstitial Tissue	Seminiferous Tubules	Intact Tissue
78	3.5	6.0

*Mean of duplicate incubations

SUMMARY AND COMMENTS

Studies on isolated seminiferous tubules from adult human
testes indicate that steroid sulfatase, 20α-reductase and 5α-re-
ductase are localized in tubules and probably are not present in
interstitial tissue. In apparent contrast to interstitial tissue,
seminiferous tubules contain very little 17-hydroxylase, C_{17}-C_{20}
lyase, or aromatizing enzymes. In our studies no difference
between seminiferous tubules and intact testicular tissue could be
discerned as regards 3β-hydroxysteroid dehydrogenase-isomerase or
17β-hydroxysteroid reductase activities. Compartmentalization of
all of these enzymic activities has not been studied in both rat
and human testes. However, from our data (3,5) and that of others
(6,8,11) the two species are similar in their testicular compartmentalization of 5α-reductase, 17-hydroxylase, C_{17}-C_{20} lyase and
aromatizing enzymes. On the other hand we have observed species
differences in compartmental localization of steroid sulfatase and
3β-hydroxysteroid dehydrogenase-isomerase. In rat testes, 3β-
hydroxysteroid dehydrogenase-isomerase appears to be present exclusively in interstitial tissue (4), while steroid sulfatase is
present in both compartments. The significance of these species
differences is not known; however, it may relate to anatomical
differences of the rat and human testis (12).

In the case of human testes the distribution of enzymes involved
in the biosynthetic pathway to dihydrotestosterone leads one to speculate that dehydroepiandrosterone sulfate or androstenediol-3-sulfate
could serve as precursors of testosterone and dihydrotestosterone in
the seminiferous tubules. Although pregnenolone sulfate is the best
substrate for the 3β-hydroxysteroid sulfatase, the very low activity
of 17-hydroxylase or C_{17}-C_{20} lyase found in seminiferous tubules,
suggests that this steroid sulfate is a less likely candidate as a
precursor of testosterone or dihydrotestosterone. In incubations
of pregnenolone with intact testicular tissue from human subjects,
dehydroepiandrosterone and androstenediol have been shown to be
intermediates in the biosynthetic pathway to testosterone (3,13).
Yanaihara and Troen (14) have also demonstrated that both dehydroepiandrosterone and androstenediol are sulfated in incubated human
testicular tissue. It is possible that these steroid sulfates
enter the seminiferous tubules where they are cleaved and then
further metabolized to testosterone and dihydrotestosterone. The
intratesticular site of sulfurylation of the Δ^5-3β-hydroxysteroids
has not been identified to date. Until this is established and until
it can be determined that the sulfate esters of Δ^5-3β-hydroxysteroids
are indeed sulfurylated in interstitial tissue and that they can be
transferred directly to the seminiferous tubules, it is difficult to
evaluate the role of these steroid sulfates in the biosynthetic
pathway to dihydrotestosterone in the human seminiferous tubule.

The demonstration in the present study that the major site of estradiol synthesis in the rat and human testis is the interstitial tissue is on conflict with a report by de Jong et al. (15) These investigators measured estradiol concentration by radioimmunoassay in isolated seminiferous tubules and isolated interstitial tissue of rat testes prior to incubation and after 3 hr incubation in Krebs-Ringer buffer. They reported that estradiol in seminiferous tubules increased from 20.2 ± 19.5 picograms/g tissue to 39.2 ± 19.5 picograms/g tissue after a 3 hr incubation. However, they could not demonstrate an increase in estradiol concentration in interstitial tissue. Since de Jong et. al. measured estradiol only in tissues any newly synthesized estradiol which was released into the media would not have been observed.

Recent studies by Chowdhury, Tcholakian and Steinberger (16, 17) indicate that estradiol can inhibit testosterone synthesis by a direct action on the testis. After a single s.c. injection of 50 µg estradiol to adult rats they observed a decrease in testosterone concentration in plasma within 1 hr and in testicular tissue within 2 hr, without a change in serum LH. Although the amount of estradiol synthesized by the testis is relatively small, the site of formation within the interstitial tissue where testosterone is synthesized, suggests that estradiol may act by inhibiting an enzyme essential for testosterorone synthesis. Further studies need to be performed to elucidate the local action of estradiol in the testis.

ACKNOWLEDGEMENTS

We are indebted to Dr. Murray R. Abell for his expert interpretation of the histologic material, and to Shirley Musich and Glen Kastelic for their excellent technical assistance. These studies were supported by USPHS Grants HD04064 and HD07690.

REFERENCES

1. Ruokonen, A., T. Laatikainen, E.A. Laitinen and R. Vihko, Biochemistry 11: 1411, 1972.

2. Payne, A.H., Biochim. Biophy. Acta 258: 473, 1972.

3. Kawano, A., A.H. Payne and R.B. Jaffe, J. Clin. Endocr. Metab. 37: 441, 1973.

4. Van der Vusse, G.J., M.L. Kalkman and H.J. Van der Molen, Biochim. Biophys. Acta 348: 404, 1974.

5. Payne, A.H., A. Kawano and R.B. Jaffe, J. Clin. Endocr. Metab. 37 : 448, 1973.

6. Rivarola, M.A., E.J. Podesta, H.E. Chemes, and D. Aguilar, J. Clin. Endocr. Metab. 37 : 454, 1973.

7. Dorrington, J.H. and I.B. Fritz, Biochem. Biophys. Res. Comm. 54 : 1425, 1973.

8. Christensen, A.K. and N.R. Mason, Endocr. 76 : 646, 1965.

9. Ruokonen, A., R. Vihko and M. Niemi, FEBS Letters 31 : 321, 1973.

10. Thompson, E.A. and P.K. Siiteri, J. Biol. Chem. 249 : 5364, 1974.

11. Rivarola, M.A. and E.J. Podesta, Endocr 90 : 618, 1972.

12. Fawcett, D.W., W.B. Neaves and M.N. Flores, Biol. Reprod. 9 : 500, 1973.

13. Yanaihara, T. and P. Troen, J. Clin. Endocr. Metab. 34 : 783, 1972.

14. Yanaihara, T. and P. Troen, J. Clin. Endocr. Metab. 34 : 793, 1972.

15. DeJong, F.H., A.H. Hey and H.J. van der Molen, J. Endocr. 60 : 409, 1974.

16. Chowdhury, M., R. Tcholakian and E. Steinberger, J. Endocr. 60 : 375, 1974.

17. Tcholakian, R.K., M. Chowdhury and E. Steinberger, J. Endocr. 63 : 411, 1974.

BIOSYNTHESIS AND METABOLISM OF TESTOSTERONE IN ISOLATED GERM CELLS

OF THE RAT AND THE RAM AND IN THE SERTOLI CELLS OF THE RAT

M.A. Drosdowsky, M. Tence, J.F. Tence and I. Barral

Laboratoire de Biochimie, Faculté de Médecine, Université

de Caen, CAEN, 14000 France

Since Christensen and Mason (1) described the wet dissection technique of the testis, the seminiferous tubule has been widely studied. It has been shown that the tubule can produce testosterone in vitro from different steroids such as pregnenolone, progesterone or dehydroepiandrosterone (1,2,3); also metabolize testosterone into 5α-reduced compounds such as 5α-dihydrotestosterone (DHT) and andro-stanediols (DIOLS) (4,5,6).

Selective destruction of the germinal epithelium allowed the study of the steroidogenic activity of the Sertoli cell. Lacy et al. (2) demonstrated that in seminiferous tubules submitted to heat, progesterone is still transformed into androgens. More recently, Dorrington and Fritz (7) showed that Sertoli cell-enriched tubules obtained from either hypophysectomized or cryptorchid or Busulphan treated rats can convert testosterone into DHT and DIOLS.

As far as germ cells are concerned, it is more difficult to study separately each cell category. Galena and Terner (8) descri-bed a method which allows the isolation of non-flagellate germ cells and showed that they can synthesize testosterone from progesterone. Dorrington and Fritz (9) isolated spermatocytes from 28 days rats and demonstrated the formation of DHT and DIOLS.

We have studied three different cell categories, Sertoli cells, round spermatids and primary spermatocytes. "Sertoli-cell only" tubules (SCO) were obtained from adult rats treated prenatally with Busulphan. Round spermatids of adult rat and round spermatids and spermatocytes of ram, were isolated using the technique of velocity sedimentation at unit gravity. In the following sections, the

results of incubations of these preparations with different steroid
precursors will be described.

MATERIALS AND METHODS

"Sertoli Cell-Only" Tubules

A) Preparation of tubules. At the 20th day of gestation,
Wistar rats are administered intraperitoneally with Busulphan (10mg/
kg body wt). As described by Gillet (10), this alkylating agent
induces gonocyte degeneration. The testes are completely deprived
of germ cells (Fig. 1). We used 90 day animals (mean weight of
the animal: 250 g; mean weight of two testes: 440 mg). Seminiferous tubules were isolated according to Christensen and Mason
(1) and rinsed several times in Krebs-Ringer bicarbonate buffer
containing 0.2% glucose (KRBG). After centrifugation, they were
sedimentated in KRBG containing 5% BSA according to Hall et al.
(11). Seminiferous tubules from normal rats were prepared the
same way to be used as controls.

B) Incubations. 200 mg of tubules were incubated in presence
of either $8x10^6$ dpm of progesterone-4-^{14}-C (S.A. 59 mCi/mM, 18 µg)
or $8x10^6$ dpm of testosterone-4-^{14}-C (S.A. 61.0 mCi/mM, 17 µg) in
2 ml of KRBG with a $NADPH_2$ generating system. A similar quantity
of undissected testis from treated animals was incubated in parallel.
Incubations were realized at 31°C in air-CO_2 (95:5) during 2 hours.
Reference steroids as well as ^{3}H-tracers were added at the end of
each incubation. Metabolites were extracted and purified by re-
petitive paper and thin layer chromatography. Identity of the
products was determined by crystallization to constant specific
activity.

C) Electron microscopy. Supporting cells examined by means
of electron microscopy look similar to normal Sertoli cells (Fig.2).
The nucleus is irregular in shape and shows several indentations.
Microtubules and lipid droplets are present as well as mitochondria
with tubular cristae. Intercellular junctions present the same
structure as normal Sertoli cells described by Flickinger and
Fawcett (12) in the adult testis. It has been shown by Fawcett et
al. (13) that these complex junctions play an important role in
the constitution of the blood-testis barrier.

D) Hormonal studies. Plasma was collected for the determination of testosterone (14).

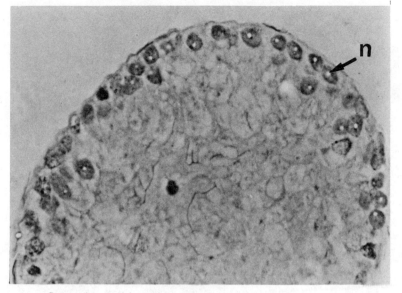

Figure 1.   Sertoli cell only-tubule.   n: refringent nucleolus
              x 150.

Germ Cells

A)   Rat germ cell preparations.   Male Wistar rats 90 days old
were used.   Seminiferous tubules were carefully dissected as described previously.   They were rinsed with phosphate buffer saline
(PBS), then incubated for 20 minutes at 33°C in 10 ml of PBSG (PBS
containing 0.1% of glucose).   Trypsin and DNase were added to obtain concentration of 0.23% (W/V) trypsin plus 20 µg/ml DNase (15).
The cell suspension was filtered through a nylon gauze.   We have
applied the Staput technique of sedimentation at unit gravity
developed by Miller and Phillips (16) with several modifications.

The sedimentation chamber was loaded at a rate of 25 ml/min
with 20 ml of PBS, followed by 8×10^7 cells suspended in 20 ml of
a 0.1% Ficoll solution in PBS and 312.5 ml of a Ficoll gradient in
PBS.   The gradient was a "buffered step gradient" with a parabolic
shape from 0.5 to 1.13% Ficoll and linear from 1.13% to 2.75% Ficoll
concentration.   It was formed by a three vessels gradient generator
and allowed to run in at the bottom of the sedimentation chamber
by gravity.   After a 90 minutes sedimentation, the chamber was
drained at a rate of 5 ml/min from the bottom through an ISCO
optical unit operating at 450 nm and connected to an absorbance
monitor.

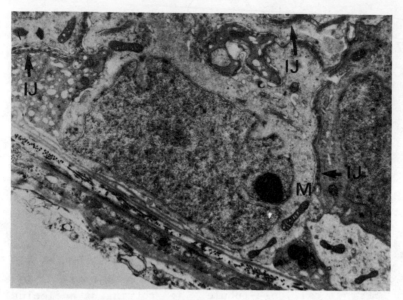

Figure 2.   Sertoli cell from Busulphan treated animal (electron
            micrograph x 4.500) (I J: Intercellular junctions; M:
            mitochondrion with tubular cristae).

Using this technique, rat germ cells can be separated into
five categories A,B,C,D and E of decreasing sedimentation velocity,
the composition of which is given in Table 1.   Peak A contains more
than 85% of primary spermatocytes (mostly pachytene).   Peak B contains an equivalent proportion (45%) of polynucleated spermatids and
early spermatids.   Peak C consists of about 88% of early spermatids
(stage 1 to 7), flagellate spermatids (6%) and unidentified cells
(5%).   Peak D contains residual bodies whereas peak E is very heterogeneous with a great number of spermatozoa.   Peak C representing
about $4x10^6$ cells was collected and centrifuged.

B) Ram germ cell preparations.   The cells were isolated according to Loir and Lanneau (17).   Two peaks corresponding respectively
to round spermatids and to primary spermatocytes were collected.
Several sets of experiments were performed of which two (rams B and
C) are described herein.

C) Incubation of germ cells.   The cells were centrifuged; the
pellet ($\simeq$ 4 mg) was homogenized with an all-glass Potter in 1 ml
of Tris buffer 0.01 M, pH 7.2.   The incubations were performed in
presence of $4x10^6$ dpm of testosterone $4-^{14}C$ (S.A. 59 mCi/mM) and of
a $NADPH_2$ generating system during 2 hours, in air, at 31°C in a
final volume of 3 ml of Tris buffer.   The metabolic products were
isolated and identified as previously described.

Table 1

Cell Distribution in Peaks A, B and C

	Primary Spermatocytes	Polynucleated Spermatids	Spermatids Stage 1-7	Other Spermatids	Other Cells	Number of Observed Cells
		Observed cell types				
Peak A	85.5%	6.8%	2.1%	2.1%	3.5%	2100
Peak B	*	44.7%	45.1%	4.0%	6.2%	500
Peak C	*	*	88.3%	6.4%	5.3%	2000

*Primary spermatocytes in Peak B and primary spermatocytes and polynucleated spermatids in Peaks B and C are very seldom encountered: they are classified in category "other cells", i.e., unidentified cells.

RESULTS

Metabolism of Progesterone in the Sertoli Cell-Only Tubules

In every incubation, progesterone is converted into 17α-hydroxyprogesterone (17α-OHP), 20α-dihydroprogesterone (20α-OHP), androstenedione and testosterone (Table 2). The precursor is weakly metabolized in the SCO tubules (80% unchanged). The main metabolites are 17α-OHP (1%) and 20α-OHP (1.6%). Androstenedione and testosterone are produced in minute quantities (0.1%). A similar metabolism is observed in normal tubules with a reduction of the yields by a factor 3 or 4. When progesterone is incubated with undissected testes from SCO animals, 17α-OHP (53%), 20α-OHP (2.3%), androstenedion (6%) and testosterone (18%) are produced.

Metabolism of Testosterone in the Sertoli Cell-Only Tubules

As shown in Table 3, testosterone is poorly metabolized. In SCO-tubules, androstenedione (3.5%) and 5α-reduced metabolites are formed: DHT (1%), 3α-androstanediol (3α-DIOL) (0.3%) and 3β-androstanediol (3β-DIOL) (0.1%). The amount of endogenous testosterone is negligible (18), when compared to the weight of precursor (17 µg). Consequently, the production of metabolites from exogenous testosterone per 200 mg tubules in 2 hours is: DHT (175 ng), 3α-DIOL (40 ng), 3β-DIOL (20 mg). In normal tubules, testosterone metabolism is nearly identical except for androstenedione (5%).

In undissected treated testes, more androstenedione is produced (9%, 1600 ng) accounting for the presence of interstitial tissue; 5α-reduced metabolites represent only 10% of the identified products. Conversion of testosterone into estrogens (17β-estradiol, estrone and estriol) was examined. No radioactivity was found associated with reference estrogens in any of the preparations studied.

Plasma Testosterone in Busulphan Treated Rats

Testosterone was determined 2 to 6 times on each plasma sample (Table 4). As it can be seen mean testosterone concentration is lower in treated animals.

Metabolism of Testosterone in Rat Spermatids

The only metabolite identified is androstenedione (2%); neither DHT nor DIOLS are detected (Table 5).

Table 2

Metabolism of Progesterone-4-^{14}C in Sertoli Cell-Only Tubules, Normal
Tubules and Undissected Testis from Treated Rats*

Percentage of initial radioactivity and ng of product formed
(number in parenthesis)

Metabolites	Sertoli Cell Only-Tubules		Normal Tubules		Undissected Treated Testis	
	Exp. 1	Exp. 2	Exp. 1	Exp. 2	Exp. 1	Exp. 2
Progesterone (unchanged)	82**	78**	89**	81**	14.0	9.2
17α-OH-progesterone	1.2 (220)	0.7 (130)	0.3 (50)	0.4 (70)	56.2 (10700)	50.8 (9650)
20α-dihydroprogesterone	2.0 (360)	1.2 (220)	0.4 (70)	0.5 (90)	2.1 (400)	2.4 (450)
Androstenedione	0.3 (60)	0.1 (20)	0.03 (<10)	***	4.7 (900)	8.3 (1600)
Testosterone	0.1 (20)	0.04 (<10)	0.05 (<10)	0.1 (<20)	17.6 (3350)	18.3 (3450)

* Details of experimental procedure as stated under Materials and Methods.
** Not crystallized.
*** Not identified.

Table 3

Metabolism of Testosterone-4-^{14}C in Sertoli Cell-Only Tubules, Normal
Tubules and Undissected Testis Treated Rats[*]

| Metabolites | Sertoli Cell-Only Tubules | | Normal Tubules | | Undissected Treated Testis |
| | Exp. 1 | Exp. 2 | Exp. 1 | Exp. 2 | |
	Percentage of initial radioactivity and ng of product formed (number in parenthesis)				
Testosterone (unchanged)	93[**]	96[**]	96[**]	95[**]	90[**]
Androstenedione	3.6 (610)	3.3 (560)	5.5 (930)	5.4 (920)	8.9 (1600)
5α-Dihydrotestosterone	0.9 (150)	1.2 (200)	0.8 (140)	0.9 (150)	0.5 (90)
3α-Androstanediol	0.3 (50)	0.2 (35)	0.1 (20)	0.2 (35)	0.2 (35)
3β-Androstanediol	0.1 (20)	0.1 (20)	[***]	0.2 (35)	0.3 (50)

[*]Details of experimental procedure as stated under Materials and Methods.
[**]Not crystallized.
[***]Not identified.

Table 4

Influence of treatment with Busulphan on
plasma testosterone levels

	n	Testosterone levels (ng/ml) (mean ± S.E.M)
Control rats	11	3.15 ± 1.00
Prenatally treated rats	6	1.36 ± 0.64*

*The difference between mean values from control and treated rats
is statistically significant at the p < 0.05 level.

Table 5

Metabolism of testosterone-4-^{14}C in round spermatids
from adult rats*

Metabolites	% of initial radioactivity		
	Exp. 1	Exp. 2	Exp. 3
Testosterone (un- changed)**	89	94	86
Androstenedione	1.9	1.8	2.4
5α-DHT	ND***	ND	ND
DIOLS	ND	ND	ND

*Details of experimental procedure as stated under Materials and
Methods.

**Not crystallized.

***Not detectable.

Table 6

Metabolism of testosterone-4-^{14}C in round
spermatids and primary spermatocytes of the ram[*]

Metabolites	% of initial radioactivity					
	Round Spermatids			Primary spermatocytes		
	Ram B		Ram C	Ram B		Ram C
	I	II		I	II	
Testosterone (un-changed)[**]	77	70	79	68	66	79
Androstenedione	1.2[***] (73)	1.1 (94)	1.6 (67)	0.6 (70)	1.2 (169)	3.2 (184)
5α-DHT	ND[****]	ND	ND	ND	ND	ND
DIOLS	ND	ND	ND	ND	ND	ND

[*]Details of experimental procedure as stated under Materials and
Methods.

[**]Not crystallized.

[***]Numbers in parenthesis: ng of product formed/mg of protein.

[****]Not detectable.

Metabolism of Testosterone in Ram Primary Spermatocytes
and Spermatids

In round spermatids, testosterone is metabolized into androstenedione (1.1%). The amount of 5α-reduced metabolites is very
low or nil (Table 6). In primary spermatocytes, the metabolism is
quite similar. Androstenedione is the only metabolite isolated
with certainty.

DISCUSSION

Steroid metabolism is seminiferous tubules is now well documented. The tubule contains the enzymatic equipment necessary for
synthesis of testosterone from progesterone and pregnenolone.

However, Cooke et al. (19) demonstrated that very little testosterone
if any is produced in the tubule from endogenous precursors.   Accordingly, since testosterone is required for completion of spermatogenesis (20), it has to come from the neighbouring Leydig cells.
The main enzymatic activity of the tubules appears to be 5α-reduction
of testosterone, leading to DHT and DIOLS with different profiles
depending on the age of the animal (5,6).   But very little is known
about the tubular components involved in this activity.

The first model we used seems suitable for the study of Sertoli
cells, since prenatal treatment with Busulphan produces an inhibition
of germ cell development.   In the other techniques employed to obtain Sertoli cell-enriched preparations, such as hypophysectomy, heat
treatment, x-ray irradiation or chronic vitamin A deficiency (21),
the germinal epithelium has been destroyed.   The cells present in
aspermatogenic tubules are mature Sertoli cells as revealed by the
electron microscopic examinations.   It is interesting to note that
their maturation has been completed in absence of germ cells.   The
same observation has been reported recently by Means (22) after irradiation of pregnant rats.   Testosterone levels in plasma of treated
rats are reduced (1.4 + 0.4 ng/ml) when compared to controls.   This
fact was already demonstrated by Hall and Gomes (23) and seems to
indicate that the interstitial tissue is not functioning normally.
However, the weight of seminal vesicles at 90 days (10) is nearly
normal which is in favour of sufficient production of androgens
for maintenance of target tissues.

Our experiment using SCO tubules confirms the view that progesterone is a poor precursor for testosterone in the tubule.   Less
than 10 ng of testosterone is produced from the exogenous substrate,
the main metabolite being 20α-OHP.   20α-OHP has been found previously
by Lacy et al. (2) in Sertoli cell-enriched tubules, but its possible
role was not explained.   Jenkins and MacCaffery (24) have shown in
the human prostate that progesterone inhibits DHT formation from
testosterone.

It might be possible, therefore, that conversion of progesterone
into 20α-OHP diminishes the inhibiting activity of progesterone on
5α-reductase which could have an important role in spermatogenesis.

Comparison of progesterone metabolism in SCO-tubules and in undissected SCO testis indicates the contribution by interstitial
cells.   If we suppose that testosterone synthesis is due to contaminating interstitial cells, contamination could be evaluated to
0.5%.   This amount of interstitial cells in the tubular preparations
could not account for the quantity of 17α-OHP, 20α-OHP and androstenedione found.   Therefore, these metabolites must be formed by
the tubules.

The yield of progesterone metabolites is lower in normal tubules when compared with SCO tubules. This fact can account for a relative reduction of metabolizing cells and favours the Sertoli cells for being the main site of progesterone metabolism.

Feminizing testicular tumors composed of Sertoli cells have been showed to contain estrogens (25). In vitro, DHA conversion to estrone and estradiol has been demonstrated (26). In our experimental conditions, SCO-tubules fail to convert testosterone into estrogens. Identical results are obtained with undissected treated testis and in normal tubules as already reported (27). SCO-tubules contain 5α-reductase activity; they convert testosterone into DHT as well as 3α- and 3β-DIOLS. These results confirm those of Dorrington and Fritz (7).

The association of SCO-tubules with interstitial tissue does not enhance the production of 5α-reduced metabolites as revealed by incubation of undissected SCO testis. This fact is in agreement with a low 5α-reductase activity in the interstitial tissue of the mature rat (27). Our data on the testosterone metabolism in normal tubules confirm the findings of several authors (4,5,6). However, in those experiments, DIOLS were produced in larger amounts than DHT. In our present work, DHT is the main 5α-reduced metabolite. Lloret and Weisz (27) have shown that a high concentration of testosterone inhibits 3α-reductase activity. Since in our experimental procedure, testes preparations were incubated with 17 µg of testosterone, an inhibition of 3α-reductase is possible.

In round spermatids of adult rat and ram, 5α-reductase activity seems absent or very low. This data confirm the view of Dorrington and Fritz (9). However, contrary to their findings on primary spermatocytes of rat, ram spermatocytes fail to convert testosterone into 5α-reduced metabolites.

If we know at the present time, how 5α-reduction evolves during tubular maturation, much remain to be done to get more precise information on the right localization of this activity and its role on germ cell differentiation.

ACKNOWLEDGEMENTS

This investigation was supported by DGRST (Grant 72-704-81) and by Foundation pour la Recherche Medicale Francaise. We are indebted to Doctor Laporte and Doctor Gillet for treatment of rats with Busulphan and to Doctor Loir for the separation of ram germ cells. The valuable technical assistance of M.J. Liegard is gratefully acknowledged.

REFERENCES

1. Christensen, A.K. and Mason, N.R., Endocrinology, 76: 379, 1965.
2. Lacy, D., Vinson, G.P., Collins, P., Bell, J., Fyson, P., Pudney, J. and Pettit, A.J. In: Gual, C., ed. Progress in Endocrinology, (Proceedings of the Third International Congress of Endocrinology), Mexico, Excerpta Medica Foundation, Amsterdam, 1054: 1019, 1969.
3. Richards, G. and Neville, A.M., Nature, 244: 359, 1973.
4. Rivarola, M.A. and Podesta, E.J., Endocrinology, 90: 618, 1972.
5. Folman, Y., Ahmad, N., Sowell, J.G. and Eik Nes, K.B., Endocrinology, 92: 41, 1973.
6. Matsumoto, K. and Yamada, M., Endocrinology, 93: 253, 1974.
7. Dorrington, J.H. and Fritz, I.B., J. Steroid Biochem., 5: 385, 1974.
8. Galena, H.J. and Terner, C., J. Endocrinol., 60: 269, 1974.
9. Dorrington, J.H. and Fritz, I.B., Biochem. Biophys. Res. Comm. 54: 1425, 1973.
10. Gillet, J., These de 3eme cycle, Poitiers, 1972.
11. Hall, P.F., Irby, D.C. and de Kretser, D.M., Endocrinology, 84: 488, 1969.
12. Flickinger, C. and Fawcett, D.W., Anat. Rec., 158: 207, 1967.
13. Fawcett, D.W., Leak, L.V. and Heidger, P.M., J. Reprod. Fert., Suppl. 10, 105, 1970.
14. Leymarie, P., Strauss, N. and Scholler, R., Path. Biol. 22: 877, 1974.
15. Meistrich, M.L., J. Cell. Physiol., 80: 299, 1972.
16. Miller, R.G. and Phillips, R.A., J. Cell. Physiol., 73: 191, 1969.
17. Loir, M. and Lanneau, M., Exp. Cell. Res., 83: 319, 1974.
18. Podesta, E.J. and Rivarola, M.A., Endocrinology, 95: 455, 1974.
19. Cooke, B.A., De Jong, F.H., Van Der Molen, H.J. and Rommerts, F.F.G., Nature New Biology, 237: 255, 1972.
20. Steinberger, E., Physiol. Reviews, 51: 1, 1971.
21. Kruger, P.M., Hodgen, G.D. and Sherins, R.J., Endocrinology, 95: 955, 1974.
22. Means, A.R., Life Sciences; 15: 371, 1974.
23. Hall, R.W. and Gomes, W.R., J. Reprod. Fert. 35: 131, 1973.
24. Jenkins, J.S., and McCaffery, V.M., J. Endocrinol., 63: 517, 1974.
25. Huggins, C. and Moulder, P.V., Cancer Research, 5. 510, 1945.
26. Pierrepoint, C.G., Galley, J., Mc, I., Griffiths, K. and Grant, J.K., J. Endocrinol., 38: 61, 1967.
27. Lloret, A.P. and Weisz, J., Endocrinology, 95: 1306, 1974.

TESTICULAR ENZYMES RELATED TO STEROID METABOLISM

Bun-ichi Tamaoki, Hiroshi Inano and Keiko Suzuki

National Institute of Radiological Sciences

Anagawa-4-chome, Chiba-shi 280, Japan

INTRODUCTION

Androgen biosynthesis and metabolism in the testis occur in a well defined cellular and subcellular localization. This paper examines the distribution of various enzymes among different testicular cells, as well as the subcellular localization of some of these enzymes.

Distribution of the Enzyme Activities Related to Testosterone Formation Between Seminiferous Tubules and Interstitial Tissue

The seminiferous tubules and interstitial cells were isolated from decapsulated testicular tissue of adult rats by microdissection as described previously (1). The activities of the enzymes related to progesterone and 17α-hydroxyprogesterone metabolism (17α-hydroxylase, C_{17}-C_{20} lyase, 20α-hydroxysteroid dehydrogenase) were quantitated in the seminiferous tubule fraction and interstitial tissue. As shown in Table 1, 17α-hydroxylase and C_{17}-C_{20} lyase activities were much higher in the interstitial tissue than in the seminiferous tubules (2).

123

Table 1

Distribution of 17α-Hydroxylase, C_{17}-C_{20} lyase, and
20α-Hydroxysteroid Dehydrogenase, Between Seminiferous Tubules and
Interstitial Tissues of Adult Rat Testis (2)

Enzyme Activity	Interstitial Tissue	Seminiferous Tubules
17α-Hydroxylase	0.48[*]	0.05
C_{17}-C_{20} Lyase	0.37	0.04
20α-Hydroxysteroid dehydrogenase	0.02	0.09

[*] nmol of product per mg protein

$[4-^{14}C]$-Progesterone (32 nmol, 4 X 10^4 cpm) and $[4-^{14}C]$-17 –
hydroxyprogesterone (30 nmol, 3.2 x 10^4 cpm) were incubated with the
homogenates of seminiferous tubules (54 mg of protein per flask)
and interstitial tissue (38 mg protein per flask), in the presence
of NADPH for 60 min, respectively.

Effect of X-Irradiation on Enzyme Activities

By local x-irradiation of the testes of adult rat, the weights
of the testes were reduced to some 60% of controls (from 2.7 to
1.4 g) whereas the weights of accessory sex organs remained unchanged.
No histological changes were observed in the prostate or seminal
vesicles at one month post-irradiation. Among all the enzymes
assayed, total enzyme activities of only Δ^5-3β-hydroxysteroid
dehydrogenase and 20α-hydroxysteroid dehydrogenase were elevated,
whereas specific activities of 17α-hydroxylase, 20α-hydroxysteroid
dehydrogenase and C_{17}-C_{20} lyase were reduced. When Human Chorionic
Gonadotropin (HCG) was administered to the normal rat for 14 days
before sacrifice, the total and specific activities of C_{17}-C_{20} lyase
and the specific activity of 17α-hydroxylase were elevated, while
those of 17α-hydroxysteroid dehydrogenase and 20α-hydroxysteroid
dehydrogenase were reduced (3). Gonadotropin treatment (HCG, 68
i.u., daily for 15 days) of the x-irradiated rat resulted in an
increase in total and specific activities of 17α-hydroxylase and
C_{17}-C_{20} lyase and a decrease of 17β-hydroxysteroid dehydrogenase.

The effect of local x-irradiation on accessory sex glands and
testes of immature rats was also examined. As shown in Table 2, a

Table 2

Influence of X-Irradiation and HCG Treatment on
Organ Weights of Immature Rat (5)

Group	Bilateral Weight (g)		
	Testes	Seminal Vesicles	Prostates
Control	2.6	0.5	0.5
Control + HCG	2.4	1.2	1.1
X-irradiated	0.4	0.1	0.2
X-irradiated + HCG	0.5	0.4	0.4

Immature rats of the Wistar strain (about 27 days of age) were
locally irradiated to the testes with 1,000 R of x-ray   (X-
irradiated group), while X-irradiated + HCG group was irradiated
in the same manner and then injected with HCG 50 i.u. daily for 15
days before sacrifice.   Control group was not irradiated and
treated with no HCG, and Control + HCG group was not irradiated,
but injected with the same amount of HCG.   The animals were
killed at 73 days of age.

reduction in the weight of the accessory sex organs was observed
in the X-irradiated rats, indicating a decrease in androgen biosynthesis in vivo.   The effect of x-irradiation on enzyme activities
is shown in Table 3.   In contrast to the adult testis, x-irradiation
resulted in increased specific activities of most enzymes assayed.

Histochemical Detection of the Hydroxysteroid
Dehydrogenase Related to Androgen Formation

Hydroxysteroid dehydrogenases were localized histochemically in
various testicular compartments. Δ^5-3β-Hydroxysteroid dehydrogenase
was clearly demonstrated in the interstitial tissue of rat testis.
However, 17β-hydroxysteroid dehydrogenase was almost undetectable,
even though this enzyme was seen in hepatic tissue by this technique
(10).   Significant activity of the enzyme was evident after incubation of androstenedione with testicular microsomes in the presence of
NADPH (11).   Since it has been previously shown that it is difficult

Table 3

Influence of Local X-Irradiation and HCG Treatment on the Enzyme
Activity of Immature Rat Testes (5)

Group*	Enzyme Activity									
	Δ^5-3β-hydroxysteroid dehydrogenase		17α-hydroxylase		C_{17}-C_{20} lyase		17β-hydroxysteroid dehydrogenase		20α-hydroxy-steroid dehydrogenase	
	Total**	S.A.***	Total	S.A.	Total	S.A.	Total	S.A.	Total	S.A.
Control	53	6	11	1	11	1	3.4	0.4	7.3	0.2
Control+HCG	68	9	25	3	20	3	3.4	0.5	6.0	0.2
X-irradiated	31	14	10	4	8	4	0.7	0.3	8.0	1.3
X-irradiated+ HCG	59	27	20	9	16	7	2.9	1.3	10.0	1.7

*See the note of Table 4.
**Total enzyme activity expressed in nmol of products per testis.
***Specific enzyme activity expressed in nmol of products per mg protein.

The enzyme activities were determined by the assay, the principle of which was same as mentioned in Table 3.

to solubilize 17α-hydroxysteroid dehydrogenase from the microsomal
membrane of rat testes (12), it is unlikely that this dehydrogenase
is eluted during staining procedure.

Testicular 20α-Hydroxysteroid Dehydrogenase

The function of this enzyme in rat testis is to catalyze the
conversion of 17α-hydroxyprogesterone to 17α,20α-dihydroxy-4-pregnen-
3-one in the presence of NADPH; oxidation of 17α, 20α-dihydroxy-4-
pregnen-3-one was hardly demonstrable in the presence of $NADP^+$ (14).
Histochemically, the dehydrogenase activity was not demonstrable in
rat testis; however, in human testis, the dehydrogenase was stained
histochemically in interstitial cells (15).

The product of 17α, 20α-dihydroxy-4-pregnen-3-one was reported
to inhibit C_{17}-C_{20} lyase activity, competing with 17α-hydroxyproge-
sterone, and accordingly to reduce the androgen synthesis, since the
dihydroxysteroid itself was not converted to androstenedione. It
has been previously suggested that 20α-hydroxysteroid dehydrogenase
may play an important role in the intracellular regulation of
androgen production in the testis (16). The 20α-hydroxysteroid dehydrogenase activity was relatively reduced following administration
of HCG to the intact immature rat, whereas Δ^5-3β-hydroxysteroid
dehydrogenase activity was markedly enhanced (6), as shown in
Table 4. These results suggested that 20α-hydroxysteroid dehydrogenase is decreased by gonadotropin, thus allowing the activation
of androgen production pathway.

Recently, Inano has shown that 20α-hydroxysteroid dehydrogenase
activity was localized mainly in the seminiferous tubule of adult
rat (Table 1) in contrast to enzymes related to androgen synthesis
(2) which were localized primarily in the interstitial compartment.
In human testis, 20α-hydroxysteroid dehydrogenase activity remained
unchanged following treatment with a synthetic estrogen which reduced
the activities of almost all the enzymes related to testosterone
synthesis. 20α-Hydroxysteroid dehydrogenase was shown to be
diminished in human hyalinized testis (17).

INTRACELLULAR DISTRIBUTION OF ENZYMES RELATED TO
STEROID METABOLISM

Nuclear, mitochondrial, microsomal and cytosol fractions
were separated by differential centrifugation as described previously (11). Previous studies have shown that the cleavage enzyme
of the cholesterol side-chain is localized in the mitochondrial
fraction (18), while 20α-hydroxysteroid dehydrogenase activity is
in the cytosol fraction of rat, pig, man, etc. (19). On the other
hand, the enzymes related to testosterone formation from pregnenolone

Table 4

Effect of HCG Upon the Testicular Hydroxysteroid
Dehydrogenases of Immature Intact Rat (6)

Treatment	Specific Activity of Dehydrogenases[*]	
	Δ^5-3β-Hydroxysteroid dehydrogenase[**]	20α-Hydroxysteroid dehydrogenase
HCG	39	6
None	4	12

[*] μg of product x 10^{-2} per mg protein.
[**] with the Δ^5-Δ^4 isomerase

The immature rats (20 days of age) were injected subcutaneously daily
with 30 i.u. of HCG for 11 days. [4-^{14}C]-pregnenolone (20 μg, 12
x 10^4 cpm) for Δ^5-3β-hydroxysteroid dehydrogenase, and [4-^{14}C]-
17α-hydroxyprogesterone (10 μg, 10 x 10^4 cpm) for 20α-hydroxy-
steroid dehydrogenase were prepared and then were respectively
incubated with testicular microsomal and cytosol fractions in
the presence of required cofactors.

is found in the microsomal fraction of testes of several animals,
such as rat, mouse, guinea pig, boar, man, ranbow trout, etc. (19).
We have recently separated the microsomal fraction of testes into
two subfractions by centrifugation on a discontinuous sucrose density
gradient containing CsCl. One fraction contained smooth endoplasmic
reticular membranes while the other consisted of rough endoplasmic
membranes and free ribosomes (20). Chemical and electron microscopic
analyses of the two subfractions showed that these biomembrane
fractions were distinctly different from each other in ultrastructure,
RNA and cytochrome P-450 contents (Table 5). The enzyme activities
related to steroidogenesis were greater in the smooth than in the
rough-surfaced microsomal fraction (Table 5).   The intermicrosomal
concentration of the 17α-hydroxylase and C_{17}-C_{20} lyase activities
which involve cytochrome P-450 as an essential component in their
systems closely correlated with the distribution of cytochrome P-450
concentration, as determined by the CO-difference spectrum.   These
results indicated that the smooth endoplasmic reticulum of the
interstitial cell is the major site of testosterone synthesis from
pregnenolone (21).

Table 5

Intermicrosomal Distribution of RNA, Cytochrome P-450 and Enzyme
Activities Related to Steroid Metabolism (21)

Fraction	RNA[*]	P-450[**]	Δ^5-3β-hydroxysteroid dehydrogenase		17α-hydroxylase		C_{17}-C_{20} lyase		17β-hydroxysteroid dehydrogenase	
			Total[***]	S.A.[****]	Total	S.A.	Total	S.A.	Total	S.A.
Microsome	0.2	4	24	1.1	14	0.7	10	0.5	7.6	0.34
Smooth-surfaced microsome	0.1	11	12	4.2	5	1.7	3	1.1	2.7	0.94
Rough-surfaced microsome	0.4	0	3	2.0	1	0.6	1	0.6	0.6	0.37

[*] RNA mg per mg protein.
[**] Difference in optical densities at 450 and 500 nm in CO-difference spectrum per μg of protein per ml.
[***] Total enzyme activity expressed in μg products per a pair of testes.
[****] Specific enzyme activity expressed in g products per mg protein.

Table 6

Intracellular Distribution of 5α-Reductase
in the Testes of Immature Rat (8)

Subcellular Fraction	Specific Activity of 5α-Reductase[*]
Nuclear	0.2
Mitochondrial	1.5
Microsomal	3.0
Cytosol	0.1

[*]nmole product per mg protein.

[4-^{14}C]-Androstenedione (35 nmol, 3.5×10^4 cpm) was incubated with the subcellular fraction of immature rat testes (equivalent to 2 testes) for 20 min at 37°C.

In case of immature rat testis (8), the major activity of 5α-reductase was observed in the microsomal fraction but very little activity was detected in the nuclear fraction (Table 6). This is in contrast to intracellular distribution of the enzyme in accessory sex organs (22).

ENZYMOLOGICAL STUDY ON 17β-HYDROXYSTEROID DEHYDROGENASE

The 17β-hydroxysteroid dehydrogenase (E.C. 1.1.1.51) activity which catalyzes the oxido-reduction between androstenedione and testosterone was concentrated in the microsomal fraction of testis of rat, mouse, pig, man and other vertebrates. This enzyme in porcine testis has been solubilized and characterized (28,29).

Species-Specific Enzymes

From the comparative aspects of endocrinology, specific enzymes and their intracellular distribution were reported in the testes of several species. 16α-Hydroxylase was found in the microsomal fraction of human testes (23), 11α-hydroxylase in the mitochondrial fraction of rainbow trout testes (24), aromatizing enzyme system and related cytochrome P-450 in the smooth-surfaced microsomes of equine testes (25) and 7α-hydroxylase in the smooth-surfaced microsomes of rat testes (26).

In conclusion, we examined inter- and intracellular distribution of the enzymes related to androgen synthesis, and proposed smooth-surfaced endoplasmic reticula of the interstitial cell as the major site of tesosterone biosynthesis in the testes. Furthermore, we have proposed that 20α-hydroxysteroid dehydrogenase may regulate androgen production by limiting the amount of substrate to be converted via the C_{17}-C_{20} lyase.

REFERENCES

1. Christensen, A.K., and Mason, N.R., Endocrinology 76: 646, 1965.
2. Inano, H., J. Steroid Biochem. 5: 145, 1974.
3. Inano, H., and Tamaoki, B., Endocrinol. Japon. 15: 197, 1968.
4. Oshima, H., Endocrinol. Japon. 14: 75, 1967.
5. Suzuki, K., Inano, H., and Tamaoki, B., Biol. Reprod. 9: 1, 1973.
6. Inano, H., and Tamaoki, B., Endocrinology 79: 579, 1966.
7. Wilson, J.D., and Gloyna, R.E., Rec. Progr. Hormonc Res. 26: 309, 1970.
8. Oshima, H., Sarada, T., Ochiai, K., and Tamaoki, B., Endocrinology 86: 1215, 1970.
9. Moore, R.J., and Wilson, J.D., Endocrinology 93: 581, 1973.
10. Personal communication with Dr. T. Matsuzawa, Institute of Endocrinology, Gunma University.
11. Shikita, M., and Tamaoki, B., Endocrinology 76: 563, 1965.
12. Machino, A., Nakano, H., and Tamaoki, B., Endocrinol. Japon. 16: 11, 1969.
13. Inano, H., and Tamaoki, B., Eur. J. Biochem. 44: 13, 1974.
14. Shikita, M., and Tamaoki, B., Biochemistry 4: 1189, 1965 and 6: 1760, 1967.
15. Baillie, A.H., Ferguson, M.M., and Hart, D.McK., Developments in Steroid Histochemistry, p. 55, Academic Press, London, 1966.
16. Inano, H., Nakano, N., Shikita, M., and Tamaoki, B., Biochim. Biophys. Acta 137: 540, 1967.
17. Oshima, H., Sarada, T., Ochiai, K., and Tamaoki, B., Invest. Urol. 12: 43, 1974.
18. Menon, K.M.J., Drosdowsky, M., Dorfman, R.I., and Forchielli, E., Steroids Suppl. 1: 95, 1965.
19. Tamaoki, B., Inano, H., and Nakano, H., The Gonads (Ed. by K.W. McKerns), p. 547, Appleton-Century-Crofts, New York, 1969.
20. Inano, H., Inano, A., and Tamaoki, B., J. Steroid Biochem. 1: 83, 1970.
21. Tamaoki, B., J. Steroid Biochem. 4: 89, 1973.
22. Nozu, K., and Tamaoki, B., Biochim. Biophys. Acta 348: 321, 1974.
23. Oshima, H., Sarada, T., Ochiai, K., and Tamaoki, B., J. Clin. Endocrinol. Metab. 27: 1249, 1967.
24. Suzuki, K., and Tamaoki, B., Gen. Comp. Endocrinol. 18: 319, 1972

25. Oh, R., and Tamaoki, B., Acta Endocrinol. $\underline{72}$:   366, 1973.
26. Inano, H., and Tamaoki, B., Biochemistry $\underline{10}$: z1503, 1971.
27. Tamaoki, B., and Inano, H., Proc. Inter. Cong. on Hormonal
     Steroids, Mexico City, 1974. J. Steroid Biochem., in press.
28. Inano, H., and Tamaoki, B., Eur. J. Biochem. $\underline{44}$:   13, 1974.
29. Inano, H., and Tamaoki, B., Eur. J. Biochem, in press.

Steroid Synthesis and Metabolism:

Perfusion and Superfusion Studies

PERFUSION OF THE MALE RAT REPRODUCTIVE TRACT: A MODEL FOR THE STUDY OF ANDROGEN SECRETION AND ACTION

H.W.G. Baker, C.W. Bardin, G.J. Eichner, L.S. Jefferson
and R.J. Santen

Departments of Medicine and Physiology
The Milton S. Hershey Medical Center of The Pennsylvania
State University, Hershey, Pennsylvania 17033

INTRODUCTION

The feasibility of perfusion of the testis has been established by the development and characterization of methods for the testes of dogs, rabbits, rams and boars (1-3). However, these methods require considerable technical expertise to cannulate the internal spermatic artery and to establish adequate perfusion without a long period of ischemia. Although a method for short term perfusion of rat testes has been reported (4), a critical evaluation of such a system has not been undertaken previously. A technique for perfusion of the male rat reproductive tract would allow performance of replicate experiments under defined conditions in a species in which the knowledge of reproductive physiology is extensive.

This report contains a description of a method for in situ perfusion of rat testes and accessory sex organs using the hemicorpus preparation previously developed for studies of skeletal muscle by Jefferson (5,6). To demonstrate the value of the method, preliminary results of studies of testosterone secretion and androgen binding in the nuclei of the accessory sex organs are also presented.

MATERIALS AND METHODS

Male Sprague-Dawley rats 60-120 days old were obtained from Charles River Breeders. The rats were used for perfusion between 1000 and 1200 hr without prior restriction of food.

Testosterone-1α, 2α-^{3}H (S.A. 50 or 59 Ci/mM), testosterone-4-^{14}C

(57.5 Ci/M) and 5α-dihydrotestosterone-4-^{14}C (50.6 Ci/M) were obtained from New England Nuclear and used after purification on thin layer chromatography.

The antiserum and method of Nieschlag and Loriaux (7) were used for radioimmunoassay of testosterone but without chromatography. The validity of this simplified assay for testosterone in samples of perfusate was established by comparing results with and without chromatographic purification of testosterone and demonstrating that the levels of the major cross-reacting steroids, 5α-dihydrotestosterone and the 5α-androstanediols were low.

Hemicorpus preparations were perfused with 20 μCi ^{3}H-testosterone to examine the uptake of androgens into the nuclei of the ventral prostate and seminal vesicles. Preparation of the nuclei was performed as follows: at the end of perfusion, the hemicorpus was flushed with 20-30 ml of 0.25 M sucrose in 0.5 M Tris buffer, pH 7.5, with 0.25 M KCl and 0.1 M MgCl$_2$ (TKM buffer). The ventral prostate and emptied seminal vesicles were homogenized in 4 volumes of 0.25 M sucrose TKM buffer with a polytron and teflon-glass homogenizer at 4ºC. The homogenate was filtered through organza, centrifuged at 800 x g for 5 min and the supernatant discarded. The pellet was washed twice by resuspension in 0.25 M sucrose TKM buffer and centrifuged at 20,000 x g for 10 min. A final wash of the nuclear pellet was 0.2% Triton-X 100 in TKM buffer was performed and after centrifugation at 800 x g for 5 min, steroids were extracted into ethanol and the precipitate stored frozen in 0.3 M perchloric acid for DNA assay by the diphenylamine reaction. Testosterone and 5α-dihydrotestosterone were isolated by thin layer chromatography on silica gel plates in methylene chloride: diethylether (4:1) using ^{14}C-labeled steroids to correct for procedural losses (8).

TECHNIQUE OF PERFUSION

Perfusion Apparatus and Medium

The perfusion apparatus described in detail by Jefferson (5,6) and constructed by Vanderbilt University Apparatus Shop, consists of a plexiglass box maintained at 37ºC with a thermostat and lamps. Inside the box, there are duplicate drum oxygenators, preparation trays, bubble traps and connecting plastic tubing. Perfusate is circulated with Harvard peristaltic finger pumps (Model 1201) situated outside the box. A gas mixture (95% O$_2$, 5% CO$_2$) is delivered into the revolving drum oxygenators after humidification. Oxygenated perfusate is pumped through a wire mesh filter in the drum and passes through the bubble trap to a teflon cannula (ID 1.48 mm; OD 2.09 mm) placed in the descending aorta of the

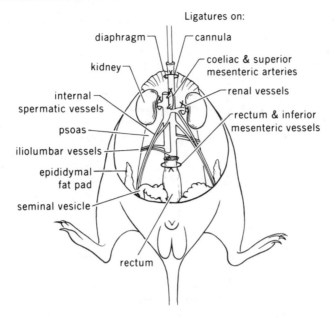

Figure 1.   The hemicorpus preparation.

CHARACTERIZATION OF THE PERFUSED HEMICORPUS

Studies by Jefferson (5,6) have indicated the viability and utility of the perfused hemicorpus preparation for studies of skeletal muscle. Normal constant water content, sorbital space and high energy phosphate levels have been demonstrated in muscle during perfusions of up to 3 hours duration. Experiments with the preparation have established its usefulness for the study of protein synthesis in skeletal muscle (5,10).

An examination of the adequacy of perfusion of the testes and accessory sex organs is in progress and the results will be reported in detail in the future. The electrolyte, pH and gas composition of the perfusate remains constant for up to 3 hours of perfusion and the glucose levels, while falling by half, still remain above 9 mM. Hemolysis is minimal or absent. The water content of the testes does not increase indicating the absence of edema. Intra-scrotal temperature is maintained between 32 and 34ºC.

hemicorpus preparation. The venous effluent drips from the cut inferior vena cava, through a wire mesh tray to a collecting trough
and is pumped back into the oxygenation drum. A T-tube in the re-
turn line permits collection of samples of the venous perfusate.

The perfusate consists of Krebs-Henseleit bicarbonate buffer
(9) modified by an increase in calcium concentration to 3.0 mM and
the addition of 0.5 mM disodium ethylenediaminetetracetic acid,
17 mM glucose, 30 gm/l bovine serum albumin (Pentex, Cohn fraction V)
and 28% washed bovine erythrocytes (5,6). This medium is freshly
prepared for each perfusion. For the studies to be described below, 250 ml of perfusate was placed in each oxygenation drum and
allowed to equilibrate with the gas mixture before perfusion was
commenced.

Preparation of the Hemicorpus

The rat is heparinized with an intraperitoneal injection of
sodium heparin, 100 mg/kg, 30 min before anesthesia with intraperitoneal sodium pentobarbital, 50 mg/kg. The abdomen is opened
with a semicircular incision below the costal margins and the
coeliac and superior mesenteric arteries, renal vessels and inferior
mesenteric vessels together with the rectum are ligated. Care is
taken to leave the internal spermatic vessels undisturbed. The
chest is opened by cutting through the left dorsal costal angles
and around the costal insertion of the diaphragm. A ligature is
passed around the aorta above the diaphragm and tied loosely.
Blood flow is stopped by a second ligature below the arch of the
aorta. A small hole is cut in the aorta approximately 1 cm above
the diaphragm and the teflon cannula inserted so that its tip is
above the origins of the renal arteries. The cannula is then se-
cured by tightening the lower ligature. Perfusion at a rate of
7 ml/min is started immediately after placement of the cannula.
The time from opening the chest to commencement of perfusion is
less than 90 sec. The upper half of the animal is cut off above
the cannula, the intestine, liver and adrenal glands are removed
and the inferior vena cava is cut at the level of the right crus
of the diaphragm. The abdominal cavity is flushed with physiological saline and covered with a plastic sheet. The rate of perfusion may then be increased, usually to 35 ml/min. The first 50 ml
of perfusate is allowed to flow out the T-tube in the venous line
and discarded. The T-tube may be closed and perfusate permitted
to recirculate or it may remain open for a single flow-through or
non-recirculating procedure. The hemicorpus preparation and the
position of the ligatures is shown diagrammatically in Figure 1.

The testicular content of ATP and GTP is normal for up to 90 min of
perfusion but falls to 5-40% at 3 hours. The cause of this decrease
in high energy phosphate levels is being examined.

The distribution of perfusate to the testes and accessory sex
organs has been determined using a method involving injection of
radioactively labeled microspheres and was found to be dependent
upon both the overall rate of perfusion and the size of the animals.
With rats weighing about 300 gm and a perfusion rate of 35 ml/min,
the flow to the testes was approximately half (0.1 ml/min/gm) the
testicular blood flow in intact rats (0.2 ml/min/gm) (11).

Continuous monitoring of caudal artery pressure during aortic
cannulation and commencement of perfusion showed a transient rise
in pressure over the first 2-3 min, presumably due to vasoconstric-
tion resulting from the anoxia associated with opening the chest.
For this reason, perfusion is started at a slow rate (7 ml/min)
and later increased. Subsequent measurements revealed constant
arterial pressure for up to 3 hr of perfusion and injection of
potent vasodilators which act directly on smooth muscle (sodium
nitroprusside and sodium nitrite) failed to alter the pressure or
the distribution of injected microspheres to the testes and accessory
sex organs. These results suggest that there is full vasodilata-
tion and no significant vasospasm in the hemicorpus preparation.

STUDIES OF THE FUNCTIONAL CAPACITY OF THE PERFUSED RAT REPRODUCTIVE
TRACT

Testosterone Secretion

The change in testosterone levels over 3 hours of recirculating
perfusion of hemicorpus preparations from 90 day old rats is shown
in Fig. 2. Without tropic hormone in the perfusate, a low and constant testosterone concentration was achieved after 30 min. The
addition of hCG was associated with increasing levels which reached
a plateau after 90 min. Why testosterone secretion stopped after
the first 90 min is uncertain but it may be linked to the low
testicular ATP levels found at 3 hours. Because the perfusion
medium contains glucose as the only intermediary metabolite, depletion of other substrates from the Leydig cells is possibly a
cause. Alternatively, toxic substances or other inhibitors of
steroidogenesis may accumulate in the recirculating perfusate.
A similar cessation of testosterone secretion has not been observed
in the flow-through perfusion system for rabbit testis by Ewing (2)
or in the canine testis preparations of Eik-Nes (1).

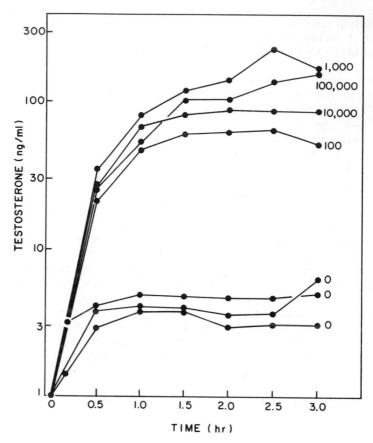

Figure 2. Testosterone levels in perfusate in response to various doses of hCG (mIU/ml).

The dose-response relationship of hCG stimulated testosterone secretion is shown in Fig. 3. The testosterone levels were measured in samples taken after 90 or 180 min of perfusion with medium containing different concentrations of hCG. The curve is approximately logarithmic over the range 50-1000 IU/ml hCG. With the present recirculating technique, calculation of secretion rates requires correction for loss of testosterone into the plastic tubing, metabolism by the hemicorpus preparation and changes in volume of perfusate due to withdrawal of samples. Preliminary studies have demonstrated the value of following the disappearance of a tracer dose of ^{3}H-testosterone from the perfusate to correct for losses. Using this method, maximally stimulated testosterone secretion rates averaged over 3 hours were 30 µg/hr. This value is 40 times greater than the unstimulated secretion rate (0.8 µg/hr) in the perfused hemicorpus, 3-4 times greater than the testosterone production rate of intact mature rats (7 µg/hr) and considerably greater than the testosterone secretion rate of 1.65 µg/gm/hr calculated by Hall (12) for whole rat testis incubated with gonadotropins in vitro.

Androgen Binding to Nuclei of Accessory Sex Organs

Figures 4 and 5 show the ^{3}H-androgens contained in the nuclei of the ventral prostate and seminal vesicles of hemicorpus preparations from 90 day old rats castrated for 24 hours, and perfused for different times with media containing 20 µCi of ^{3}H-testosterone. The results of two preparations perfused for 15 and 120 min with a 1000-fold excess of radioinert testosterone are also shown to demonstrate the specificity of binding. It can be seen that the

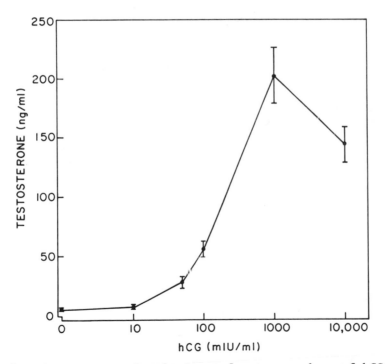

Figure 3. Testosterone levels in perfusate vs. dose of hCG, mean (±SEM) results for 3-8 experiments.

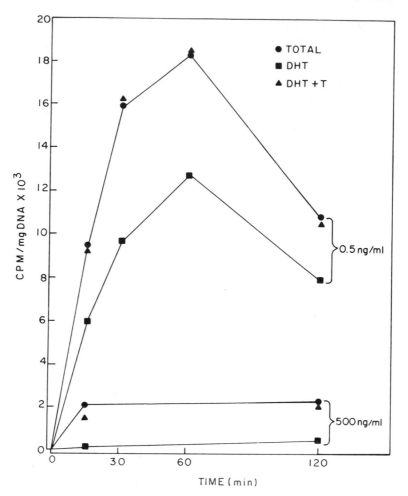

Figure 4. Time course of binding of androgens to prostate gland
nuclei. Mass of testosterone perfused 0.5 ng/ml or 500 ng/ml.
● Total tritium, ■ ^{3}H-dihydrotestosterone, ▲ ^{3}H-dihydrotes-
tosterone + ^{3}H-testosterone.

nuclear content of androgens becomes relatively constant by 30-60
min. After correction for non-specific binding, 5α-dihydrotesto-
sterone accounted for 68-87% and 68-81% of the radioactivity in
prostate and seminal vesicle nuclei respectively and most, if not
all, the remaining radioactive steroid was testosterone. These
results are similar to those generally accepted for the nuclear
androgens of rat accessory sex organs although the proportion of
5α-dihydrotestosterone is slightly lower (13,14).

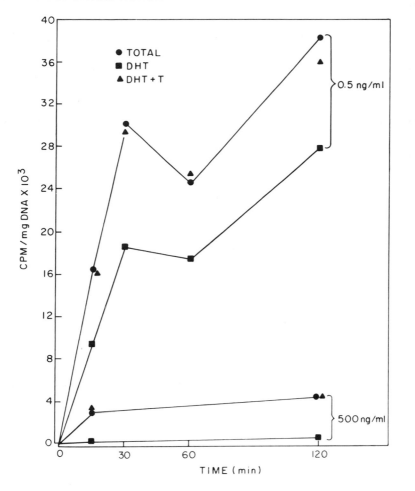

Figure 5. Time course of binding of androgens to seminal vesicle
nuclei. Symbols as for Fig. 4.

SUMMARY

        A method for perfusion of the male rat reproductive tract
in situ has been described and its applicability to studies of androgen secretion and action demonstrated. While full characterization of the system is as yet incomplete, it promises to be a useful tool in the investigation of male reproductive physiology.

ACKNOWLEDGEMENTS

The authors thank Dr. D. L. Loriaux for the gift of the testosterone antiserum, Amel P. French and James W. Robinson for their
technical assistance and Mrs. Marlene Brinser for typing.

This investigation was supported in part by a Public Health
Service International Research Fellowship No. F05 TW02118-01
by Grant No. AM-15658 from the National Institutes of Health,
and PHS Grant No. HD-05276.

REFERENCES

1. Eik-Nes, K.B., Rec. Progr. Horm. Res. 27: 517, 1971.

2. Ewing, L.L. and Eik-Nes, K.B., Can. J. Biochem. 44: 1327,
    1966.

3. Linzell, J.L. and Setchell, B.P., J. Physiol. (Lond.) 201: 129,
    1969.

4. Frederik, P.M. and van Doorn, L.G., J. Reprod. Fert. 35: 117,
    1973.

5. Jefferson, L.S., Koehler, J.O., and Morgan, H.E., Proc. Nat.
    Acad. Sci. USA 69: 816, 1972.

6. Jefferson, L.S., Methods in Enzymology, 1975, in press.

7. Nieschlag, E. and Loriaux, D.L., Z. Klin. Chem. 10: 164, 1972.

8. Djoseland, O., Hansson, V. and Haugen, H.N., Steroids 21: 773,
    1973.

9. Krebs, H.A. and Henseleit, K., Hoppe-Seyler's Z. Physiol. Chem.
    210: 33, 1932.

10. Jefferson, L.S., Rannels, D.E., Munger, B L., and Morgan, H.E.,
    Federation Proc. 33: 1098, 1974.

11. Setchell, B.P., Testicular Blood Supply, Lymphatic Drainage and
    Secretion of Fluids, In The Testis, Johnson, A.D. et al. (eds.),
    Vol. 1, p. 101, Academic Press, New York, 1970.

12. Hall, P.F., Endocrinology of the Testis, In The Testis, Johnson,
    A.D. et al. (eds.), Vol. 2, p. 1, Academic Press, New York, 1970.

13. Bruchovsky, N. and Wilson, J.D., J. Biol. Chem. 243: 5953, 1968.

14. Anderson, K.M. and Liao, S., Nature (Lond.) 219: 277, 1968.

SOME FACTORS AFFECTING TESTOSTERONE, DIHYDROTESTOSTERONE, 5α-ANDRO-
STAN-3α,17β-DIOL AND 5α-ANDROSTAN-3β,17β-DIOL SECRETION BY IN VITRO
PERFUSED RABBIT TESTES

Larry L. Ewing

Division of Reproductive Biology, Department of Population
Dynamics, Johns Hopkins School of Hygiene, 615 N. Wolfe
Street, Baltimore, Maryland 21205

Dihydrotestosterone[*] and 5α-androstan-3α,17β-diol are present
in the peripheral circulation of several vertebrate species (1-11).
Although considerable quantities of these 5α-reduced androgens are
derived via the peripheral conversion of blood borne precursors
(5,12,13) it is now clear that significant amounts of 5α-reduced
androgens originate from the gonads of two species, namely, dogs
(6,14) and rabbits (15,16). The most likely explanation for
gonadal derivation of these androgens is that testicular and epididymal function are testosterone dependent (17,18) and that testosterone probably exerts its regulatory effects only after conversion
to DHT (19,20) which subsequently is metabolized to androstanediols
(3α-androstanediol and 3β-androstanediol) in the male gonad. Thus,
testosterone secretion might represent a balance between intratesticular biosynthesis on one hand and intratesticular metabolism
on the other. In fact, such a scheme has been proposed to explain
the transient changes in net testosterone biosynthesis in maturing
guinea pig (21) and rat (22-28) testis. Significant metabolism of

---

[*]The following trivial names and abbreviations are used in this
paper: dihydrotestosterone, DHT = 5α-androstan-17β-ol-3-one;
testosterone, T = 17β-hydroxy-androst-4-en-3-one; 3α-androstane-
diol = 5α-androstan-3α,17β-diol; 3β-androstanediol = 5α-andro-
stan-3β,17β-diol; pregnenolone = 5-pregnen-3β-ol-20-one; Δ5-
androstendiol = 5-androsten-3β,17β-diol; medrogestone = 6,17-
dimethylpregnan-4,6-diene-3,20-dione; progesterone = 4-pregnen-3,20-
dione; cyproterone acetate = 1,2α-methylene-6-chloro-Δ⁶-17α-hydroxy-
progesterone acetate.

a steroidal hormone prior to its secretion from the biosynthetic
source is not without precedent since Kitay and co-workers (29-32)
showed that corticosterone secretion by the rat adrenal depends not
only upon the rate of corticosterone synthesis but also upon its
conversion to 5α-reduced metabolites.

We recently observed a discrepancy (33) in testosterone secretion rate by in vitro perfused rabbit testes depending upon
whether testosterone was quantified by a highly specific gas liquid
chromatographic (34) or a nonspecific radioligand assay (35).
Testosterone secretion was invariably higher when measured by the
radioligand rather than the gas liquid chromatographic method.
This suggested to us the presence of unidentified 17β-hydroxy-
steroids in rabbit spermatic vein blood since the sex hormone
binding globulin present in third trimester pregnancy plasma used
in the radioligand assay possessed an avidity for several 17β-
hydroxysteroids including DHT, 3α-androstanediol and 3β-
androstanediol.

Herein are reviewed our experiments proving that testosterone
gives rise intratesticularly to DHT, 3α-androstanediol and 3β-
androstanediol which are secreted into the venous effluent of the
in vitro perfused rabbit testis. Additionally, new results are
presented showing the effect of: medium flow, gonadotrophin infusion, inhibition of testosterone synthesis, and experimental
cryptorchidism upon in vitro secretion of DHT, 3α-androstanediol
and 3β-androstanediol by the perfused testis.

MATERIALS AND METHODS

Most of the materials used in these experiments were described
elsewhere (15,16). Pregnenolone was purchased from Steraloids, Inc.,
Pawling, New York and crystallized to constant melting point prior
to use. Medrogestone was a gift from Drs. Coffey and Heston of
the Brady Laboratory for Reproductive Biology at The Johns Hopkins
School of Medicine. NIH-LH-S17 was obtained from The National
Institute of Arthritis and Metabolic Diseases.

New Zealand white rabbits (6-12 months) purchased from
Bunnyville in Altoona, Pennsylvania were housed in an air con-
ditioned (20±2°C) and light controlled (14 hr light:10 hr dark)
room and supplied daily with 120 gms Rabbit Checkers, Rulston
Purina Co., St. Louis and water ad libitum.

Rabbit testes with seminiferous tubules containing normal
spermatogenesis but which were incapable of secreting testosterone
when perfused in vitro were produced by the subcutaneous implanta-

tion for 90 days of testosterone filled polydimethylsiloxane implants providing 25,600 mm^2 surface area (36). Rabbits were rendered cryptorchid by a surgical technique described elsewhere (37,38).

The perfusion method has been discussed previously (39–41). One additional technique used in some experiments described herein was the perfusion of the rabbit testis minus the epididymis. This was accomplished by carefully dissecting the epididymis and fat pad from the testis. Since the testicular artery of the rabbit makes three complete revolutions around the long axis of the testis prior to entering the parenchyma it was a simple matter to incise the tunica albuginea over the artery on the dorsal aspect of the testis and to cannulate the artery. The effluent from this preparation contained not only venous perfusion medium but also rete testis fluid.

The Sephadex LH–20 column chromatography and recrystallization to constant specific activity were completely described in an earlier publication (15). The extraction, paper and thin layer chromatographic separation, gas chromatographic measurement and mass spectrometric identification of testosterone, DHT, 3α–androstanediol and 3β–androstanediol were also described earlier (16).

RESULTS

Formation of Dihydrotestosterone, 5α–Androstan–3α,17β–Diol and
5α–Androstan–3β,17β–Diol by Perfused Rabbit Testis–Epididymis

We (15) infused testosterone-1,2,6,7-^{3}H into the perfused rabbit testis-epididymis, collected the spermatic venous effluent, extracted free steroids from the venous effluent plasma with dichloromethane and developed the residue of the extract on a Sephadex LH–20 column. As expected, several peaks of radioactivity were observed in the column eluate (Fig. 1).

We (15) subsequently proved that the four peaks of radioactivity were not red blood cell testosterone metabolites, that the four radioactive peaks accounted for nearly 90% of the radioactivity in the sample and that the same four peaks were forthcoming when an extract of testicular effluent from a testis-epididymis infused with acetate-1-C^{14} was similarly chromatographed. Elution volumes from the Sephadex LH–20 column, Rf's in four thin layer chromatographic systems, retention times on the gas liquid chromatograph and crystallization of the unknown radioactive compounds from the Sephadex column to constant specific activity proved that peaks A,B,C and D in Figure 1 were DHT, testosterone, 5α–androstan–3α, 17β–diol and 5α–androstan–3β,17β–diol, respectively.

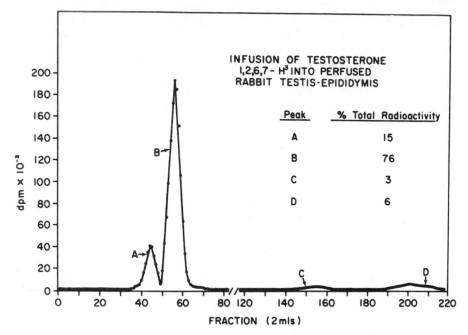

Figure 1.   Peaks of radioactivity eluted from Sephadex LH-20 column.
The radioactive mixture eluted from the column was a dichloromethane extract of venous effluent obtained from two rabbit testes-
epididymides perfused for two hours with an artificial medium containing testosterone-1,2,6,7-^{3}H (1x10^6 dpm/hr).   By courtesy of
the editor of Endocrinology.

Secretion of Testosterone, Dihydrotestosterone, 5α-Androstan-3α,
17β-Diol and 5α-Androstan-3β,17β-Diol by the Perfused Rabbit
Testis-Epididymis

        Ewing et al. (16) developed a gas chromatographic assay that
permitted the simultaneous measurement of T, DHT, 3α-androstanediol
and 3β-androstanediol concentration in one rabbit spermatic vein
sample.   The specificity of the assay method was attested to by
the fact that each compound exhibited an Rf similar to the appropriate steroid standard in a Bush A$_2$ paper chromatographic system,
and after acetylation Rf's and retention times similar to the
appropriate steroid acetate standards in a thin layer and gas
chromatographic system, respectively.   Moreover, the mass spectra
of the samples of suspected testosterone acetate, dihydrotestosterone acetate, 5α-androstan-3α,17β-diacetate and 5α-androstan-
3β,17β-diacetate were identical to corresponding steroid standards
(16).   Using this measurement technique Ewing and co-workers (16)
found that perfusion of the rabbit testis-epididymis with a physiological concentration of LH resulted in a T, DHT, 3α-andro-
stanediol and 3β-androstanediol secretion of 3.1, 0.7, 0.4 and 0.6
μg/hr, respectively (Fig. 2).   The testosterone/5α reduced androgen

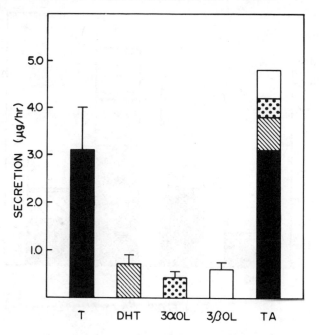

Figure 2. Secretion of testosterone (T) dihydrotestosterone (DHT), 5α-androstan-3α,17β-diol (3αol) and 5α-androstan-3β,17β-diol (3βol) by rabbit testes-epididymides perfused in vitro with artificial medium containing 2.5 ng/ml of NIH-LH-S17, ovine. TA represents a composite of testosterone, dihydrotestosterone, 3α-androstanediol and 3β-androstanediol secretion. The testosterone/5α-reduced androgen ratio is 1.9+0.3. The T above each bar denotes the standard error of the mean. (N=6). By courtesy of the editor of Endocrinology.

ratio was 1.9. Similar secretion rates were obtained for each steroid when spermatic venous effluent was collected from anesthetized rabbits in situ (16).

Some Factors Effecting the Secretion of Testosterone Dihydrotestosterone, 5α-Androstan-3α,17β-diol and 5α-Androstan-3β,17β-diol by the Perfused Rabbit Testis

Results in Figure 3 show that testosterone and 5α reduced-androgen secretion were optimal when testes-epididymides were

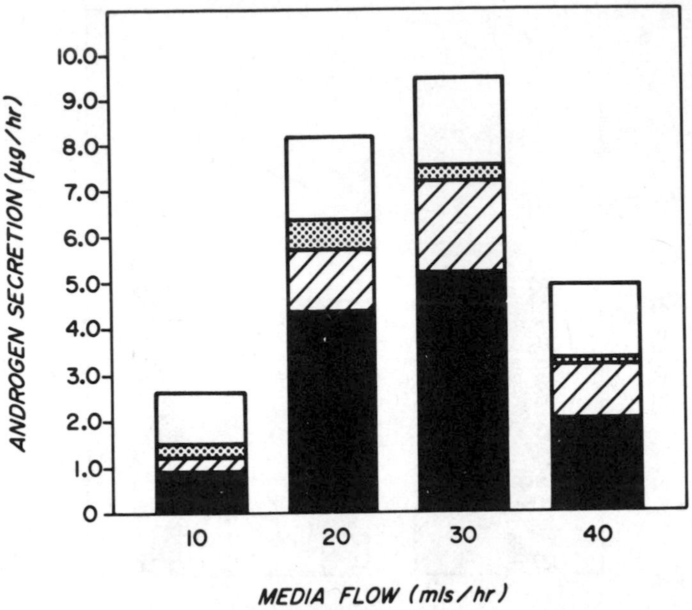

Figure 3. The effect of medium flow upon testosterone, [solid black box] ; dihydrotestosterone, [hatched box] ; 5α-androstan-3α,17β-diol [dotted box] and 5α-androstan-3β,17β-diol [open box] secretion by in vitro perfused rabbit testes-epididymides. The artificial medium contained 100 ng/ml of NIH-LH-S17, ovine. Each bar represents the mean total of the four androgens secreted during the second hour of perfusion by five testes-epididymides. The actual secretion of each steroid is denoted by the code above.

perfused in vitro with 20 or 30 mls of artificial medium/hr. The results in Figure 4 show that increasing the artificial medium LH concentration increased androgen secretion. There was little increase in androgen secretion when LH was increased from 10 to 100 ng/ml of artificial medium.

Next the testis minus the epididymis was perfused with artificial medium containing 100 ng/ml LH at 20 ml/hr. The results in Figure 5 show that the secretion rates of DHT, 3α-androstanediol and 3β-androstanediol by the testis alone were identical to that seen when the testis-epididymis was similarly perfused at either 20 or 30 ml/hr (Fig. 3). Surprisingly, testosterone secretion was elevated when testes were perfused in the absence of the epididymis and fat pad (Fig. 5).

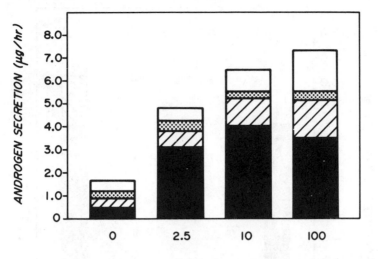

Figure 4. The effect of LH concentration upon testosterone ████, dihydrotestosterone, ▨▨▨ ; 5α-androstan-3α,17β-diol; ▨▨▨ and 5α-androstan-3β,17β-diol ▭ secretion by in vitro perfused rabbit testes-epididymides. Medium flow was maintained at 10 ml/g testis/hr. Each bar represents the mean total of the four androgens secreted during the second hour of perfusion by five testes-epididymides. The actual secretion of each steroid is denoted by the code above.

In the next experiment rabbit testes were perfused at 20 ml/hr with artificial medium containing 100 ng/ml LH either in the absence or presence of Medrogestone. We suspected that inhibition of testosterone biosynthesis by Medrogestone would result in diminished DHT, 3α-androstanediol and 3β-androstanediol secretion. The results in Figure 6 show a dose dependent inhibition of testosterone secretion by Medrogestone. As expected, the inhibition of DHT, 3α-androstanediol and 3β-androstanediol secretion was proportional to the reduction in testosterone secretion.

Desjardins et al. (36) recently showed that rabbit testes from animals treated with large doses of testosterone failed to secrete testosterone when perfused in vitro despite the fact that Sertoli and germ cell morphology, sperm production and fertility appeared normal. Consequently, rabbits were similarly treated with testosterone for 90 days and their androgen secretion in vitro was compared with that of testes from control rabbits. The results in Figure 7 proved that rabbits which failed to secrete testosterone also failed to secrete

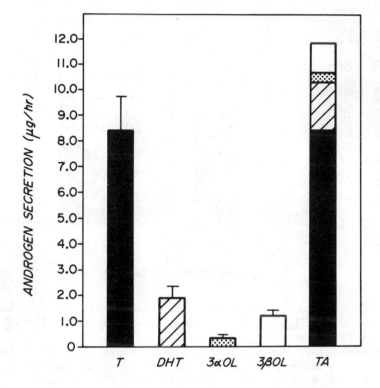

Figure 5. Secretion of testosterone (T), dihydrotestosterone (DHT),
5α-androstan -3α,17β-diol (3αol) and 5α-androstan-3β,17β-diol (3βol)
by rabbit testes perfused in vitro with artificial medium containing
100 ng/ml of NIH-LH-S17, ovine. TA represents a composite of
testosterone, dihydrotestosterone, 3α-androstanediol and 3β-andro-
stanediol secretion. The T above each bar denotes the standard
error of the mean (N=8).

DHT, 3α-androstanediol and 3β-androstanediol even though the Sertoli
and germ cells were intact.

It occurred to us that Sertoli and germ cells might lack some
critical biosynthetic intermediate, other than testosterone, normally diffusing from the secretory Leydig cells. Consequently,
we once again compared the secretion of testosterone and 5α-reduced
androgens by testes from control versus testosterone treated rabbits.
However, this time the testes received no LH but were infused instead with artificial medium containing zero or 20 μg/ml of
pregnenolone. The results in Figure 8 show that control testes
perfused with artificial medium (no LH; no pregnenolone) produced

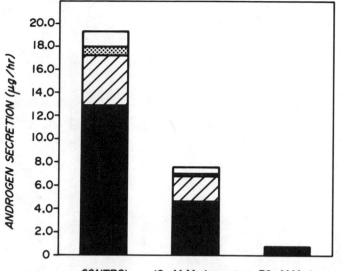

Figure 6. The effect of Medrogestone upon testosterone, ▰ ;
dihydrotestosterone, ⧄ ; 5α-androstan-3α,17β-diol, ▨ and
5α-androstan-3β,17β-diol ▭ secretion by in vitro perfused
rabbit testes. The artificial medium contained 100 ng/ml of NIH-LH-
S17, ovine and was perfused through the testis at 10 ml/g testis/hr.
Each bar represents the mean total of the four androgens secreted
during the second hour of perfusion by eight testes. The actual
secretion of each steroid is denoted by the code above.

less than 2 μg/hr of androgens. In contrast, control testes receiving no LH but instead 20 μg/hr of pregnenolone secreted over
10 μg/hr of the four androgens measured. Finally, testes derived
from animals receiving massive doses of testosterone for 90 days
prior to the perfusion experiment similarly perfused with pregnenolone failed to secrete testosterone, DHT, 3α-androstanediol and
3β-androstanediol.

     Lastly, the effect of germinal epithelium destruction by
heat upon the secretion of testosterone, DHT, 3α-androstanediol
and 3β-androstanediol was tested. Individual testes from rabbits
rendered experimentally cryptorchid for 18 days weighed approximately 0.8 compared to 2.5 g for testes taken from control rabbits.
As expected, this loss of weight reflected a dramatic disappearance
of advanced germ cell types from the rabbit testis (Table 1).

     We perfused 8 control and 8 cryptorchid rabbit testes with
10 ml of artificial medium/g testis/hr containing 100 ng/ml LH.

Table 1

Comparison of the Relative Number of Germ and Sertoli Cells Per Cross-Section of Seminiferous Tubule at Stage VI of the Cycle of the Seminiferous Epithelium in Normal Rabbits, Rabbits Subjected to Sham Operation and Those Rendered Cryptorchid for 18 Days

GERM CELL NUMBERS

Treatment	N	Type A Spermatogonia	Preleptotene Spermatocytes	Pachytene Spermatocytes	Step 6 Spermatids	No. of Sertoli cells with a nucleolus
Normal rabbits	15	1.0 ± 0.10	15.4 ± 0.7	15.9 ± 0.8	56.2 ± 4.1	3.2 ± 0.4
Sham operated rabbits	6	0.91 ± 0.11	15.2 ± 0.7	15.5 ± 0.7	58.8 ± 3.8	3.0 ± 0.5
18 day cryptorchid rabbits	7	0.8 ± 0.14	none present	none present	none present	5.7 ± 0.6

Each value represents the mean ± standard error determined by counting the indicated cells in 20 "round" tubular cross-sections at Stage VI. All cell counts were corrected for differences in nuclear diameter by Abercrombie's formula and germ cell counts were corrected for tubular shrinkage by a Sertoli cell correction factor (calculated by dividing the average number of Sertoli nuclei per tubular cross-section in testes of control animals by the corresponding number of Sertoli nuclei in testes of cryptorchid animals).

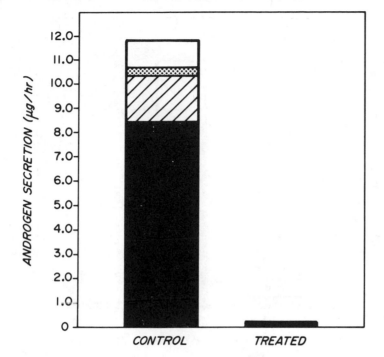

Figure 7. Secretion of testosterone, ▆▆▆ ; dihydrotestosterone, ▨▨▨ ; 5α-androstan-3α,17β-diol ▨▨▨ and 5α-androstan-3β,17β-diol ☐ by rabbit testes from control and rabbits receiving testosterone filled polydimethylsiloxane implants for ninety days which provided 25,600 mm^2 surface area (treated). The artificial medium contained 100 ng/ml of NIH-LH-S17, ovine and was perfused through the testis at 10 ml/g testis/hr. Each bar represents the mean total of the four androgens secreted during the second hour of perfusion by eight testes. The actual secretion of each steroid is denoted by the code above.

The rate of secretion of each androgen by control and cryptorchid testes is shown in Table 2. Surprisingly, drastic depopulation of the seminiferous tubules by experimental cryptorchidism did not significantly alter the secretion of T, DHT, and 3α-androstanediol. In contrast, the secretion of 3β-androstanediol was significantly ($P<0.05$) reduced in cryptorchid compared to control testes.

DISCUSSION

It now seems clear that mature rabbit testes metabolize

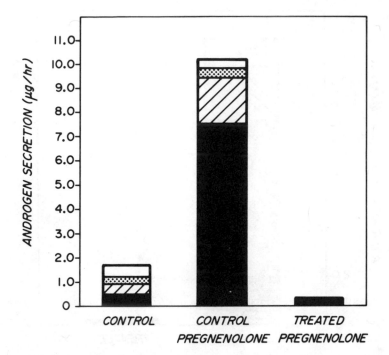

Figure 8.   The effect of pregnenolone upon the secretion of testosterone, ██████ ; dihydrotestosterone, ▨▨▨ , 5α–androstan–3α,17β–
diol, ▨▨▨▨ and 5α–androstan–3β,17β–diol ▭ by control rabbits
and rabbits receiving testosterone filled polydimethylsiloxane implants for ninety days which provided 25,600 mm^2 surface area
(treated).   The artificial medium was perfused through the testis
at 10 ml/g testis/hr.   No exogenous LH was added to the artificial
medium.   Instead the artificial medium contained zero or 20 μg/ml
of pregnenolone.   Each bar represents the mean total of the four
androgens secreted during the second hour of perfusion by eight
testes.   The actual secretion of each steroid is denoted by the
code above.

testosterone prior to its escape into the peripheral circulation
to dihydrotestosterone, 5α–androstan–3α,17β–diol and 5α–androstan–
3β,17β–diol.   Since the intratesticular testosterone concentration
is about 20 times that of peripheral blood plasma in the rabbit
(36) it was not surprising that even modest gonadal conversions of
testosterone result in the secretion of DHT, 3α–androstanediol and
3β–androstanediol.

        Rabbit testicular–epididymal secretion of testosterone relative
to DHT (T/DHT) both in vitro and in situ (16) was similar to that

Table 2

The Effect of Experimental Cryptorchidism for 18 Days Upon
Testosterone (T), Dihydrotestosterone (DHT), 5α–Androstan-
3α,17β-diol (3αdiol) and 5α–Androstan-3β,17β-diol (3βdiol)
Secretion by in vitro Perfused Rabbit Testes

Androgen Secretion (µg/hr)

TREATMENT	T	DHT	3α Diol	3β Diol
Control	8.4 + 1.3	1.9 + .40	.34 + .07	1.2 + .18
Cryptorchid	9.0 + 1.5	2.3 + .34	.30 + .10	0.31 + .22*

Each value represents the mean + standard error for eight testes
perfused in vitro.   * (P<0.05). Each testis was perfused without
the epididymis for two hours with artificial media containing 100
ng/ml NIH LH–S17, ovine. Media flow was maintained at 10 ml/g
testis/hr.

reported for the dog (6,14). Although reports of the secretion of
DHT, 3α–androstanediol and 3β–androstanediol are scanty or non-
existent, considerable evidence exists documenting that these and
other testosterone metabolites are formed in vitro by testes of
several species (6,22,24,42–46). Many of the aforementioned experiments were conducted with the rat and the consensus of opinion
is that while the rate of testosterone metabolism to ring A reduced
androgens is high in the immature, it is low in mature rat testes
(21–28). It was difficult to reconcile this concept with our observation (16) suggesting that 35% of testosterone biosynthesized
within adult rabbit testes was metabolized to 5α–reduced androgens
prior to its release into the peripheral circulation. However,
this apparent discrepancy may simply reflect species variation in
intratesticular testosterone metabolism since Falvo and Nalbandov
(47) showed that the rabbit was the only one of eight species
showing a discrepancy between the apparent testosterone concentration in peripheral blood plasma when measured by a radioimmunoassay with and without Sephadex LH-20 chromatography. Predictably,
the apparent testosterone concentration in rabbit peripheral blood
plasma was always higher in the unchromatographed samples. We
recently confirmed Falvo and Nalbandov's (47) findings for the
rabbit. Moreover, we also found that the discrepancy in apparent
testosterone concentration in unchromatographed versus chromatographed samples of rabbit peripheral blood plasma was totally
accounted for by the presence of DHT, 3α–androstanediol and
3β–androstanediol.

In discussing some factors effecting the secretion of testosterone dihydrotestosterone, 5α-androstan-3α,17β-diol and 5α-
androstan-3β,17β-diol by the perfused rabbit testis we are assuming
that testicular steroid secretion reflects testicular steroid
metabolism.   This assumption is probably valid since there appears
to be little storage of testosterone in rabbit testicular tissue
(40).

Several important questions remained unanswered at outset of
this investigation.   Does the testis produce significant quantities
of the 5α-reduced androgens or do they originate largely from the
epididymis?   Is the production of DHT, 3α-androstanediol and 3β-
androstanediol dependent upon the intratesticular biosynthesis of
testosterone?   Can the Sertoli and germ cells produce DHT, 3α-
androstanediol and 3β-androstanediol when testicular testosterone
biosynthesis is inhibited?   Finally, what is the effect of germinal
epithelium destruction by heat upon the secretion of testosterone,
DHT, 3α-androstanediol and 3β-androstanediol?

Prior to designing experiments to answer the above questions,
it was imperative to establish optimum and carefully controlled
in vitro perfusion conditions.   Since the rate of medium flow (Fig.
3) and medium LH concentrations (Fig. 4) altered androgen secretion,
subsequent perfusions were performed at a flow rate of 10 ml/g
testis/hr with artificial medium containing 100 ng/ml of NIH-LH-
S17, ovine, unless otherwise noted.

Although difficult to quantify the testicular and epididymal
contribution to secreted T, DHT, 3α-androstanediol and 3β-androstane-
diol, it was possible to prove whether the testis secreted measure-
able quantities of the androgens in question.   The results in
Figure 5 prove that when the testis itself was perfused, the secretion of the 5α-reduced androgens was equivalent to that seen when
the testis-epididymis was similarly perfused (Fig. 3).   We have
no explanation for the apparent increase in testosterone secretion
when the epididymis was removed.   It is worthy of mention at this
juncture that when the testis is perfused in the absence of the
epididymis, the venous effluent contains some contribution from
the rete testis fluid.   Spermatic vein flow is several hundred
times more than rete testis fluid flow (48) while testosterone concentrations in the two fluids are similar (49) in the ram.   Assuming that the same relationship exists between fluid volumes and
steroid concentrations in the rabbit it seems likely that the rete
testis fluid contribution to androgen secretion by the in vitro
perfused rabbit testis must be small compared to that from the
spermatic vein.

Results from at least two publications (50,51) suggest that
DHT can be formed by a pathway that does not require testosterone

as an intermediate. We reasoned that if DHT is formed by a pathway
independent of testosterone we should be able to inhibit testosterone
but not 5α-reduced androgen secretion. Consequently, we infused
Medrogestone into the perfused testis since Medrogestone is a potent
inhibitor of the Δ^5-3-ketosteroid isomerase enzyme (52) and should
therefore inhibit testosterone biosynthesis. The results in Figure 6
show that the inhibition of testosterone biosynthesis resulted in a
corresponding and dose dependent loss of DHT, 3α-androstanediol and
3β-androstanediol secretion. Similar concentrations of other progestins such as progesterone and cyproterone acetate failed to inhibit the secretion of any of the androgens measured. The secretion
of the last known intermediate (Δ^5-androstenediol) on the Δ^5 biosynthetic pathway to testosterone was measured to substantiate that
Medrogestone inhibited the Δ^5-3-ketosteroid isomerase. Predictably,
Δ^5-androstenediol secretion was increased 20 fold in testes receiving
Medrogestone when compared to control testes. Unfortunately, this
experiment was inconclusive since the possibility existed that
Medrogestone may have inhibited some unknown enzyme required for
the intratesticular formation of DHT via a biosynthetic pathway
not involving testosterone.

     Desjardins et al. (36) recently showed that Sertoli and germ
cell morphology, sperm production and fertility were maintained in
male rabbits receiving large dosages of testosterone for 90 days.
Paradoxically, these same testes failed to secrete testosterone when
perfused in vitro with FSH and LH for four hours (36) suggesting
that the Leydig cells were non-secretory. Although seminiferous
tubular function appears normal in these animals we predicted that
testicular DHT, 3α-androstanediol and 3β-androstanediol secretion
in vitro would be greatly reduced since testosterone biosynthesis
is inhibited by the previous exposure to exogenous testosterone for
90 days. The results in Figure 7 proved this prediction to be
correct. Taken together, the results of the last two experiments
suggested but did not prove that intratesticular DHT, 3α-andro-
stanediol and 3β-androstanediol formation depended upon the prior
formation of testosterone by the perfused rabbit testis.

     Some authors (53,54) ascribe steroidogenic functions to the
seminiferous tubule. It occurred to us that the Sertoli and germ
cells in the testosterone treated testis described above might
have failed to produce testosterone and/or 5α-reduced androgens because of the lack of some biosynthetic intermediate normally diffusing from secretory Leydig cells (55,56). Consequently, testes
from control and testosterone treated rabbits were next perfused
with artificial media containing either 0 or 20 μg/ml of pregnenolone but devoid of LH. The five fold increase in androgen
production (Fig. 8) by control testes receiving pregnenolone compared to those receiving only artificial media suggested that
pregnenolone infused via the arterial vasculature was readily

available to the steroid biosynthesizing enzymes of the testis.
Pregnenolone was probably available to all steroid synthesizing
compartments within the testis since the androgen secretion by
control testes receiving pregnenolone was identical to that obtained when saturating LH concentrations were infused into other
control testes (Fig. 5). Finally, the failure of testosterone
treated testes to secrete any of the androgens measured, suggested
that the seminiferous tubular components lacked the enzymes required to synthesize testosterone, DHT, 3α-androstanediol or 3β-
androstanediol from pregnenolone. Thus these data coupled with
the effect of Medrogestone and pituitary suppression upon 5α-
reduced androgen secretion as well as the incorporation of testo-
sterone-^{3}H into the 5α-reduced androgens (15) strongly suggested
that DHT, 3α-androstanediol and 3β-androstanediol are formed
intratesticularly from testosterone.

We hypothesized that depopulation of germ cells in the seminiferous tubule by experimental cryptorchidism would result in a
diminution of 5α-reduced androgen but not testosterone secretion
since numerous authors suggest that testosterone is formed in
Leydig cells (57-61) and that DHT and androstanediols are probably
formed by some seminiferous tubular cells (42-46) probably spermatocytes (62,63). As expected, experimental cryptorchidism for 18
days caused a dramatic disappearance of advanced germ cell types
from the rabbit testis (Table 1). While achieving our goal of de-
populating the seminiferous tubules of germ cells, the resultant
size differential between control and cryptorchid testes created the
dilemma of how much artificial medium to perfuse through the
respective testes since androgen secretion was altered by medium
flow (Fig. 3). Fortunately, considerable data was available regarding the relationship between testicular weight and in situ
blood flow in rats (64,65) and rabbits (66). Typical of these data
is that of Jones (65) who showed that x-irradiated rat testes
declined both in weight and total blood flow during a six week post-
irradiation period. Surprisingly, the blood flow per gram of
testis was similar to unirradiated control rats and constant over
the entire six week period. Similar results have been reported
for cryptorchid rat testes (64) and for rabbit testes during the
growth period associated with sexual maturation (66). Armed with
this information we perfused 8 control and 8 cryptorchid rabbit
testes with 10 ml artificial medium/g testis/hr containing 100 ng/
ml of LH. As expected, experimental cryptorchidism for 18 days did
not alter testosterone secretion (Table 2). We were surprised that
this drastic testicular depopulation of advanced germ cell types did
not affect DHT or 3α-androstanediol secretion. Obviously, there
are many possible explanations for this observation but it is
tempting to speculate that the enzymes converting testosterone to
DHT and 3α-diol within the seminiferous tubule are sequestered in
heat resistant testicular cells (perhaps Sertoli cells). It also

remains likely that considerable amounts of these metabolites are
formed by interstitial cells. Since testosterone, DHT and 3α-
androstanediol secretion were unaffected by experimental cryptorchidism, it was surprising to see the significant (P<0.05) reduction
of 3β-androstanediol secretion in cryptorchid as compared to control testes (Table 2). It was possible that the differential effect
of temperature upon the secretion of testosterone, DHT, 3α-andro-
stanediol and 3β-androstanediol in some way resulted from our deci-
sion to perfuse testes at flow rates based upon testicular weight
(10 ml/g/hr). Consequently, the entire experiment was repeated with
another 16 rabbits but this time the control and cryptorchid testes
were perfused at identical flow rates of 20 ml/hr. In this instance
the testosterone and DHT secretion were significantly (P<0.05) elevated, 3α-androstanediol secretion unchanged but once again 3β-
androstanediol secretion was significantly (P<0.05) reduced in the
18 day cryptorchid compared to the control testes. The diminution
of 3β-androstanediol secretion by cryptorchid testes suggests that
its formation may take place in temperature sensitive testicular
cells. Alternatively, the enzyme(s) responsible for 3β-androstane-
diol formation may be deleteriously affected by the heat treatment.

Taken together these data prove that the rabbit testis secretes
significant quantities of biologically potent androgens other than
testosterone. We estimated (16) that DHT plus 3α-androstanediol
plus 3β-androstanediol contributed 48% of the rat ventral prostate
bioassayable androgenic activity secreted hourly by the rabbit
testis-epididymis. This argument followed to its logical conclusion
suggests that these same three steroids might exert similar effects
upon the control of gonadotrophin secretion or epididymal sperm
maturation in rabbits. Even more intriguing is the idea that DHT,
3α-androstanediol and 3β-androstanediol might exert some steroid
specific regulatory influence upon androgen target tissues. This
concept is not without precedent since Lubicz-Nawrocki (67) suggested a specific role for 3α-androstanediol in promoting epididymal
sperm survival in hamsters. Similarly, Robel et al. (68) and
Lasnitzki (69) suggested an effect of 3β-androstanediol upon the
promotion of secretion but not cell division of prostatic epithelia.
Finally, it has not escaped the author's attention that the androgen
profile in spermatic vein blood and in peripheral blood plasma
might reflect not only steroidogenic but also spermatogenic function
of rabbit testes.

SUMMARY

Intra-arterial infusion of testosterone-^{3}H gave rise to
tritiated dihydrotestosterone, 5α-androstan-3α,17β-diol and 5α-
androstan-3β,17β-diol in spermatic venous effluent of the perfused
rabbit testis-epididymis. Mass spectrometric measurements confirmed that these four androgens were present in spermatic venous

effluent of the perfused rabbit testis-epididymis. Gas liquid
chromatographic measurement showed that testosterone, dihydrotestosterone, 5α-androstan-3α,17β-diol and 5α-androstan-3β,17β-diol were
secreted in similar amounts by the in vitro perfused and in situ
rabbit testis-epididymis. Results obtained by perfusing the testis
minus the epididymis suggested that the bulk of these androgens
originate from the catabolism of testosterone within the testis
rather than the epididymis. Surprisingly, germinal epithelium
destruction by heat failed to alter the testosterone, dihydrotestosterone and 5α-androstan-3α,17β-diol secretion by the in
vitro perfused rabbit testis. In contrast, the secretion of 5α-
androstan-3β,17β-diol was significantly (P<0.05) reduced in the same
cryptorchid compared to control testes.

ACKNOWLEDGEMENTS

The assistance of Dan Irby, Elizabeth Higginbottom and
Curtis Chubb is gratefully acknowledged. NIH-LH-S17, ovine was
a gift from the Pituitary Hormone Distribution Program of the
National Institute of Arthritis and Metabolic Diseases. This author
expresses his deepest gratitude to Dr. Claude Desjardins for
estimating the effect of cryptorchidism upon spermatogenesis in
rabbits. The research was supported in part by NICHD Contract
No. 3-2745, Research grant No. 07204, Training Grant No. 00109
and Population Center Grant No. 06268.

REFERENCES

1. Mauvais-Jarvis, P., Floch, H.H. and Bercovici, J.P., J. Clin.
     Endocr. 28: 460, 1968.
2. Murphy, B.E.P., Rec. Prog. Horm. Res. 25: 563, 1969.
3. Murphy, B.E.P., Acta Endocr. (KBH) 64 Suppl. 147: 37, 1970.
4. Ganjam, V.K., Murphy, B.E.P., Chan, I.H., and Currie, P.A.,
     J. Steroid Biochem. 2: 155, 1971.
5. Mahoudeau, J.A., Bardin, C.W. and Lipsett, M.B., J. Clin.
     Invest. 50: 1338, 1971.
6. Trembley, R.R., Forest, M.G., Shalf, J., Martel, J.G.,
     Kawarski, A. and Migeon, C.J., Endocrinology 91: 556, 1972.
7. Mauvais-Jarvis, P., Charronansol, G. and Bobas-Masson, F.,
     J. Clin. Endocr. 36: 452, 1973.
8. Strickland, A.L., Apland, M. and Bruton, J., Steroids 21:
     27, 1973.
9. Gupta, D., McCafferty, E. and Roger, K., Steroids 19: 411,
     1972.
10. Haltmeyer, G.C. and Eik-Nes, K.B., Anal. Biochem. 46: 45, 1972.
11. Ito, T. and Horton, R.J., J. Clin. Endocr. 31: 362, 1970.

12. Ito, T. and Horton, R.J., J. Clin. Invest. 50: 1621, 1971.
13. Bird, C.E., Choong, A., Knight, L. and Clark, A.F., J. Clin. Endocr. 38: 372, 1974.
14. Folman, Y., Haltmeyer, G.C. and Eik-Nes, K.B., Am. J. Physiol. 222: 653, 1973.
15. Ewing, L.L. and Brown, B., Endocrinology 96: 479, 1975.
16. Ewing, L.L., Brown, B., Irby, D.C. and Jardine, I., Endocrinology 96: 610, 1975.
17. Steinberger, E., Physiol. Rev. 51: 1, 1971.
18. Orgebin-Crist, M.C., Davies, J. and Tichenor, P., In Regulation of Mammalian Reproduction, Charles C. Thomas, Springfield, Ill., 1972, p. 224.
19. Bruchovsky, N. and Wilson, J.P., J. Biol. Chem. 243: 5953, 1968.
20. Anderson, K.M. and Liao, S., Nature 219: 277, 1968.
21. Snipes, C.A., Becker, W.G. and Migeon, C.J., Steroids 6: 771, 1965.
22. Nayfeh, S.N., Barefoot, S.W. Jr. and Baggett, B., Endocrinology 78: 1041, 1966.
23. Inano, H. and Tamaoki, B.I., Endocrinology 79: 579, 1966.
24. Ficher, M. and Steinberger, E., Steroids 12: 491, 1968.
25. Steinberger, E. and Ficher, M., Biol. Reprod. Suppl. 1: 19, 1969.
26. Coffey, J.C., French, F.S. and Nayfeh, S.N., Endocrinology 89: 865, 1971.
27. Steinberger, E. and Ficher, M., Endocrinology 89: 679, 1971.
28. Ficher, M. and Steinberger, E., Acta Endocrinol. 68: 285, 1971.
29. Kitay, J.I., Coyne, J.I. and Swygert, N.H., Endocrinology 87: 1257, 1970.
30. Witorsch, R.J. and Kitay, J.I., Endocrinology 91: 764, 1972.
31. Colby, H.D. and Kitay, J.I., Endocrinology 91: 1247, 1972.
32. Colby, H.D. and Kitay, J.I., Endocrinology 91: 1523, 1972.
33. Ewing, L.L., Irby, D.C., Johnson, B.H. and Chubb, C., Fed. Proc. 32: 298, 1973.
34. Brownie, A.C., van der Molen, H.J., Nishizawa, E.E. and Eik-Nes, K.B., J. Clin. Endocr. 24: 1091, 1964.
35. Murphy, B.E.P., In Steroid Assay by Protein Binding, Diczfalusy, E. (Ed.), Supplementum No. 147 of Acta Endocrinologica, Bagtrykkeriet Forum, Denmark, 1970, p. 32.
36. Desjardins, C., Ewing, L.L. and Irby, D.C., Endocrinology 93: 450, 1973.
37. Ewing, L.L. and VanDemark, N.L., J. Reprod. Fert. 6: 9, 1963.
38. Ewing, L.L. and Schanbacher, L.M., Endocrinology 87: 129, 1970.
39. VanDemark, N.L. and Ewing, L.L., J. Reprod. Fert. 6: 1, 1963.
40. Ewing, L.L. and Eik-Nes, K.B., Can. J. Biochem. 44: 1327, 1966.
41. Johnson, B.H. and Ewing, L.L., Science 173: 635, 1971.

42.   Folman, Y., Ahmad, N., Sowell, J.G. and Eik-Nes, K.B.,
      Endocrinology 92: 41, 1973.
43.   Rivarola, M.A., Podesta, E.J., Chemes, H.E. and Aguilar, D.,
      J. Clin. Endocr. 37: 454, 1973.
44.   Rivarola, M.A. and Podesta, E.J., Endocrinology 90: 618, 1972.
45.   Payne, A.H., Kawano, A. and Jaffee, R.B., J. Clin. Endocr.
      37: 448, 1973.
46.   Kasai, H., Mizutani, S. and Matsumoto, K., Acta Endocrinol. 74:
      177, 1973.
47.   Falvo, R.E. and Nalbandov, A.V., Endocrinology 95: 1466, 1974.
48.   Waites, G.M.H. and Setchell, B.P., In The Gonads, McKerns,
      K.W. (ed.), Appleton-Century-Crofts, N.Y., 1969, p. 649.
49.   Cooper, T.G. and Waites, G.M.H., J. Endocr. 62: 619, 1974.
50.   Baulieu, E.-E. and Robel, P., Steroids 2: 111, 1936.
51.   Yamada, M. and Matsumoto, K., Endocrinology 94: 777, 1974.
52.   Givner, M.L. and Dvorny, D., Experientia 28: 1105, 1972.
53.   Lacy, D. and Pettit, A.J., Brit. Med. Bull. 26: 87, 1970.
54.   Bell, J.B.G., Vinson, G.P. and Lacy, D., Proc. R. Soc. Lond.
      B. 176: 433, 1971.
55.   Eik-Nes, K.B., In The Androgens of the Testis, Eik-Nes, K.B.
      (ed.), Marcel Dekker, Inc., N.Y., 1970, p. 7.
56.   Van der Molen, H.J. and Eik-Nes, K.B., Biochim. Biophys. Acta
      248: 343, 1971.
57.   Wattenberg, L.W., J. Histochem. Cytochem. 6: 225, 1958.
58.   Levy, H., Deane, H.W., and Rubin, B.L., Endocrinology 65:
      932, 1959.
59.   Christensen, A.K. and Mason, N.R., Endocrinology 76: 646,
      1965.
60.   Cooke, B.A., DeJong, F.H., Van der Molen, H.J. and Rommerts,
      F.F.G., Nature New Biol. 237: 255, 1972.
61.   Van der Vusse, G.J., Kalkman, M.L. and Van der Molen, H.J.,
      Biochim. Biophys. Acta 297: 179, 1973.
62.   Rivarola, M.A., Podesta, E.J. and Chemes, H.E., Endocrinology
      91: 537, 1972.
63.   Dorrington, J.H. and Fritz, I.B., Biochim. Biophys. Res.
      Comm. 54: 1425, 1973.
64.   Glover, T.D., Acta Endocr. (Kbh.) Suppl. 100: 38, 1965.
65.   Jones, T., Brit. J. Radiol. 44: 841, 1971.
66.   Larson, L.L. and Foote, R.H., Proc. Soc. Exptl. Biol. Med.
      147: 151, 1974.
67.   Lubicz-Nawrocki, C.M., J. Endocr. 58: 193, 1973.
68.   Robel, P., Lasnitzki, I. and Baulieu, E.-E., Biochimie 53:
      81, 1971.
69.   Lasnitzki, I., In Male Accessory Sex Organs, Brandes, D.
      (ed.), Academic Press, N.Y., 1974, p. 348.

METABOLISM AND SECRETION OF ANDROGENS BY RAT SEMINIFEROUS TUBULES:

TRACER SUPERFUSION STUDIES

P.G. Satyaswaroop and Erlio Gurpide[*]

Departments of Obstetrics and Gynecology and Biochem-
chemistry, Mount Sinai School of Medicine of the City
University of New York, New York, N.Y.   10029

INTRODUCTION

Although the seminiferous tubules are known to possess enzymes involved in the synthesis and metabolism of androgens, it is unclear whether they are capable of producing steroid hormones independently of precursors supplied by the interstitial cells.

Regardless of the source of androgens, the tubules can be expected to influence strongly the overall secretory pattern of the whole testes. The relatively large mass of tubules and their anatomical relation to the interstitial tissue calls for the study as to how they handle major androgens, like androst-4-ene-3,17-dione (androstenedione) and testosterone, either produced by the tubules or presented to them by the Leydig cells.

The purpose of the present investigation was to compare the metabolism and secretion of androstenedione and testosterone in whole testes and tubules, in vitro, and to attempt the estimation of rates of synthesis of these compounds in seminiferous tubules in the absence of exogenous precursors.

As the continuous flow incubation method, which provides steady state isotopic data, is well suited for such a study, decapsulated whole testes and teased seminiferous tubules from immature and mature rats were superfused with ^{3}H- and ^{14}C-labeled androstenedione and testosterone. Kinetic parameters of metabolism of these hormones were estimated from measurements of concentrations and specific activities in tissue and superfusates, using formulas published elsewhere (1).

----

*Career Scientist, Health Research Council of the City of New
 York

MATERIALS AND METHODS

1,2-^{3}H-testosterone (50 Ci/mmole), 1,2-^{3}H-androstenedione (50 Ci/mmole), 4-^{14}C-testosterone (57.5 mCi/mmoles) and 4-^{14}C-andro-stenedione (57.5 mCi/mmole) were purchased from New England Nuclear Corp. and purified by paper chromatography using the system hexane-90% aq. methanol before use. Non-radioactive, testosterone, andro-stenedione, 5α-dihydrotestosterone (DHT), 3α,17β-dihydroxy-5α-androstane (3α-androstanediol), 5α-androstane-3,17-dione (andro-stanedione), were supplied by Steraloids, Inc. (Pawling, N.Y.).

Tubules were isolated from testes of decapitated Sprague-Dawley rats, of ages 21 to 25 days (immature) and 90 to 100 days (mature), by the weight dissection method of Christensen and Mason (2). After dissection in oxygenated normal saline containing 1 mg/ml glucose at 0-4°C, the tubules were separated from adhering inter-stitial cells by sedimentation through 5% albumin in Krebs-Ringer bicarbonate buffer containing 1 mg/ml glucose (KRBG), pH 7.4, 0-4°C, as suggested by Hall et al. (3). The tubules were washed twice in the above medium, filtered through a nylon mesh, and resuspended in KRBG. These preparations or decapsulated whole testes were super-fused at 20 ml/hr, 37°C, with a KRBG medium saturated with 5% CO_2 and 95% O_2 containing the labeled steroids, as described previously (4). In experiments aiming to determine rates of synthesis, two superfusions were conducted in parallel, one with a mixture of testosterone or ^{14}C-androstenedione (or ^{3}H-androstenedione and ^{14}C-testosterone) and the other with unlabeled steroids. The concentrations of androstenedione and testosterone in the medium were the same in each of the two superfusion media. Combination of data from both runs were used to determine the specific activities of the steroids isolated from the tissue. Superfusates were collected separately every 20 minutes in tubes chilled in ice. At the end of 100 minutes of superfusion, the tissue was rapidly washed with 10 ml cold saline and transferred to a homogenizer containing 6 ml of a methanolic solution of testosterone and androstenedione (200 μg each). After homogenization, the pre-cipitated proteins were centrifuged and the protein estimated by Lowry's method (5). The supernatant was evaporated to dryness and the steroids were purified by TLC on Silica Gel GF-254 (Merck, Darmstadt) using the system chloroform: acetone:hexane (4:1:3, v/v). The zones corresponding to testosterone and androstenedione were localized under ultraviolet light, eluted and further purified by high pressure liquid chromatography (6000 psi HPLC equipped with U6K injector, Waters Associates), using a 0.25" x 12" microporasil column and the solvent system chloroform:isooctane (6:4, v/v). Baseline separations of androstanedione, andro-stenedione, dehydroisoandrosterone, dihydrotestosterone (DHT), 3α- and 3β-androstanediol were achieved. The superfusion medium and the superfusate fractions were similarly analyzed.

Recoveries of the added carriers were estimated by measuring the absorption at 240 nm with a Beckman DU2 spectrophotometer. Radioactivity was measured with a Nuclear Chicago Isocap 300 liquid scintillation spectrophotometer. Some of the purified compounds were crystallized from methanol-water after addition of 10 mg of authentic carriers.

Testosterone and androstenedione levels in tissue superfused with unlabeled steroids were measured by radioimmunoassay.

Calculations

Data from the superfusions with labeled steroids, viz, concentrations of ^{3}H and ^{14}C-labeled testosterone (T) and androstenedione (A) in superfusage (in cpm/ml), and in tissue (in cpm/g) were used to calculate the fractions of tracers that entered the tissue (α_A, α_T), were converted to the other superfused compound (ρ_{AT}, ρ_{TA}), and were released to the medium either without change (β_A, β_T), after conversion to the other compound (γ_{AT}, γ_{TA}) or to other metabolites (γ_{AX}, γ_{TX}). The isotopic data also served to estimate intracellular clearance rates (IC), which denote the fractions of the compounds in tissue removed irreversibly per unit of time, at the steady state. This parameter represents the ratio between the rate at which the compound appears de novo in the tissue (e.g., the production rate, PR) and the amount of compound present in the tissue (IC = PR $\div$ W x c), where W and c are weight of tissue and intracellular concentration of the compound. These calculations have been discussed in detail elsewhere (1).

Various parameters can be used to evaluate the preferred direction in the reversible conversion of androstenedione to testosterone (ρ's and intracellular ratios of labeled androstenedione and testosterone derived from either of the two superfused tracers). However, the ratio of the rate constants characterizing the reductive and oxidative directions, may be the most meaningful. If the rate constant k_{AT} is defined as the ratio of the rate of conversion of androstenedione (A) to testosterone (T) per g of tissue and the intracellular concentration of androstenedione, with a similar definition for k_{TA}, then

$$\frac{k_{AT}}{k_{TA}} = \frac{v_{AT}}{v_{TA}} \cdot \frac{c_{T,tissue}}{c_{A,tissue}}$$

The ratio of rate constants can be estimated from isotopic data. For instance, if ^{3}H-androstenedione (A) and ^{14}C-testosterone (T) are superfused,

$$\frac{k_{AT}}{k_{TA}} = \frac{c_{T,\ tissue}^{^3H}/c_{A,\ medium}^{^3H}}{c_{A,\ tissue}^{^{14}C}/c_{T,\ medium}^{^{14}C}}$$

This equation includes the experimentally verified assumption that $\alpha_A = \alpha_T$.

Data from superfusion with unlabeled androstenedione and testosterone serve to estimate the total intracellular concentration of these hormones achieved during the superfusions ($c_{A,total}$, $c_{T,total}$). The contribution of exogenous androstenedione and testosterone to these total concentrations can be estimated from the data obtained from superfusions with labeled steroids. For instance, if ^3H-androstenedione (^3H-A) and ^{14}C-testosterone (^{14}C-T) were superfused,

$$c_{A,\ exogenous} = \frac{c_{A,\ tissue}^{^3H}}{Sp\ act\ ^3H\text{-}A\ superfused} + \frac{c_{A,\ tissue}^{^{14}C}}{Sp\ act\ ^{14}C\text{-}T\ superfused}$$

$$c_{T,\ exogenous} = \frac{c_{T,\ tissue}^{^3H}}{Sp\ act\ ^3H\text{-}A\ superfused} + \frac{c_{T,\ tissue}^{^{14}C}}{Sp\ act\ ^{14}C\text{-}T\ superfused.}$$

The contribution of endogenous precursors can then be calculated as follows:

$$c_{A,\ endogenous} = c_{A,\ total} - c_{A,\ exogenous}$$

$$c_{T,\ endogenous} = c_{T,\ total} - c_{T,\ exogenous.}$$

The rate of endogenous production of androstenedione and testosterone can be estimated by multiplying these concentrations by the corresponding intracellular clearances, i.e.,

$$\frac{PR_{A,\ endogenous}}{W} = IC_A \times c_{A,\ endogenous}$$

$$\frac{PR_{T,endogenous}}{W} = IC_T \times c_{T,\ endougenous.}$$

On the basis of values for PR_A, PR_T, ρ_{AT} and ρ_{TA}, the rates at which androstenedione (A) and testosterone (T) are interconverted, are formed from other precursors, and are irriversibly metabolized can be estimated using formulas already published (1,6). Furthermore,

the fraction of the endogenously produced hormone which is secreted
to the medium can be estimated from isotopic data, i.e.,

$$SR_A = (\frac{\beta}{\alpha})_A \ PR_A$$
$$SR_T = (\frac{\beta}{\alpha})_T \ PR_T.$$

RESULTS

Figure 1 shows the fraction of each tracer that enters the
tissue and is released back to the medium (β/α), by tubules and
whole testes of immature and mature rats. These data make apparent
that a larger fraction of testosterone is released to the medium from
preparations obtained from mature than from immature rats, both by
whole testes and tubules. Thus, in tissues from immature rats about
20% of the testosterone formed de novo in the tissue appeared in
the medium, whereas a value of more than 50% is found in tissues
from mature animals. Such an increase is not observed for androstenedione. Actually, a decrease in the fraction of androstenedione
released to the medium is noted in whole testes from mature rats.
As a consequence, the ratio of rates of secretion of testosterone
and androstenedione could be expected to be higher in mature than
immature testes, in agreement with results obtained by direct
measurement of testosterone/androstenedione ratios in spermatic
vein and peripheral plasma (7,8).

Consistent with this observation is the finding, illustrated
in Figure 2, that the fraction of superfused androstenedione released as testosterone (γ_{AT}/α_A) is larger in preparations from
mature than from immature animals, both for tubules and whole testes.
In contrast, the fraction of testosterone released as androstenedione
is low and rather constant in all cases.

The lower fractional release of testosterone observed in immature tubules and whole testes is likely due to the high 5α-
reductase activity demonstrated in testes from immature rats (9-19).
Figure 3 presents the fractions of androstenedione and testosterone
converted to other metabolites (γ_{AX}/α_A, γ_{TX}/α_T) by tubules and whole
testes   The larger fractional rate of metabolism of the androgens
in immature testicular preparations is evident from these data.

Whether androstenedione is metabolized directly or after conversion to testosterone can be evaluated from the isotopic data as
described in a previous publication (4). Apparently, most of the
metabolism occurs via testosterone to form 5α-reduced metabolites
such as dihydrotestosterone, 3α-androstandiol and androstandione,
as is evident from Table 1. In most cases, the isotope ratios of

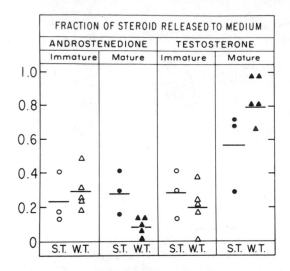

Figure 1. Teased seminiferous tubules and decapsulated whole testes from immature (21 to 26 days old) and mature (90 to 100 days old) rats were superfused with a 5% CO_2 and 95% O_2 saturated KRBG (1 mg/ml) buffer medium, pH 7.4, containing ^{3}H-T and ^{14}C-A (or ^{3}H-androstenedione and ^{14}C-testosterone) at 37°C for 100 minutes. The fractions of androstenedione (A) and testosterone (T) released to the medium (β_A/α_A, β_T/α_T) were determined from concentrations of the labeled hormones in tissue, superfusate and superfusion medium.

metabolites, isolated from tissue at the isotopic steady state, were similar to the ^{3}H/^{14}C ratios of testosterone and significantly different from the isotope ratios of androstenedione.

The extent of interconversion between androstenedione and testosterone, relative to other metabolic processes involving these hormones, is reflected by the values of the conversion factors (ρ_{AT}, ρ_{TA}), determined by comparing the ^{3}H/^{14}C ratios in the androgens isolated from the tissue with the isotope ratio in the superfusion medium. Considerable interconversion between androstenedione and testosterone, both in whole testes and tubules, is observed. About 80% of androstenedione is converted to testosterone, in all groups. The conversion of testosterone to androstenedione is about 30% in immature tubules and whole testes, but increases after puberty. This is clearly evidenced when whole testes are used. Again, the explanation for this increased fractional conversion of testosterone to androstenedione may be found in a reduced metabolism of testosterone after puberty.

Table 1

^{3}H:^{14}C Ratios in Androstenedione, Testosterone and Metabolites Isolated from Superfused Tissues

Steroid	Immature Seminiferous Tubules			Immature Whole Testis				Immature Seminiferous Tubule	
	#5C	#51	#53	#33	#44	#43	#62	#52	#54
Androstene-dione	4.0	26	1.6	1.4	21	13	1.8	20	2.4
Testosterone	8.4	7.0	9.0	4.6	4.5	5.0	8.0	9.1	7.6
Adiol	10.0	-	7.1	4.8	6.4	6.4	5.0	10.4	6.6
DHT	8.7	6.5	8.3	4.3	6.2	5.9	4.2	6.9	4.0
Adione	-	9.8	-	-	-	-	4.0	-	5.7

Androstenedione (A), testosterone (T) and the metabolites 3α-androstenediol (Adiol) dihydrotestosterone (DHT) and androstanedione (Adione) isolated from the superfused tissues were chromatographed and twice crystallized in methanol-water.

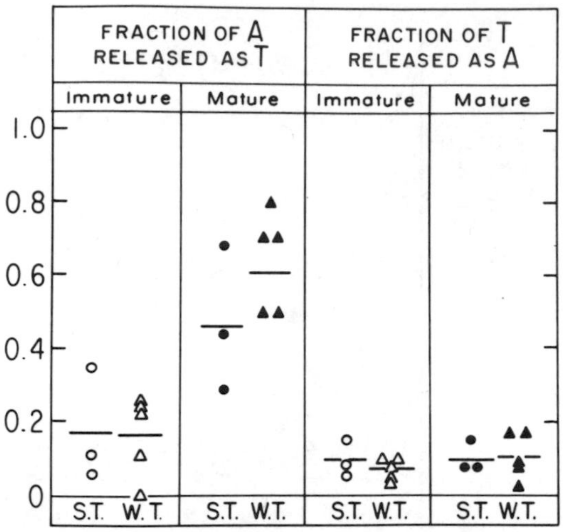

Figure 2. The fraction of androstenedione (A) released as testosterone (T), or vice versa (γ_{AT}/α_A, γ_{TA}/α_T) determined as described in the legend to Figure 1.

Another indicator of the extent of interconversion is the ratio of intracellular concentrations of labeled testosterone and androstenedione with respect to the isotope superfused either of the two hormones. As shown in Figure 4, it was found that, regardless of the precursors, there is always predominance of labeled testosterone over labeled androstenedione. The ratio derived from androstenedione is about 2 in immature tubules and whole testes and goes up to about 7 in the mature preparations. The ratio derived from testosterone is about 9 in immature whole testes and tubules and is as high or higher in preparations from mature rats.

The most direct parameter reflecting the preferred direction in the reversible conversion of androstenedione to testosterone is the ratio of the rate constants of each of these processes, as described in the section on Calculations. On an average, the rate constant of conversion of androstenedione to testosterone is about 10 times larger than the rate constant of conversion of testosterone to androstenedione, both in tubules and whole testes.

Figure 5 shows the values for intracellular clearances of androstenedione and testosterone seminiferous tubules and whole testes from immature and mature rats. A large dispersion of values is noted in some groups. However, the intracellular clearance of testosterone in mature preparations, both of whole testes and tubules,

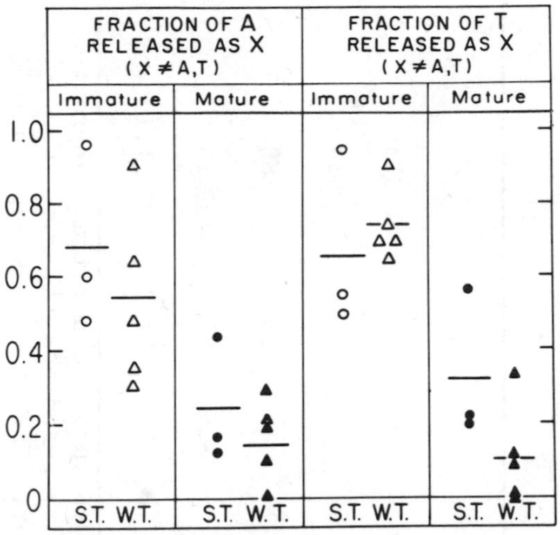

FRACTION OF A RELEASED AS X $(X \neq A,T)$		FRACTION OF T RELEASED AS X $(X \neq A,T)$	
Immature	Mature	Immature	Mature

Figure 3.   The fractions of androstenedione (A) released as metabolites X $-(\frac{\gamma_{AX}}{\alpha_A} = 1 - \frac{\beta_A}{\alpha_A} - \frac{\gamma_{AT}}{\alpha_A})$ or of testosterone (T) released as metabolites X $(\frac{\gamma_{TX}}{\alpha_T} = 1 - \frac{\beta_T}{\alpha_T} - \frac{\gamma_{TA}}{\alpha_T})$ were calculated from data presented in Figures 1 and 2.

seems to be significantly smaller, as expected from a lower metabolism of testosterone after puberty. This parameter serves to calculate production rates of the androgens from data on the intracellular concentrations of androstenedione and testosterone. The proper values of concentrations to be used in these calculations are those corresponding to the estimated concentrations derived from endogenous production during the superfusion period.

We have found a large variability in the endogenous concentration of androstenedione and testosterone, as has been the experience of other workers. We have not assessed as yet the extent and causes of such variations and therefore cannot draw conclusions regarding synthesis of the two hormones in tubules. However, the results from one experiment are shown in order to illustrate our experimental approach. Table 2 shows the calculations of endogenous concentrations and Figure 6 the rates of synthesis, interconversion, metabolism and secretion estimated from the values of PR's, ρ's and (β/α)'s. According to the results from this experiment, tubules seem to synthesize testosterone and androstenedione in the absence of exogenous precursors. Furthermore, the

Table 2

Rates of "de novo" Synthesis of Androstenedione and Testosterone by
Seminiferous Tubule of Immature Rat Testes

Parameter	Estimation	Values	
		A	T
Intracellular concentration			
• after superfusion (ng/g)	c_{total} by RIA	51	333
• from superfused A and T	c_{exo} from isotopic data	35	245
• from endogenous sources	$c_{endo} = c_{total} - c_{exo}$	16	88
Intracellular clearance (hr^{-1})	$IC = \dfrac{\phi\alpha}{W(T/M)}$	83	13
Endogenous rate of production (µg/gxh)	$PR_{endo} = IC \times c_{endo}$	1.3	1.1

Seminiferous tubules obtained from two 24 day old rats were divided into two portions (approximately 70 mg each). One was superfused with a solution of ^{3}H-androstenedione (A) and ^{14}C-testosterone (T) in oxygenated KRBG buffer for 100 min at 20 ml/hr. The other was superfused in parallel under identical conditions with unlabled androgens. The concentration of androstenedione and testosterone were the same in both superfusion media (1.25 and 51.8 ng/ml, respectively). The following symbols are used in the formula for intracellular clearances: φ, flow rate; α, fraction of superfused tracer entering tissue; W, weight of tissue; T/M, ratio of concentrations of labeled compound in tissue and superfusion medium.

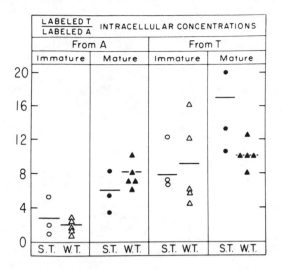

Figure 4.   Ratios of intracellular concentrations of labeled testosterone and androstenedione with respect to the isotope superfused
either as testosterone or androstenedione.

predominant biosynthetic pathway appears to lead to the direct
formation of androstenedione, from 17-hydroxyprogesterone or dehydroisoandrosterone, followed by conversion of androstenedione to
testosterone.

DISCUSSION

In evaluating the results of these studies, a distinction
should be made between data involving measurements of radioactivity,
used to estimate parameters of metabolism, and those involving
measurements of endogenous concentrations of androstenedione and
testosterone, necessary for the calculation of rates and pathways
of synthesis.

The isotopic data appear to be reliable; consistent patterns
are obtained in all experiments.   Inversion of isotopes in the
tracers did not influence the results.   This test was of importance
since the specific activities of the two tracers differ by a factor
of about 1000.   The results yielded by these experiments may be
useful to interpret not only in vitro experiments but also the in
vivo situation since tissue integrity has been preserved.

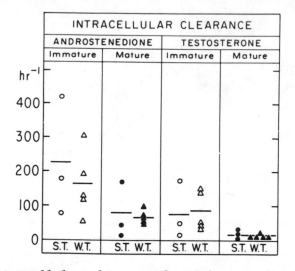

Figure 5.   Intracellular clearance for androstenedione and testosterone were calculated using the formula given in Table 2.

The heterogeneity of cell populations in the testes creates
special problems. We chose to study decapsulated whole testis, in
which the anatomic relation between interstitial cells and tubules
is maintained, and seminiferous tubules prepared by methods which,
according to published reports (20), almost completely eliminate
contaminating Leydig cells. Superfusion of interstitial cells was
not attempted since preparations enriched in this cell type by
currently available methods contain a large proportion of germ
cells.

The results obtained with whole testes preparations were
approximately the same as those obtained with seminiferous tubules.
This finding is not surprising since the tubules constitute the
bulk of the testicular tissue. There are, however, differences in
some of the parameters of metabolism of testosterone in whole
testes and seminiferous tubule preparations from mature rats. These
differences can be explained considering the fact that enzymes responsible for the metabolism of testosterone are preferentially
located in seminiferous tubules. Localization of 5α-reductase
activity in tubules has been demonstrated in several laboratories
(14,18). Germ cells have been shown to possess this enzymatic
activity (21). Therefore, it could be predicted that the metabolism
of testosterone per g of tissue would be higher in seminiferous tubules than in whole testes, in agreement with the experimental
findings (Fig. 3). Consequently, it could also be expected that

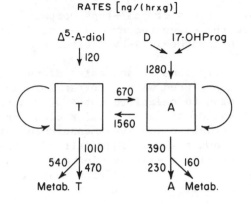

RATES [ng/(hrxg)]

SEMINIFEROUS TUBULES FROM IMMATURE RAT

Figure 6. Rates of synthesis, interconversion, metabolism and
secretion of androstenedione (A) and testosterone (T) in an immature seminiferous tubule preparation, estimated from the data
shown in Table 2 and the values ρ_{AT} = 0.8, ρ_{TA} = 0.4, $(\beta/\alpha)_A$ = 0.2
and $(\beta/\alpha)_T$ = 0.4 determined from superfusion with labeled androstenedione and testosterone.

the fraction of the total metabolism of testosterone contributed
by its conversion to androstenedione would be larger in whole testes,
as was found experimentally (average values for conversion factors:
0.9 and 0.5 in whole testes and tubules of mature rats, respectively). The relatively lower metabolic rate of testosterone noted
in whole testis would result in a higher concentration of diffusible
testosterone and explain the observed larger fractional release of
this hormone to the medium (Fig. 1). Consistent with this pattern
is the finding that a larger fraction of androstenedione is released
to the medium as testosterone in whole testis than in seminiferous
tubule preparations (Fig. 2).

The failure to see these differences in preparations from immature rats may be due to their lower content of Leydig cells in
the whole testis (22,23) and to the higher 5α-reductase activity
present in the immature tubule (14,18).

Calculated endogenous production rates of androstenedione and
testosterone may be imprecise since their sensitivity to small
variations in the values for each of the parameters used was found
to be great. Further studies of the precision and accuracy of the

data, as well as of problems of cell-type compartmentalization
are necessary before the suggested experimental design for the
estimation of rates of synthesis is validated.

Endogenous concentrations of androstenedione and testosterone
measured in tissues superfused with a buffer solution containing
no steroids, can be used to calculate rates of synthesis when used
in conjunction with values of intracellular clearance and conversion
factors. Another alternative involves measurement of concentrations
of both hormones in fresh tissue. This latter choice, is however,
objectionable since the intracellular clearances and conversion
factors prevailing under in vivo conditions may be different from
those determined from in vitro experiments.

The results shown in Fig. 6 suggest that seminiferous tubules
from immature testis are capable of androgen synthesis in the
absence of precursors provided by Leydig cells and that testosterone
is formed mainly by the intermediacy of androstenedione. However,
the issue of independent tubular steroidogenesis remains unsettled
(24,25).

ACKNOWLEDGEMENTS

Mrs. Milagros M. de la Pena conducted the testosterone and
androstenedione assays.

This work was supported by grants HD 7197 of the National
Institutes of Health, and 680-0798 from the Ford Foundation.

REFERENCES

1. Gurpide, E., Methods in Enzymology 36: 75, 1974.
2. Christensen, A.K. and Mason, N.R., Endocrinology 65: 646, 1965.
3. Hall, P.F., Irby, D.C. and De Kretser, D.M., Endocrinology
    84: 488, 1969.
4. Satyaswaroop, P.G. and Gurpide, E., J. Steroid Biochem. 5:
    Oct., 1974.
5. Lowry, O.H., Rosebrough, N.J., Farr, A.L. and Randall, R.J.,
    J. Biol. Chem. 193: 265, 1951.
6. Gurpide, E., "Tracer Methods in Hormone Research", Monographs
    on Endocrinology, Vol. 8, Springer-Verlag, N.Y., Heidelberg,
    1975.
7. Hashimoto, I. and Suzuki, Y., Endocrinol. Japan 13: 326, 1966.
8. Resko, J.A., Feder, A.H. and Goy, R.W., J. Endocrinol. 40:
    485, 1968.
9. Inano, H., Hori, Y. and Tamaoki, B.I., Ciba Found. Coll.
    Endocrinol. 12: 105, 1967.

10. Nayfeh, S.N., Barefoot, S.W., Jr. and Baggett, B., Endocrinology
     78: 1041, 1966.
11. Ficher, M. and Steinberger, E., Steroids 12: 491, 1968.
12. Steinberger, E. and Ficher, M., Endocrinology 89: 679, 1971.
13. Rivarola, M.A. and Podesta, E.J., Endocrinology 90: 618, 1972.
14. Rivarola, M.A., Podesta, E.J. and Chemes, H.E., Endocrinology
     91: 537, 1972.
15. Strickland, A.L., Nayfeh, S.N. and French, F.S., Steroids, 15:
     373, 1970.
16. Coffey, J.C., French, F.S. and Nayfeh, S.N., Endocrinology
     89: 865, 1971.
17. Folman, Y., Sowell, J.G. and Eik-Nes, K.B., Endocrinology
     91: 702, 1972.
18. Folman, Y., Ahmed, N., Sowell, J.G. and Eik-Nes, K.B.,
     Endocrinology 92: 41, 1973.
19. Oshima, H., Sarada, T., Ochiai, K. and Tamaoki, B.I.,
     Endocrinology 86: 1215, 1970.
20. Rommerts, F.F.G., Van Doorn, L.G., Galjaard, H., Cooke, B.A.
     and Van der Molen, H.J., J. Histochem. Cytochem. 21:
     572, 1973.
21. Matsumoto, K. and Yamada, M., Endocrinology 93: 253, 1973.
22. Niemi, M. and Ikonen, M., Endocrinology 72: 433, 1963.
23. Knorr, D.W., Vannha-Pertula, T. and Lipsett, M.B.,
     Endocrinology 86: 1298, 1970.
24. Lacy, D. and Petitt, A.J., Brit. Med. Bull. 26: 87, 1970.
25. Cooke, B.A., De Jong, F.H., Van der Molen, H.J. and
     Rommerts, F.F.G., Nature New Biol. 237: 255, 1972.

LOCAL INCREASE IN CONCENTRATION OF STEROIDS BY VENOUS-ARTERIAL TRANSFER IN THE PAMPINIFORM PLEXUS

Michael J. Free

Biology Department, Batelle, Pacific Northwest
Laboratories, Richland, Washington 99352

Stephen A. Tillson

Alza Research, Palo Alto, California 94304

The ability of the pampiniform plexus to exchange respiratory gases was recognized by Cross and Silver (1) and examined by Setchell and Hinks (2) in conscious and anesthetized rams and marsupials. Transfer of oxygen and CO_2 was found only in anesthetized rams breathing oxygen-rich gas mixtures and amounted to a 5% rise in pCO_2 and a 22% fall in pO_2 of arterial blood as it passed through the plexus. Other than countercurrent exchange of heat (3) this was the first demonstration of exchange in the pampiniform plexus.

We obtained indirect evidence of venous-arterial transfer of other substances in the pampiniform plexus of the rat when vaso-active substances injected into the internal spermatic vein brought about a marked reduction in lateral pressure and volume flow in the testis artery without changing central blood pressure. This response was observed following injections of epinephrine and norepinephrine (4), prostaglandins (5) and serotonin (6). Apparently these substances were able to pass from vein to artery within the pampiniform plexus and cause constriction of the coiled internal spermatic artery, increasing the arterial pressure drop across the pampiniform plexus up to two-fold.

More recently several studies have demonstrated that at least five types of labeled molecules infused into the testis vein appear at higher concentrations in the testis artery blood than in the general circulation (Table I). This venous-arterial short circuit takes place in the pampiniform plexus since it occurred when the

181

TABLE I

SUMMARY OF STUDIES DEMONSTRATING TRANSFER OF LABELED TRACER MOLECULES
BETWEEN VEIN AND ARTERY IN THE PAMPINIFORM PLEXUS

Tracer Molecule	Species	Route and Form of Administration	% Transfer from Spermatic Vein to Spermatic Artery	Ref.
Testosterone-^{3}H	Rat	a	1.5-9.0	7
Testosterone-^{3}H	Rat	b	1.0-6.0	8
Testosterone-^{3}H	Rat	c	46	8
Testosterone-^{3}H	Rat	d	(1)	9
Testosterone-^{3}H	Baboon	a	(2)	unpubl.
Testosterone-^{14}C	Ram	a	2	10
Testosterone-^{14}C	Wallaby	a	10	10
Prostaglandin-F$_{2\alpha}$-^{3}H	Ram	a	11	10
Prostaglandin-F$_{2\alpha}$-^{3}H	Wallaby	a	1	10
^{3}H$_2$O	Ram	a	9	10
^{3}H$_2$O	Wallaby	a	21	10
^{3}H$_2$O	Rat	a	(3)	6
Xenon-133& Krypton-85	Rat	d	(4)	11

(1) More label appeared in ipsilateral than contralateral corpus epididymis even after ligation of efferent ducts.

(2) Label appeared in testis artery at maximum of 2.5 times the level in femoral artery

(3) Label appeared in tenfold concentrations in testis artery compared with femoral artery

(4) Label appeared in epididymis or testis even after ligation of the efferent ducts

a Infused into blood of testis vein

b Perfused with blood into testis vein

c Perfused with dextran into testis vein

d Injected into testis (testosterone), or testis and epididymis (xenon or krypton)

TABLE II

LOCAL INCREASE IN TESTOSTERONE CONCENTRATION IN THE TESTIS ARTERY OF DIFFERENT SPECIES

Except where referenced, data were obtained using the radioimmunoassay procedure described elsewhere (14). Mean ± S.E.M.

Species	n	Testis Vein (TV) Blood	Testosterone in Central Artery or Heart (CA) Blood	Testis Artery (TA) Blood	Central versus Testis Artery % Transfer $\frac{TA-CA}{TV-TA}$ x100	Ref.
Rat	11	40.5 ± 6.2	2.8 ± 0.8[1]	7.6 ± 2.5***	14.6	7
Rat	5		1.7 ± 0.2	3.1 ± 3.1†		
Rabbit	11	91.0 ± 6.5	2.7 ± 0.5	5.1 ± 0.7****	2.8	
Guinea Pig	4		3.8 ± 0.5	5.7 ± 0.7†		
Dog	7		2.5 ± 0.5	3.8 ± 1.1 (NS)		
Boar	1		4.5	5.4		
Goat	10		6.7 ± 0.64	8.0 ± 1.0 (NS)		
Ram	5		5.7 ± 1.6[2]	6.4 ± 4.3*		12
Ram	7		3.8 ± 0.7[2]	4.3 ± 0.9*		12
Rhesus Monkey	1		5.7	7.2		
Rhesus Monkey	11		4.6[2]	5.1**		13
Baboon	1		5.9	6.0		
Baboon	1		5.7	5.9		

† Testis artery was always higher than central artery, but means were not significantly different (NS)
Paired t-test of testicular versus central artery concentrations: ****$p<0.001$ ***$p<0.01$ **$p<0.02$
*$p<0.05$
[1] ng/ml blood
[2] ng/ml plasma

spermatic artery and vein were disconnected from the testis and
perfused with the tracer material in blood or dextran (7,8).

As the testicular steroid testosterone was among the substances
that pass from vein to artery in this fashion, and since a concentration gradient for testosterone normally exists between the two
vessels, there exists the potential for local concentration of
testosterone in the reproductive tract circulation. Endogenous
testosterone levels in testis artery blood compared with the
general circulation have been measured in at least nine mammalian
species (Table II). In four species, rat, rabbit, ram and rhesus
monkey, significant measurable elevation of testosterone levels
occurred in the arterial blood when it passed through the pampiniform plexus. This local increase in concentration was highest in
the rat where levels of testosterone in arterial blood entering
the testis showed a three or even four fold increase over central
arterial blood levels. In the rabbit the testosterone levels in
this system were doubled, whereas in the ram or rhesus monkey the
local increase in testosterone levels only amounted to 11-13%.
Large variation in testosterone levels within individual blood
vessels, coupled with small sample populations, probably masked
some increases in the testis arteries of other species. For example,
even though the paired t-test failed to show a significant difference,
blood from one group of rat and guinea pig testis arteries contained
more testosterone than femoral blood in every animal sampled (Table
II). Furthermore, venous-arterial transfer of tritium-labeled
testosterone was demonstrated in the baboon pampiniform plexus
(Table I) even though no difference in endogenous testosterone
levels between testis and central arterial blood could be detected
in the same animals (Table II).

Within species, the extent to which testosterone levels were
elevated in the arterial blood as it passed through the pampiniform
plexus appeared to be related to the concentration gradient for
testosterone between the testis vein and testis artery (Figure 1).
This relationship was less pronounced in the rabbit than in the rat.

In order to elucidate the mechanisms involved in venous-arterial
transfer in the pampiniform plexus, we have studied the dynamics of
transfer of radiolabeled testosterone in the pampiniform plexus
isolated from its testis in vivo. These studies were performed on
halothane/N_2O/oxygen-anesthetized rats in which the testis artery
was ligated on the surface of the testis and spermatic arterial
blood diverted to the femoral vein or to a collection reservoir
while blood from the femoral artery or from a donor reservoir was
pumped into a branch vein on the cranial pole of the same testis.
All flow rates were controlled and simultaneous blood samples were

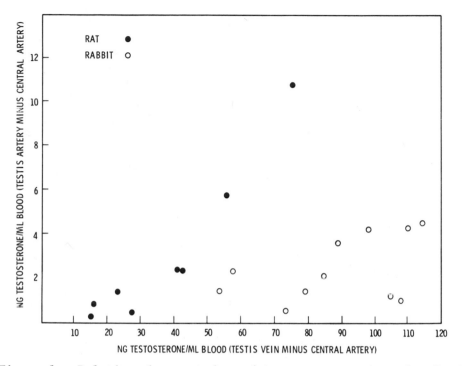

Figure 1.   Relations between the endogenous testosterone levels in the testis vein and artery of rats and rabbits. Simultaneous blood samples were drawn from the testis artery, a branch of the testis vein and the femoral artery or heart of anesthetised rats and rabbits. Samples were assayed for testosterone by radioimmunoassay.

taken from the spermatic artery outflow, the testis vein inflow and from a femoral artery. Details of the procedures have been given elsewhere (8).

Figure 2 shows the distribution of specific radioactivity between femoral and testis artery blood of a rat during perfusion of the testis vein at 0.1 ml/min with donor blood containing 27 ng/ml of testosterone-1,2,-^{3}H. Venous-arterial transfer reached a plateau after 30 minutes and declined slightly as the venous-arterial con- centration gradient diminished. When the concentration gradient is eliminated, as when unlabeled donor blood is substituted for the testosterone-1,2,-^{3}H blood perfusate, the testis arterial blood radioactivity fell rapidly to baseline levels.

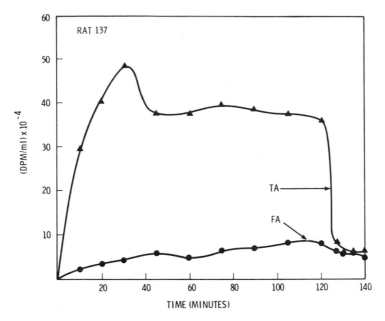

Figure 2. Specific radioactivity in testicular and femoral artery
blood during perfusion of testosterone-1,2,^{3}H into the spermatic
vein of a rat. Donor blood containing 27 ng/ml testosterone-1,2,
^{3}H was perfused at 0.1 ml/min into a branch of the testis vein
at the cranial pole of the ischemic testis for 120 minutes.
Sequential blood samples were drawn from the femoral artery and
testis artery outflow and assayed for radioactivity.

        By introducing different levels of testosterone-1,2,6,7,^{3}H
into the blood stream diverted from the femoral artery into the
testis vein we were able to construct a curve relating the
testosterone concentration in the veins of the pampiniform plexus
to the rate of venous-arterial transfer (Figure 3). The relationship appeared to be linear over the physiologic range of spermatic
vein testosterone concentrations and was reminiscent of the curve
relating endogenous testosterone levels in the spermatic vein and
artery of the rat (Figure 1). In the tracer experiments specific
radioactivity in the general circulation never exceeded 2% of
spermatic venous blood levels, thus ensuring continuous sink conditions on the arterial side of the venous-arterial barrier.
Under these conditions testosterone-^{3}H transfer is a measure of
testosterone flux across the intervening membrane barrier. The
proportionality between flux across a membrane barrier and concen-

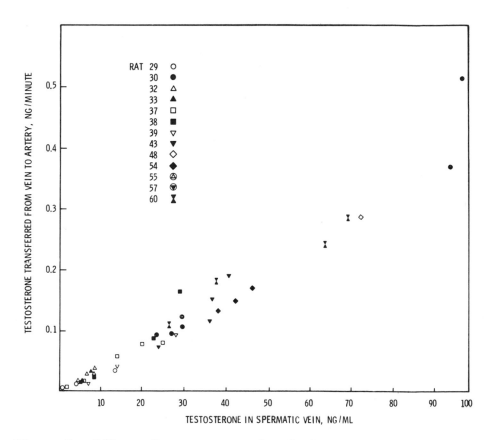

Figure 3. Effect of testosterone levels in spermatic venous blood on the rate of venous-arterial transfer of testosterone in the pampiniform plexus of the rat. In 13 rats blood was shunted from the femoral artery to the testis vein at a flow rate of 0.29-0.36 ml/min and was infused with testosterone-1,2,6,7-^{3}H to give testosterone levels of 2-100 ng/ml in the spermatic venous blood. Duplicate blood samples (5 µl) were drawn simultaneously from the femoral and testis arteries after 10 minutes of infusion and assayed for radioactivity. Venous-arterial transfer rate of testosterone was calculated from the product of the difference between testosterone-^{3}H (ng/ml) in the femoral and testis artery blood, and the volume flow of blood (ml/min) through the system. From Free and Jaffe, 1975 (8).

tration at the membrane surface indicates that the rate-limiting
membrane barriers are not saturated over the range of concentrations
employed. The testosterone transfer system in the rat pampiniform
plexus thus behaves like a passive diffusion system that is con-
centration-limited under physiologic conditions.

The passive model is also suggested by the results obtained
when the venous-arterial concentration gradient is reversed and
testosterone-4-^{14}C is infused into the rat spermatic artery central to the pampiniform plexus (8). In this case, with the testis
vascular bed closed off, 65% of the radioactivity appeared down-
stream at the level of the testis artery. The remaining 35%
appeared in the spermatic vein central to the plexus. Testosterone
thus passes down the concentration gradient between the vessels of
the pampiniform plexus, regardless of its direction.

Relations between rate of blood flow and venous-arterial transfer
rate (Figure 4) confound the picture because more testosterone was
transferred per unit time as blood flow increased. As blood flow
approached normal physiologic rates for the rat testis (0.35 ml/min/
testis) this relationship became less marked in most animals tested.
The fraction of spermatic venous testosterone transferred (testosterone transferred per unit volume of spermatic venous blood) was
2-5% and remained relatively constant for rates of blood flow between
0.01 and 0.02 ml/min. These findings are compatible with the passive
diffusion model of venous-arterial transfer if it is assumed that
testosterone concentration declined along the surface of the diffusion
membrane; i.e., if a significant reduction in diffusible testosterone occurred in the venous blood as it passed along the spermatic
vein. Characteristically in a diffusion system the transfer rate
across the membrane will continue to increase with increased flow
until the testosterone concentration is uniform over the entire surface of the membrane. At this point diffusion rate becomes independent of flow.

If this interpretation is correct, then the membrane barriers
permitting testosterone transfer in the pampiniform plexus of the
rat are not fully utilized under physiologic conditions. In addition
there must be a significant reduction in the concentration of
testosterone "seen" by the membrane as the blood passes from the
testis to the central portion of the pampiniform plexus. Clearly
the 2-5% reduction in total testosterone would not qualify as a
significant reduction in this type of system. However, it is
possible that all blood testosterone is not diffusible, only the
testosterone that is not bound to blood proteins. Assuming that
the rate of exchange between bound and diffusible testosterone is
small compared to the rate of diffusion across the membrane, it is
possible that a significant reduction in unbound testosterone
could occur along the membrane surface.

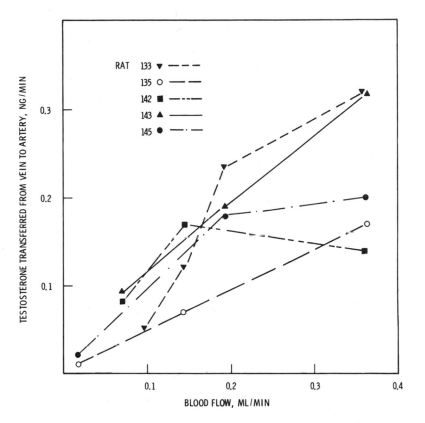

Figure 4. Effect of blood flow on venous-arterial transfer of testosterone in the pampiniform plexus of rat. Blood containing 25-35 ng/ml testosterone-1,2,-^{3}H was perfused into a testicular vein of five rats at different rates with 5 μl blood samples were drawn at 5-10 minute intervals from the femoral and testis arteries and assayed for radioactivity. Each rat was perfused at three or four different flow rates in random sequence. Rate of transfer was calculated from the product of the difference between testosterone-^{3}H (ng/ml) in the femoral and testis artery blood and the volume flow of blood (ml/min) through the system. From Free and Jaffe, 1975 (8).

The implication that the relation between free and bound
testosterone in blood has an influence on the testosterone transfer system is supported by the markedly higher transfer rate in
rats which the spermatic vein was perfused with dextran instead
of blood (Figure 5). Under these conditions presumably none of
the steroid was bound and so all of it was diffusible. Thus
testosterone-1,2,-^{3}H was able to approach equilibration across the
membrane barriers of the pampiniform plexus even at maximum flow
rates. Although these results are not conclusive because of the
unknown effect of dextran on the membrane barrier, they do nevertheless suggest that the transfer system involves only unbound
testosterone. Furthermore, the tenacity of testosterone binding
is suggested by the observation that the fraction of testosterone
transferred was relatively constant throughout the flow range
(Figure 4) and that this fraction increased sharply only when flow
approached zero (8). Individuals, species or molecules with
different blood binding characteristics should therefore exhibit
different transfer rates. Additionally, conditions which decrease
binding of a molecule in blood should increase the transfer of that
molecule across the membrane.

Diverse small molecules can transfer from vein to artery in the
pampiniform plexus. In addition to those listed in Table 1, we have
shown that dihydrotestosterone, dehydroepiandrosterone, estradiol,
progesterone, pregnenolone and cholesterol can transfer from dextran
across the vessels of the pampiniform plexus (15). The relative
rates of transfer of these steroids from blood have not yet been
determined. The molecular size limit in this system is not known
at present but methoxyinulin-^{3}H (M.W. 5000-5500) did not transfer
from vein to artery or vice versa in the pampiniform plexus of the
rat (8).

We can conclude from the studies to date that a countercurrent
exchange of testosterone and other substances can occur in closely
juxtaposed and convoluted veins and arteries of the pampiniform
plexus in many species and that because of the high level of testosterone in the spermatic vein a net increase in arterial blood
testosterone normally occurs as the blood courses through that region. However, the physiologic significance of all this is unclear
at the present. Einer-Jensen (9) has demonstrated that higher
specific radioactivity can be found in the ipsilateral than the
contralateral epididymis after injection of testosterone-^{3}H into the
rat testis even when the efferent ducts and associated lymphatics
are ligated. Additionally, we have found specific radioactivity
at a higher level in epididymal artery than in femoral artery blood
during perfusion of the ipsilateral spermatic vein of two rats with
blood containing testosterone-^{3}H. Additional studies are needed to

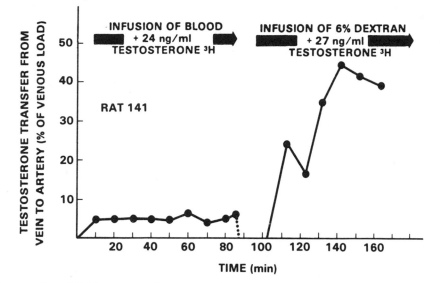

Figure 5. Differences between venous-arterial transfer of testosterone 1,2,-³II from whole blood and from 6% dextran in the pampiniform plexus of the rat. Blood or dextran containing 24 and 27 ng/ml of testosterone-1,2,-³H respectively was perfused into a testis vein at 0.36 ml/min while 5 μl blood samples were drawn at 10 min. intervals from the femoral and testis artery and assayed for radioactivity. The fraction of spermatic venous blood testosterone transferred to the spermatic artery, expressed as a percentage, was calculated by dividing the difference between specific radioactivity in the testis artery and femoral artery blood by the specific radioactivity in the testicular vein perfusate.

quantitate this contribution to the epididymis and compare it with contributions from the testis tubular fluid. Contribution of this elevated arterial testosterone to the germinal epithelium seems unlikely in view of the proximity of the Leydig cells and high level of that steroid in the peritubular lymph (16,17); however, it is possible that the contents of the rete testis may benefit from higher testosterone levels in the arterial blood supply.

From the practical standpoint a local concentration mechanism may serve to concentrate drugs in the target organ, thereby improving the drug's therapeutic ratio. Clearly, in the case of the

TABLE III

Distribution of Radioactivity 6 and 12 Hours After Implantation of Silastic Capsules Containing Progesterone 1,2,^{3}H Between the Left Testis and Cauda Epididymidis. dpm/g x 10^{-2} Mean ± S.D.

Time After Implantation

	6 hr		12 hr	
	Left	Right	Left	Right
Testes	30 ± 16	33 ± 12	33 ± 6	28 ± 9
Cauda Epid.	---	---	1728 ± 1708	38 ± 15
Caput Epid.	520 ± 432	47 ± 15	136 ± 50	51 ± 16
Epid. Fat Pad	220[1] ± 117	109[2] ± 76	---	---
Kidney	116 ± 43	105 ± 44	152 ± 66	110 ± 37
Liver	313 ± 140		312 ± 156	
Blood (dpm/ml)				
Fem. Artery	23 ± 10		23 ± 4	
Test. Artery	23 ± 10		23 ± 4	
Test. Vein	19[3] ± 6		23 ± 5	

[1] 8 samples from 4 animals (one rat omitted because of high (192 x 10^5 dpm/g) counts indicated capsule leakage into fat).

[2] 10 samples from 5 animals.

[3] 4 animals.

scrotal testis, it would be advantageous if the access to the
concentration mechanism could be gained through the tunica albuginea or vaginalis, in which case sustained release devices
containing antispermatogenic or antisperm maturation agents could
be placed in the scrotal cavity. To test this route of drug delivery, silastic capsules 15 mm long by 1.96 mm OD, filled with
progesterone-1,2,-^{3}H (13.3 µCi) with an in vitro release rate of
0.643 µCi/hr, were placed between the tunica vaginalis and tunica
albuginea adjacent to the left cauda epididymis and testis in 10
rats. Distribution of radioactivity was measured in groups of 5
rats at 6 hours and 12 hours after implantation (Table III). Although the route of administration was effective for general
distribution of the drug, there was no evidence of diffusion across
the tunica albuginea into the testis vascular bed, and no differential distribution between the blood vessels of the general circulation and those entering and leaving the pampiniform plexus.
However, the epididymis did appear to receive high local concentrations of the steroid, probably by diffusion, but also, possibly,
through a local recirculation between the common epididymal artery
and vein which are closely intertwined in the rat. Differences may
exist that would render the testis vascular bed more accessible
from the scrotum in other species. In dog and human, for example,
anastomoses have been observed between the testicular and scrotal
circulation (18). However, in the rat it appears as if only the
epididymis can be selectively treated through sustained release
vehicles implanted in the scrotum.

REFERENCES

1. Cross, B.A. and Silver, I.A. J. Reprod. Fertil. 3: 377, 1962.

2. Setchell, B.P. and Hinks, N.T. J. Reprod. Fertil. 20: 179, 1969.

3. Waites, G.M.H. and Moule, G.R. J. Reprod. Fertil. 2: 213, 1961.

4. Free, M.J. and Jaffe, R.A. Am. J. Physiol. 223: 241, 1972a.

5. Free, M.J. and Jaffe, R.A. Prostaglandins 1: 483, 1972b.

6. Free, M.J. and Kien, N.D. Proc. Soc. Exp. Biol. Med. 143: 284,
    1973.

7. Free, M.J., Jaffe, R.A., Jain, S.K. and Gomes, W.R., Nature New
    Biol. 244: 24, 1973.

8. Free, M.J. and Jaffe, R.A. Endocrinology, 1975 (in press).

9.   Einer-Jensen, N.   J. Reprod. Fertil. 37: 145, 1974a.

10. Jacks, F. and Setchell, B.P.   J. Physiol. 233: XVIIP, 1973.

11. Einer-Jensen, N. J. Reprod. Fertil. 37: 55, 1974b.

12. Ginther, O.J., Mapletoft, R.J., Zimmermann, N., Meckley, P.E.
     and Nuti, L.   J. Animal Sci. 38: 835, 1974.

13. Dierschke, D.J., Walsh, S.W., Mapletoft, R.J., Robinson, J.A.,
     Ginther, D.J.   Proc. Soc. Exp. Biol. Med. 148: 236, 1975.

14. Free, M.J. and Tillson, S.A.   Endocrinology 93: 874.   1973.

15. Free, M.J. and Jaffe, R.A.   7th Ann. Meeting Soc. Study of
     Reproduction, Ottawa, Canada, 1974.

16   Linder, H.R., In Participation of Lymph in the Transport of
     Gonadal Hormones, Proc. 2nd Intern. Congr. Hormonal Steroids,
     Excerpta Med. Found. Intern. Congr. Ser. No. 132, A 821.
     Excerpta Med. Found., Amsterdam, 1966.

17. Fawcett, D.W., Neaves, W.B. and Flores, M.N.   Biol. Reprod. 9:
     500, 1973.

18. Joranson, Y., Emmel, E. and Pilka, H.J.   Anat. Rec. 41: 157,
     1929.

Steroid Hormones
in the
Seminiferous Tubule

REGULATION OF TESTOSTERONE AND DIHYDROTESTOSTERONE LEVELS IN RETE
TESTIS FLUID. EVIDENCE FOR ANDROGEN BIOSYNTHESIS IN SEMINIFEROUS
TUBULES IN VIVO

A. Bartke, M. E. Harris and J. K. Voglmayr

Worcester Foundation for Experimental Biology

Shrewsbury, Massachusetts 01545

INTRODUCTION

The lumen of the seminiferous tubules is filled with a fluid
which is distinctly different in its composition compared to blood
plasma and testicular lymph. Seminiferous tubular fluid is apparently secreted by the Sertoli cells (1-3). This fluid flows from
the tubules through the rete testis and efferent ducts into the
caput epididymidis where most of it is resorbed (1,4,5). Studies
in the ram (1) and in the rat (5-8) have shown that the concentration of testosterone (T) in rete testis fluid (RTF) is much higher
than peripheral blood although not as high as in testicular venous
blood. These findings provide strong support to the concept that
high androgen levels in the seminiferous tubules and in the proximal portion of the epididymis may plan an important role in the
maintenance of spermatogenesis as well as in the survival and
maturation of spermatozoa in the epididymis.

This review brings together our recent work on hormonal regulation of androgen levels in the RTF using techniques for acute
collection of RTF from anesthetized rats (6,9) and for continuous
collection of RTF from conscious rams (4,5). In the rat, we have
examined the effects of hypophysectomy, human chorionic gonadotrophin (hCG) and testosterone propionate (TP) on the concentration
of T and dihydrotestosterone (DHT) in RTF. In the ram, we have
studied changes in T and DHT concentration in serial samples of
RTF after a single dose of hCG, Luteinizing Hormone (LH), Follicle
Stimulating Hormone (FSH), or LH + FSH.

In addition, the effects of pregnenolone and other C-21
steroids on the concentration of T and DHT in the RTF, peripheral
blood and testicular venous blood of hypophysectomized rats have
also been studied. Administration of these compounds to hypophysectomized rats was previously shown to maintain spermatogenesis
without preventing the atrophy of accessory reproductive glands
(10). We now have measured T and DHT levels in the RTF of such
animals to determine whether maintenance of spermatogenesis can be
explained by the conversion of non-androgenic C-21 steroids to
androgens in vivo. Using this experimental model we have also obtained information on the relative role of various compartments of
the testis in the biosynthesis of androgens from exogenous C-21
steroids.

MATERIALS AND METHODS

Animals

Rats. Intact and hypophysectomized adult male CD rats were
obtained from Charles River Breeding Laboratories. Acute collection of RTF was carried out in the rats according to the technique
of Tuck and colleagues (9) with minor modifications (6). Immediately after RTF collection, blood was obtained by cardiac puncture.
The weight of the testes, the ventral prostate, the seminal vesicles
and the caput epididymides were also recorded. For collection of
testicular venous blood, the animals were anesthetized with Nembutal
(Abbot), the testes were exteriorized through a scrotal incision and
blood was collected from several cut surface veins (11).

Rams. Catheters were placed into the rete testis (4,5) and
jugular vein of three adult rams. This allowed collection of serial
samples of RTF and peripheral blood at short time intervals from
conscious animals.

Hormones. The rats were injected s.c. with TP in sesame oil
(Lilly) or hCG (Follutein, Squibb) in aqueous solution. The last
injections were made 24 hours before the collection of RTF and
plasma. Schedules of treatments and dose levels are given in the
tables. In the C-21 steroid experiments, pregnenolone, 17-hydroxy-
pregnenolone, progesterone and 17-hydroxyprogesterone (Searle) were
injected s.c. in 0.2 ml of sesame oil at a dose of 2 mg/day, and
RTF and plasma were collected on the day of the last hormone injection.

The rams were given a single i.v. injection of 1 mg of ovine
LH (NIH-LH-S17), 5 or 10 mg of ovine FSH (NIH-FSH-S10), 1 mg LH +
5 mg FSH or 750 IU hCG dissolved in sterile saline. Series of
samples from RTF and blood were taken at intervals ranging from 15

to 60 minutes over a period of 1 1/2 hours before the injections and for up to 6 hours afterwards.

All samples of RTF and plasma were stored frozen until used for measurement of T and DHT by radioimmunoassay.

Assay of Testosterone and 5α-Dihydrotestosterone

Testosterone in rat RTF and plasma was measured by radioimmuno-assay (12). In this method, DHT, androstenedione, and TP do not interfere with T measurement. Dihydrotestosterone was separated from T by chromatography on Sephadex LH-20 columns (12) and measured in the same radioimmunoassay since the antibody to T-Bovine Serum Albumin used crossreacts completely with DHT. The T content of all rat RTF samples fell within the range of the T assay, and within each group, T and DHT concentration did not vary with the volume of RTF assayed.

In the experiments with rams, the assay procedure was the same except that chromatography of the ether extract was omitted. Since the antibody used does not distinquish between T and DHT, the re-sults represent the sum of concentrations of both hormones. Ram RTF contains DHT at a concentration approximately 10% that of T (Bartke and Voglmayr, unpublished) whereas ram peripheral plasma appears to contain no detectable DHT (13,14).

Histological Studies

Spermatogenesis in hypophysectomized rats was evaluated quantita-tively by enumerating the nuclei of Sertoli cells, type A sper-matogonia, preleptotene and pachytene primary spermatocytes and step 7 spermatids on histological cross sections of the testes (15, 16).

RESULTS

Intact Animal Model

In the acute RTF collection experiments with adult intact rats, the concentration of T in the RTF was approximately 20 times greater than that found in plasma (Table I). Administration of hCG (200 IU/day) produced a significant increase in T concentration in the RTF as well as in plasma ($P < 0.001$). In contrast, administration of TP (1 mg/day) produced a decrease in T concentration in RTF ($P < 0.001$).

Table I

Effect of testosterone propionate (TP) or human chorionic
gonadotrophin (hCG) on testosterone concentration in
rete testis fluid (RTF) and plasma in the intact rat (mean $\pm$ SE)

Treatment (no. of rats)		Testosterone RTF	(ng/ml) Plasma	Fluid/plasma
Control	(17)	31.7±2.1	1.7±0.2	21.4±1.8
hCG 200 IU/day for 3 days	(8)	64.0±7.6*	14.9±2.7*	4.7±0.4*
TP 1 mg/day for 4 days	(8)	17.7±1.4*	13.1±1.2*	1.4±0.2*

*Different from controls (P<0.001).

Plasma T levels, however, were elevated in the TP-treated animals,
resulting in an RTF to plasma ratio of about 1.

In the chronic RTF collection experiments with the adult rams,
basal androgen levels in the plasma and in RTF varied markedly between animals and between series of samples collected from the
same animal on different days. However, basal androgen levels were
quite stable during the 1 1/2 hour control period (Fig. 1). The
ratio of mean pretreatment T + DHT concentration in RTF to mean
pretreatment T concentration in the plasma ranged from 4.2 to 40.0.
The concentrations of T in the plasma and RTF of rams observed in
the present study were similar to the values reported earlier (1,7,
13,14,17-19).

Administration of a single dose of LH or hCG usually produced
a significant increase in androgen concentration in both plasma
and RTF (Fig. 1). In contrast, i.v. administration of 5 or 10 mg
ovine FSH produced no elevations in T concentration in plasma or T
+ DHT concentration in RTF. The increase in plasma T levels after
an injection of 1 mg LH + 5 mg FSH was nearly identical to that observed after treatment with LH alone. However, in the RTF, the concentration of T + DHT was increased to a level significantly higher
than that observed after administration of LH alone to the same
animal. A similar difference between the effect of LH + FSH and
LH alone was seen in another ram (not shown).

Hypophysectomized Animal Model

Hypophysectomy caused a decrease in the level of T in RTF and
plasma. The course of T disappearance in RTF (Fig. 2) was much
slower than that seen in the plasma (Fig. 3). Administration of

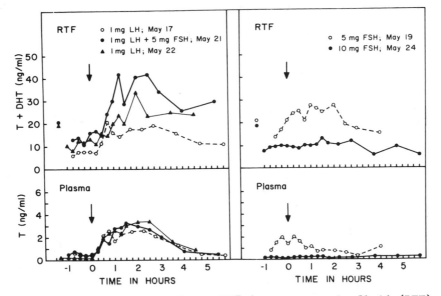

Figure 1. Concentration of T + DHT in rete testis fluid (RTF) and concentration of T in the plasma in a ram after administration of LH or LH + FSH (left panel) and after administration of FSH (right panel). Note different scale for RTF and plasma. Details and significance of responses in the text. Arrow indicates time of injection. Separate symbols represent concentration of T + DHT in overnight collections of RTF.

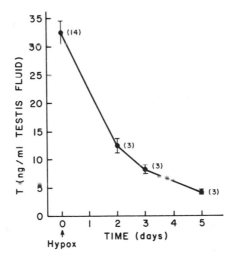

Figure 2. Disappearance of testosterone (T) from rat testis fluid after hypophysectomy. Each point represents the Mean ± SE of T concentration in the testis fluid. Number of rats per group is indicated in parentheses. From Harris and Bartke 1974 (6).

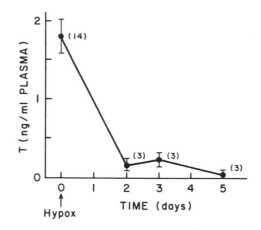

Figure 3. Disappearance of testosterone (T) from rat plasma after
hypophysectomy. Blood was collected by cardiac puncture under
ether anesthesia. Different groups of rats were used at each of
the times indicated. Each point represents the Mean + SE of T
concentration in the plasma. Number of rats per group is indicated
in parentheses. From Harris and Bartke 1974 (6).

hCG to hypophysectomized rats resulted in an increase in both fluid
and plasma T levels (Fig. 4). A daily dose of 0.5 IU hCG restored
fluid and plasma T to levels close to those seen in the intact controls. Note that increasing the daily dose of hCG beyond 5 IU did
not result in a further increase in the concentration of T in RTF
and plasma.

    Treatment of hypophysectomized rats with pregnenolone main-
tained the T concentration in the RTF at a level which was not
significantly different from that in the intact animal (Table II).
The three remaining C-21 steroids were not as effective as pregnenolone but did increase the T concentration in RTF significantly
above the levels observed in hypophysectomized controls. Dihydrotestosterone concentrations in RTF were generally maintained at
approximately 10% of T, a relationship similar to that seen in the
intact controls. Plasma levels of T in these rats were however, not
distinguishable from the level of T seen in the plasma of oil-
treated hypophysectomized control rats. Dihydrotestosterone was
nondetectable in the peripheral plasma of hypophysectomized rats
treated with C-21 steroids.

    The low peripheral androgen levels in C-21 steroid treated hy-
pophysectomized rats were consistent with the low weight of ventral
prostate and seminal vesicles in these animals (8). In contrast,

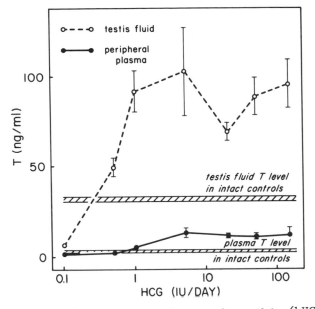

Figure 4.   Effect of human chorionic gonadotrophin (hHG) on testosterone (T) concentration in rete testis fluid and peripheral plasma
in hypophysectomized rats.   HCG was injected sc daily for 4 days
starting on the 4th or 5th day after hypophysectomy.   Each point
represents the Mean ± SE of 6-10 rats.   Control bars represent
Mean ± SE of 17 intact control rats.

the weight of the caput epididymidis in hypophysectomized rats
treated with pregnenolone, 17-hydroxypregnenolone, or 17 hydroxyprogesterone were significantly increased over hypophysectomized
controls.   Similarly, the testis weight in C-21 steroid treated
hypophysectomized rats were significantly higher than those of the
hypophysectomized controls.   On the other hand, treatment of intact
rats with pregnenolone did not produce a statistically significant
alteration in the weights of the sex accessories or of the testes.

Table III shows T concentrations in the testicular venous
plasma, RTF, and peripheral plasma in two additional groups of hypophysectomized rats which were treated with pregnenolone or TP.
Although the mean T concentration in the testicular venous plasma
of intact rats was 148.4 ng/ml, the mean T concentration in the
testicular venous plasma of hypophysectomized rats treated with
pregnenolone was only 17.5 ng/ml.   Histological examination of the
testes revealed that administration of pregnenolone maintains essentially normal seminiferous tubules without altering the atrophied
state of Leydig cells.

Table II

Effect of C-21 steroids (2 mg/day for 14 days) on testosterone (T) and dihydrotestosterone (DHT) concentrations in rete testis fluid (RTF) of hypophysectomized rats (Mean ± SE)

Treatment		T (ng/ml)		DHT (ng/ml)	
		RTF	Plasma	RTF	Plasma
Intact	(4)	46.5+3.6	1.2+0.5	4.9+1.5	0.04+0.02
Intact + preg	(5)	37.7+3.4	1.2+0.2	2.3+0.8	0.02+0.02
Intact + TP	(5)	39.2+4.8	18.5+2.9[a]	1.7+0.4[a]	0.15+0.07
Hypox	(4)	4.9+0.4	0.5+0.08	–	–
Hypox + preg	(7)	35.2+4.8	0.4+0.04	3.3+1.0	n.d.
Hypox + 17 preg	(3)	29.5+3.3[a]	0.4+0.1	0.4+0.4[a]	n.d.
Hypox + prog	(3)	22.9+1.5[b]	0.3+0.05	2.4+1.0	n.d.
Hypox + 17 prog	(4)	30.9+1.8	0.7+0.08	2.0+1.6[a]	n.d.
Hypox + TP	(8)	47.2+4.1	37.3+5.1[c]	4.2+0.8	3.6+1.9

preg = Pregnenolone; 17 preg = 17α-hydroxypregnenolone; prog = Progesterone; 17 prog = 17α-hydroxyprogesteron; TP = Testosterone Propionate; n.d. = non-detectable. Significance of difference vs intact control: a = P <.05; b = P <.01; c = P <.001. From Harris and Bartke 1975 (8).

Table III

Testosterone concentrations in rat rete testis fluid (RTF) testicular vein plasma and peripheral plasma (mean ± SE)

Treatment		Testosterone (ng/ml)		
		RTF	Testicular venous plasma	Peripheral plasma
Intact	(4)	46.5+3.6	148.4+11.4	4.1+ 0.7
Hypox	(4)	4.9+0.4	1.0+ 0.2	0.7+ 0.1
Hypox + preg*	(6)	35.2+4.8	17.5+ 4.8	0.6+ 0.2
Hypox + TP*	(4)	47.2+4.1	96.0+ 8.0	118.0+18.4

preg = pregnenolone; TP = testosterone propionate; * 2 mg steroid/-day for 14 days. From Harris and Bartke 1975 (8).

DISCUSSION

The concentration of T in RTF in both the intact adult rats and the intact adult rams was much greater than the concentration of T in peripheral plasma of these animals in agreement with an earlier report (1). The ratio of RTF to plasma T was around 20 in the rat and ranged from 4 to 40 in the ram. Since most of the RTF appears to originate in the seminiferous tubules, these findings indicate that divisions and differentiation of germinal cells take place in an environment rich in T. The ability of T to maintain spermatogenesis is well documented in many species, including man (20-29).

In intact rats a large dose of TP inhibits release of gonado-trophins from the pituitary and produces atrophy of the Leydig cells (30). One might therefore assume that little endogenous T is produced in TP-treated animals. Therefore the level of T in the RTF and plasma seen in the intact adult rat treated with 1 mg TP (Table I) in our study probably reflects an equilibrium of ex-ogenous T between RTF and plasma, suggesting a transfer from blood to RTF. The reduction in testicular T concentration and the inc-rease in plasma T level in response to TP administration has re-cently been reported also in the human using testicular biopsies for T determinations (28).

Injection of hCG or LH to intact adult rats (Table I) and rams (Fig. 1) resulted in a significant increase in T concentration in both RTF and plasma. The increase in androgen concentration in RTF is in all probability due to the stimulation of Leydig cells. The rates of increase in the levels of T in the plasma and in the levels of T + DHT in RTF after gonadotropin administration was usually elevated approximately two-fold 15 minutes after the administra-tion of hCG or LH (Fig. 1). It continued to increase for about 1 hour, so that the mean plasma T concentration 1 - 3 hours after treatment was approximately 6-10 fold greater than pre-treatment levels. In contrast, the concentration of T + DHT in RTF was never elevated earlier than 30 minutes, and usually not until 45-60 min-utes, after gonadotrophin injection. Furthermore the elevation in RTF concentration of T + DHT was more persistent and the decline more gradual than in plasma T levels. The magnitude of the in-crease in mean T + DHT concentration in ram RTF after administra-tion of hCG, LH or LH + FSH was always less than 3 fold and con-siderably smaller than the concomitant increase in T concentration in the peripheral blood. These differences in response may be partially due to differences in the flow rate of blood and RTF. Blood flows through the ram testis at a rate of approximately 1200 ml/hour (2). It is understandable, therefore, that the increased activity of Leydig cells would be reflected within minutes in an elevated T concentration in peripheral blood. In contrast, RTF is secreted by the testis at a rate of approximately 2 ml per hour (2)

so that there may be an appreciable time lag before the elevation
of T levels in the lumen of seminiferous tubules is reflected in
the samples collected through the rete testis catheter. Thus the
androgen concentration in RTF does not fluctuate as readily as in
the plasma, and the concentration of T in RTF probably corresponds
to the average rate of T release over a certain time period rather
than to short-term changes in Leydig cell activity.

The more gradual decline in T concentration in RTF than in
peripheral plasma was also observed in the rat in response to hypophysectomy (Fig. 2,3). If T levels are a true reflection of
Leydig cell activity, one might expect a similar course of disappearance of T in both plasma and RTF. However, the slower rate of
disappearance of T from RTF after hypophysectomy is probably the
result of the retention of T in RTF due to binding. This explanation is consistent with the presence of androgen-binding protein
(ABP) in the rat RTF (31,32) and in the non-flagellate germ cells
(34) as well as by the absence of testosterone binding globulin
(TeBG) in rat plasma (33).

Of particular interest was the observation that, in the ram,
treatment with a combination of LH and FSH caused a greater elevation of T + DHT concentration in RTF than was observed after the
administration of LH alone (Fig. 1). In contrast, plasma T levels
after treatment with LH + FSH or with LH alone were nearly identical. This raises the intriguing possibility that FSH may have a
specific role in the regulation of androgen levels in RTF. Follicle stimulating hormone (FSH) increases the uptake of labeled T
by rat seminiferous tubules (35), binds to Sertoli cells (36,37),
and increases cyclic AMP levels in Sertoli cells (38). Furthermore, the synthesis of testicular androgen binding protein (ABP)
depends on FSH (32,39). One could also speculate that a combination of LH and FSH stimulates the conversion of non-androgenic
steroids to androgens in the seminiferous tubules which are capable of converting pregnenolone and progesterone to androgens (40-
42). It has been suggested that the action of FSH on spermatogenesis could be explained, in part, by its effect on the concentration
of androgenic steroids in the immediate vicinity of the dividing
and differentiating germinal cells (39,43).

Studies in hypophysectomized rats have shown that hormone
treatment could restore the levels of T in RTF and in plasma to
those seen in the intact rat (Fig. 4). Increasing doses of hCG
produced a gradual increase in plasma T. On the other hand, fluid
T levels reached a maximum with a dose of 1.0 IU hCG/day and did
not increase further in response to higher doses of hCG. These observations indicate that regulation of the T concentration in RTF
and plasma in the intact rat is under pituitary control, although
the exact role that endogenous T plays in maintaining testis fluid
T concentration is yet to be elucidated.

The concentration of T found in the RTF depends not only on the amount of T produced by the testis but also on the flow of RTF. Hypophysectomy is known to cause a reduction in fluid secretion (44,45), and in the present study, the volume of fluid collected from untreated hypophysectomized animals was less than 50 µ1 as compared to more than 150 µ 1 collected from intact animals. Administration of hCG to the hypophysectomized rat increased but generally did not restore fluid volume to that seen in the intact animal. Thus, the high concentration of T in RTF of hypophysecto-mized animals receiving hCG may be a consequence of incomplete re-storation of flow of fluid combined with stimulation of endogenous T production. However, it is important to keep in mind that ef-ferent duct ligation could alter the permeability characteristics of the basement membrane resulting in altered transport of T (46). In this connection it should be noted that the responses to hCG seen in the RTF collected from anesthetized rats after efferent duct ligation were in general agreement with those seen in the con-scious rams from which RTF was continually collected. This suggests the reliability of the acute rat preparation.

The finding that C-21 steriods maintained T + DHT levels in RTF of hypophysectomized rats suggests that T and/or DHT rather than the C-21 steroid itself maintained the testis weight and spermatogenesis in these animals. It appears that relatively little of the T present in the testes of C-21 steroid treated hy-pophysectomized rats is released into the peripheral circulation since levels of T in the testicular venous plasma and peripheral plasma were low. In addition, ventral prostates and seminal ves-icles were atrophied despite the fact that testis weights were maintained, as shown previously (10, 47-52). High levels of T and DHT in the RTF of these animals were due to the conversion of exogenous C-21 steroids to androgens within the testis.

Where, then, in the testis does the conversion of pregnenolone to androgen occur? In hypophysectomized rats treated with pregnen-olone or other C-21 steroids, the Leydig cells were atrophic (6, 53). Decreased activity of the Leydig cells was also reflected in the low levels of T in the testicular venous plasma. These observa-tions, and particularly the normal T levels in RTF together with the drastically reduced T levels in testicular venous blood, suggest that in the hypophysectomized C-21 steroid treated rat, unlike in the intact animal, most of the T does not originate in the Leydig cell. Cells within or in close proximity to the tubules apparently possess the capacity for the in vivo conversion of C-21 steroids to T.

The possibility that C-21 steroids enter the seminiferous tu-bule and are converted there to T is supported by previous results showing that exogenous pregnenolone and progesterone readily enter the rat and rabbit seminiferous tubules (54-56). Non-flagellate germ cells from rat testis will bind progesterone as well as T and DHT (57) and the isolated seminiferous tubules can convert progesterone or pregnenolone to T in vitro (40-42). Haltmeyer and Eik-Nes (58) have suggested that the DHT in the spermatic lymph of the dog may be produced outside the Leydig cells. The production of T in the seminiferous tubules would provide a local source of T for the developing germinal epithelium. Bubenick and colleagues (59) working with rats and squirrel monkeys have immunohistochemically localized significant amounts of androgen in the seminiferous tubules in the layer adjacent to the tubular wall, and suggest that the restricted localization in the tubules might indicate de novo synthesis of steroids in the seminiferous tubules. Thus, it seems possible that seminiferous tubules usually convert non-androgenic steroids, derived either from the Leydig cells or from extratesticular sources, into T and DHT and contribute to the high concentration of these androgens in the immediate vicinity of the dividing and differentiating germinal cells.

SUMMARY

The testosterone occurring in relatively high concentrations in rete testis fluid (RTF) may play an important role in the maintenance of spermatogenesis and survival of spermatozoa in the epididymis. In the present study we have used preparations for the acute collection of RTF from anesthetized rats and for the continuous collection of RTF from conscious rams to determine the effects of gonadotrophins on testosterone (T) and dihydrotestosterone (DHT) concentration in the fluid. Administration of hCG and LH caused a pronounced and rapid elevation of T concentrations in peripheral blood plasma but a more gradual increase in the concentration of T + DHT in RTF. Follicle stimulating hormone (FSH) did not affect the concentration of T + DHT in RTF or peripheral plasma, but when administered together with LH it augmented the effect of LH in RTF but not in peripheral blood plasma. Pregnenolone and other C-21 steroids known to support spermatogenesis maintained normal concentrations of T + DHT in RTF in hypophysectomized rats despite atrophy in testicular venous blood. These results are indicative of bioconversion of steroids in the seminiferous tubules and this activity may contribute to the relatively high androgen concentrations in RTF. It is suggested that measurements of androgens in RTF provide a valid estimate of the hormonal milieu in the seminiferous tubules and useful information on compartmentalized steroidogenesis in the testis.

ACKNOWLEDGEMENTS

This work was supported by PHS Fellowship 1 F22 HD01219, by Steroid Training Program NIH 5 TO 1AM-05564-17, by the Elijah

Romanoff Assistance Program, by NICHD Research Career Development Award 5 K04 HD70369 (A.B.) and by NICHD grant 1 R01 HD06867. We thank Ms. Susan Dalterio for her excellent technical assistance (Mr. Laurence Underwood) in the experiments with rams, NIAMDD for generously supplying ovine LH and FSH, Dr. D. W. Hamilton for demonstrating the RTF collection technique in the rat, D. L. Ewing for helpful suggestions and Dr. B. V. Caldwell for the testosterone antiserum.

REFERENCES

1. Voglmayr, J., Waites, G. and Setchell, B., Nature, Lond. 210: 861, 1966.

2. Setchell, G., Scott, T., Voglmayr, J. and Waites, G., Biol. Reprod. 1: 40, 1969.

3. Setchell, B., Reprod. Fertil. 19: 391, 1969.

4. Voglmayr, J., Scot, T., Setchell, B. and Waites, G., J. Reprod. Fertil 14: 87, 1967.

5. Voglmayr, J., In Handbook of Physiology, ed. Hamilton, D. W. and Greep, R. O., Am. Physiol. Society, Washington, D. C., vol 5, section 7, 437, 1975.

6. Harris, M. and Bartke, A., Endocrinology 95: 701, 1974.

7. Cooper, T. and Waites, G., Endocrinology 62: 619, 1974.

8. Harris, M. and Bartke, A., Endocrinology 96: 1975, (in press).

9. Tuck, R., Setchell, B., Waites, G. and Young, J., Pflugers Arch. 318: 225, 1970.

10. Steinberger, E. and Chowdhury, A., Endocrinology 92: A-97, (Suppl) 1973.

11. de Jong, F., Hey, A. and van der Molen, H., J. Endocrinol. 57: 277, 1973.

12. Bartke, A., Steele, R., Musto, N. and Caldwell, B., Endocrinology 92: 1223, 1973.

13. Purvis, K., Illius, A. and Haynes, N., Endocrinology 61: 241, 1974.

14. Falvo, R. and Nalbandov, A., Endocrinology 95: 1466, 1974.

15.   Clermont, Y. Morgentaler, H., Endocrinology 57: 369, 1955.

16.   Clermont, Y., and Harvey, S. C., Ciba Fdn. Colloq. Endocr. 16: 173, 1967.

17.   Katongole, C., Naftolin, F. and Short, R., Endocrinol. 60: 101, 1974.

18.   Sanford, L., Winter, J., Palmer, W. and Howland, B., Endocrinology 95: 627, 1974.

19.   Ginther, O., Mapletoft, R., Zimmerman, N., Meckley, P and Nuti, L., J. Anim. Sci. 38: 835, 1974.

20.   Nelson, W. and Merckel, C., Proc. Soc. Exp. Biol. Med. 36L 825, 1937.

21.   Nelson, W., Anat. Rec. 79: 48, 1941.

22.   Albert, A. In Sex and Internal Secretions, ed. Young, Williams and Wilkins, Co., Baltimore, 305, 1961.

23.   Hall, P., In The Testis, ed. Johnson, A. D., Gomes, W. R. and Van Demark, N. L., Academic Press, New York, 2: 1, 1970.

24.   Wells, L., Endocrinology 32: 455, 1943.

25.   Bartke, A., Endocrinology 49: 311, 1971.

26.   Desjardins, C., Ewing, L. and Irby, D., Endocrinology 93: 450, 1973.

27.   Van Wagenen, G. and Simpson M., Anat. Rec. 118: 231, 1954.

28.   Morse, H. and Heller, C., Biol. Reprod. 9: 102, 1973.

29.   Steinberger, E., Root, A., Ficher, M. and Smith, K., J. Clin. Endocr. Metab. 37: 746, 1973.

30.   Shay, H., Gershon-Cohn, J., Paschkis, K. and Fells, S., Endocrinology 28: 485, 1941.

31,   French, F. and Ritzen, E., J. Reprod. Fertil. 32: 479, 1973.

32.   Hansson, V., Trygstad, O., Franch, F., McLean, W., Smith, A. Tindall, D., Weddington, S., Petrusz, P., Nayfeh, S. and Ritzen, E., Nature 250: 387, 1974.

33.   Corvol, P. and Bardin, C., Biol. Reprod. 8: 277, 1973.

34. Galena, H., Pillai, A. and Terner, C., Biol. Reprod. 9: 63, 1973.

35. Seilicovich, A., Declercq de Perez Bedes, G., Monastirsky, R., Gonzalez, N. and Rosner, J., Steroids Lipids Res. 4: 224, 1973.

36. Castro, A., Alonso, A. and Mancini, R., Endocrinol. 52: 129, 1972.

37. Means, A. and Vaitukaitis, J., Endocrinology 90: 39, 1972.

38. Dorrington, J and Fritz, I., Endocrinology 94: 395, 1974.

39. Hansson, V., Rensch, E., Trygstad, O., Torgersen, O., Ritzen, E. and French, F., Nature, New Biol. 246: 56, 1973.

40. Christensen, A. and Mason, N., Endocrinology 76: 646, 1965.

41. Hall, P., Irby, D. and deKretser, D., Endocrinology 84: 488, 1969.

42. Bell, J., Vinson, G. and Lacy, D., Proc. Roy. Soc. London B 176: 433, 1971.

43. Galena, H., Pillai, A. and Terner, C., J. Endocrinol. 63: 233, 1974.

44. Setchell, B., Aust. J. Biol. Med. Sci. 46: 35, 1968.

45. Setchell, B., Reprod. Fertil. 23: 79, 1970.

46. Neaves, W., Biol. Reprod. 9: 90, 1973.

47. Nelson, W., Anat. Rec. 67: 110, 1936 (Abstract).

48. Selye, H., Endocrinology 30: 437, 1942.

49. Leathem, J. and Brent, B., Proc. Soc. exp. Biol. Med. 52: 341, 1943.

50. Ruzicka, L. and Prelog, V., Helv. chim. Acta 26: 975, 1943.

51. Masson, G., Am. J. Med. Sci. 212: 1, 1946.

52. Kim, K. and Straw, J., The Physiologist 14: 171, 1971.

53. Tache, Y., Selye, H., Szabo, S. and Tache, J., J. Endocrinol. 58: 233, 1973.

54. Parvinen, M, Hurme, P. and Niemi, M., Endocrinology 87: 1082, 1970.

55. Galjaard, H., von Gaasbeek, J., De Bruyn, H. and van der Molen, H., J. Endocrinol. 48: 1i, 1970 (Abstract).

56. Cooper, T. and Waites, G., Reprod. Fertil. 31: 506, 1972.

57. Galena, H. and Terner, C., Endocrinol. 60: 269, 1974.

58. Haltmeyer, G. and Eik-Nes, K., J. Reprod. Fertil. 36: 41, 1974.

59. Bubenik, G., Brown, G. and Grota, L., Endocrinology 96: 63, 1975.

CONCENTRATION OF STEROID HORMONES AND ANDROGEN BINDING PROTEIN (ABP) IN RABBIT EFFERENT DUCT FLUID

Guerrero, R.[1], Ritzen, E. M.[2], Purvis, K.[1],

Hansson, V.[3], and French, F. S.[4]

[1]Swedish Medical Research Council, Reproductive Endo-
crinology Research Unit and [2]Pediatric Endocrinology
Unit, Dept. of Pediatrics, Karolinska sjukhuset, S-104 01
Stockholm 60, [3]Institute of Pathology, Rikshospitalet,
Oslo, and [4]Depts. of Pediatrics and Labs. for Reprod.
Biol., Univ. of N.C., Chapel Hill, N.C.

INTRODUCTION

Androgenic hormones are necessary for the completion of normal spermatogenesis (1) and may mediate the stimulatory influence of the gonadotrophins FSH and LH on germ cell development (2). Although the stimulatory effects of LH on Leydig cell secretion are well documented, the mechanism by which FSH influences the various testicular compartments has been more speculative. The demonstration of a high affinity androgen binding protein (ABP) in the testicular efferent duct fluid (EDF) of the rat (3,4) and rabbit (5) and its control by FSH (2,6,7) has raised the possibility that FSH may influence the local concentration of androgens in the immediate vicinity of the developing and maturing germ cells. In order to test this hypothesis, a radioimmuno-assay technique, which enables the simultaneous measurement of 8 steroids, including the major androgens, (8,9) was applied to a study of the steroid concentrations in rabbit EDF. It was hoped that steroid assays in conjunction with ABP measurements in the same samples would answer the following questions: (a) What is the steroid composition of the fluid bathing the testicular sperm? (b) Is there a relationship between the concentration of androgens and the levels of ABP?

MATERIALS AND METHODS

Animals and Hormones. Sexually mature New Zealand white rabbits

213

(weight 3-3.4 kg) were used. Radioactive steroids: 1,2,6,7-(^{3}H)-
Progesterone (110 Ci/mmol), 7-^{3}H)-pregnenolone (25 Ci/mmol), 7-(^{3}H)-
dehydroepiandrosterone (16 Ci/mmol), 1,2,6,7-(^{3}H)-testosterone (100
Ci/mmol), 2,4,6,7-(^{3}H) estrone (85 Ci/mmol) and 1,2-(^{3}H) dihydrotestosterone (49 Ci/mmol) were obtained from New England Nuclear Corporation. They were purified and diluted as previously described
(8). Nonradioactive steriods were purchased from Sigma Chemicals.

Collection of efferent duct fluid. Rabbits were anesthetized
with phenobarbital (100-200 mg i.v.), the inguinal canal was opened
and the proximal part of the testis and epididymis was exposed.
The efferent ducts were dissected free from the surrounding fat,
and a silk ligature was applied 1-2 mm from the testis. One to
four days later (six rabbits after 1 day; five rabbits after 3-4
days) the rabbits were killed by bleeding during phenobarbital
anesthesia, the testes were exposed, and EDF was collected by
puncture of the distended ducts. From each testis, 0.2-1.0 ml of
fluid could be collected. The fluid was received into an ice cold
test tube, centrifuged, and kept at -25ºC, until used. Blood was
allowed to clot at room temperature for 1/2 h and serum was frozen
in aliquots at -25ºC.

Assay of androgen binding protein. Aliquots of 5-10 µl EDF
or serum were diluted with buffer (Tris-HCl 10 mM, EDTA 1.5 mM,
2-mercaptoethanol 1 mM, and glycerol to make 10%, pH 7.4) to 100
µl and run in polyacrylamide gels containing 2 nM (^{3}H)-dihydrotes-
tosterone. In this system (steady state polyacrylamide gel electrophoresis or SS-PAGE), radioactive hormone is picked up by the
proteins moving into the gel, and after measuring the radioactivity
in the gel slices at the end of the electrophoresis, the hormone
binding proteins are displayed as peaks of radioactivity. The concentration of ABP was determined from dpm in the ABP peak, as described previously (10), using K_d = 1.9 x 10^{-9} (derived from fig. 6
ref. 10). In this system, ABP is well separated from other binding
proteins including corticosteroid binding globulin and albumin.

Steroid assays. The various steroids were isolated and quantitated as previously described (8, 9). Aliquots of EDF (25 µl) were
diluted to 1 ml with assay buffer (8), extracted with ether and subjected to celite column chromatography. The fractions containing
the different steroids were evaporated to dryness, dissolved in
buffer and divided into assay and recovery aliquots.

Validation of the radioimmunoassay. The recovery of the steroids
under investigation was assessed by adding known amounts of radioactive standards to the samples prior to extraction: Mean percent
recoveries ± S.D. for EDF and serum respectively were: progesterone,
73.4 ± 4.8 and 83.0 ± 3.8, pregnenolone, 52.2 ± 13.4 and 57.0 ± 6.22,
dehydroepiandrosterone, 53.6 ± 6.6 and 56.3 ± 8.0, testosterone,

68.4 ± 9.8 and 80.2 ± 3.1, estrone, 82.7 ± 7.7 and 84.1 ± 4.0,17β-estradiol, 70.4 ± 9.8 and 68.0 ± 5.6, 5α-dihydrotestosterone, 70.9
8.0 and 77.1 ± 7.0 and androstenedione 82.9 ± 6.9 and 83.2 ± 5.8.

The method blank was estimated by processing assay buffer in the
same manner as the EDF or serum samples. The cpm resulting from the
radioimmunoassay of the blank samples were compared by means of a
t-test with those in the test tubes of the standard curve which did
not contain any nonradioactive steroid. In all cases, no differences
could be detected at the 95% probability level, and thus the presence
of blanks was considered to be negligible. The chromatographic procedures and antisera used in this investigation were the same as
described previously (8, 9). Studies of the within-assay and between-
assay variation were carried out on pools of EDF and rabbit serum.
For all steroids and for both types of samples, the within and between
assay variation, expressed as coefficients of variation, were always
below 10%.

To test the parallelism between different levels of EDF or serum
and authentic hormone, increasing amounts of sample (12.5, 25 and
50 µl of EDF and 0.5, 1.0 and 2.0 ml of serum) were assayed. A complete analysis of variance (8) indicated that the relationship between increasing amounts of the sample and authentic hormone was
linear and parallel over the range studied.

RESULTS

Steroid Pattern in Serum

There was extensive variation in the concentrations of the
various steroids in serum (Table I). Of the eight steroids measured
(testosterone, dihydrotestosterone (DHT), androstenedione, pregnenolone, dehydroepiandrosterone (DHEA), progesterone, 17β-estradiol and
estrone), testosterone was the major hormone present. Lower but still
significant levels were found for the other androgenic hormones (DHT,
androstenedione and DHEA), and for progesterone, whilst estrone was
present in trace quantities and 17β-estradiol was undetectable.

Steroid Pattern in EDF

The most striking difference between steroid levels in serum and
EDF was the high concentrations of testosterone and DHT present in
the latter fluid (Table I). Androstendione, pregnenolone and DHEA
were present in EDF in approximately 10 times higher concentrations
than in the peripheral serum. As in serum, estrone was present in
only trace quantities and 17β-estradiol was not detectable. The
concentrations of testosterone in EDF showed a strong positive corre-

TABLE I

	EDF		Serum		Ratio EDF/Serum	
	ng/ml	Rel. to testost. x 100	ng/ml	Rel. to testost. x 100	$\bar{x}$	Conf. limits of $\bar{x}$
T	57.4 ± 33.4	100.0	2.75 ± 3.64	100.0	39.8	92.8–17.1
DHT	21.3 ± 9.5	37.1	.637 ± .506	23.1	56.0	126.9–24.7
Adione	5.17 ± 1.57	9.0	.432 ± .217	15.7	12.1	17.6– 8.4
DHEA	4.19 ± 1.39	7.3	.479 ± .277	17.3	9.5	13.3– 6.8
Preg	3.27 ± 1.80	5.7	.531 ± .531	19.2	8.3	14.4– 4.8
Prog	1.21 ± .555	2.1	.348 ± .211	12.6	3.8	6.0– 2.4
E_1	.027 ± .015	0.0	.015 ± 0.008	0.5	2.0	3.7– 1.1
E_2	–	–	–	–	–	–

Concentration of testosterone (T), dihydrotestosterone (DHT), androstenedione (Adione), dehydroepiandrosterone (DHEA), pregnenolone (preg), progesterone (prog), estrone (E_1) and estradiol (E_2) in efferent duct fluid (EDF) and serum of rabbits. Means ± s.d. The ratios between efferent duct fluid and serum concentrations were calculated for each individual rabbit, and the means ($\bar{x}$) of the ratios and confidence limits of means presented.

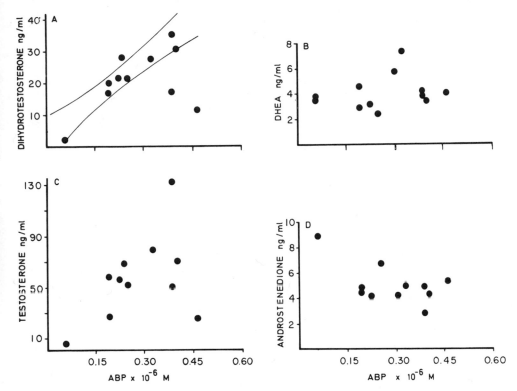

Fig. 1.   Concentration of androgenic hormones versus concentration
           of androgen binding protein (ABP) in rabbit efferent duct
           fluid.   A positive correlation is noted for dihydrotesto-
           sterone (A) and testosterone (C).   The 95% confidence
           limits of the regression line dihydrotestosterone-ABP
           for 9 rabbits is indicated, excluding two rabbits of low
           hormone but high ABP levels (see text).

lation with that of DHT (correlation coefficient r = +0.94), but
negative to androstenedione (r = -0.59).

Androgen Binding Protein in EDF

    The concentration of ABP in EDF showed equally large variations
as the steroid hormones, varying between 0.06 - 0.45 μM, assuming

one binding site per molecule of ABP. A positive correlation was
noted between ABP and both DHT (r = +0.45) and testosterone (r = +0.45)
(Fig. 1). Two animals deviated from this trend which decreased the
correlation coefficient between DHT and ABP from 0.94 to 0.45. No
technical reason could be found for this deviation, and due to the
shortage of samples, the assays could not be repeated after the initial
duplicate measurements. The 95 percent confidence limits of the regression line for 9 values is given in Fig 1 and indicates the extent
of deviation from the rest of the population.

Comparison Between 1 and 3-4 Day Ligation

A comparison of the steroid content of EDF and serum between
rabbits having their efferent ducts ligated for one day with those
maintained for 3-4 days revealed no significant difference in the
levels of androgens, although the progesterone concentration was
significantly higher (p < 0.02) in EDF collected 3-4 days after ligation, (1.6 ± 0.6 ng/ml), than after 1 day (0.9 ± 0.3 ng/ml). In
the serum of the same animals, only pregnenolone showed a significant
difference (p < 0.01); the concentration in animals killed 3-4 days
after efferent duct ligation were 1.0 ± 0.6 ng/ml, compared to 0.2 ±
0.1 ng/ml in those sacrificed after 1 day.

DISCUSSION

There are at least three different periods in the early life of
a germ cell which may be discussed in connection with its milieu of
androgenic hormones: (a) spermatogenesis, (b) the transport of sperm
from the seminiferous tubule to the epididymis and (c) the maturation
of the spermatozoa in the caput edpidiymis. During recent years, it
has become increasingly evident that androgenic hormones may mediate
the stimulatory influence of both FSH and LH on spermatogenesis (2).
Thus, spermatogenesis can be maintained in the hypophysectomized rat
by administration of large doses of testosterone or DHT (see review 1)
or by local implantation of DHT in the testes (12). Pregnenolone,
androstenedione and DHEA have also been reported to maintain spermatogenesis in hypophysectomized rats (13), most probably due to their
conversion to active androgens (14). The present study reveals that
in the intact rabbit the fluid secreted by the seminiferous tubule
is extremely rich in androgenic steroids, especially testosterone
and DHT. This observation thus supports the view that a local high
concentration of androgen is conducive to normal spermatogenesis.
Although the literature is fragmentary on this subject, the above
finding does confirm similar work in other species. The testosterone
concentration in rete testis fluid or efferent duct fluid in the
rat (14) ram (15) and bull (16) is, in all cases, much higher than
its level in peripheral blood. In the monkey, however, it has been
reported that there is no marked difference in the concentration of

testosterone in the two compartments (17). This is an important
observation which needs to be confirmed.

The origin of the large quantities of steroid in EDF is still
a matter of conjecture. It has been previously shown that the blood-
testis barrier completely excludes cholesterol from the tubular compartment (22), whereas other steroids including androgens apparently
enter freely (18). FSH exerts little effect on the secretion of
androgens by the testis. However, we have suggested that its influence on spermatogenesis may be indirect due to an effect on transport
of active androgens into the tubules (2). Thus, the spermatogenic
elements are exposed to high concentrations of androgens which, if
not for FSH, may have dissipated or been metabolized. The basis of
this concentrating mechanism may be the androgen-binding protein
(ABP) which is produced in the Sertoli cells (2,6,7,19,23) as a response to FSH (6,7). It accumulates in the seminiferous fluid in
large quantities and is transported to the caput epididymis. In the
rabbit, there is a very high concentration of ABP in EDF (2.7×10^{-7} M).
At 37°C rabbit ABP exhibits high avidity for DHT, 5α-androstandiol
and testosterone (decreasing in that order) (11) whilst androstenedione, DHEA, pregnenolone and progesterone (11, and unpublished observations) showed no detectable binding. In the present study,
the EDF/serum ratio was highest for DHT>testosterone>andostenedione>
DHEA and pregnenolone. Thus the relative steroid concentrations in
EDF appear to parallel the relative binding affinities which the
different steroids exhibit for ABP. Although the radioimmunoassay
technique used in the present communication has not yet been applied
to the measurement of 5α-androstandiol in EDF, its binding affinity
for ABP would suggest that it might be present in relatively high
amounts.

In addition to its possible role in concentrating steroids within
the tubule, ABP may also be required for transporting androgens to
the epididymis. Androgenic hormones have been shown to be necessary
for the maturation of spermatozoa in the rabbit epididymis (20, 21)
and ABP would maintain a high androgenic concentration at least in the
proximal segments of this organ. If this and its tubular role are
confirmed, ABP may prove to be one of the most important components
in the increasingly complicated process of spermatogenesis and sperm
maturation.

SUMMARY

The concentrations of eight steroid hormones in rabbit efferent
duct fluid and serum were determined by radioimmunoassay following
celite column chromatography, and the concentrations of androgen
binding protein (ABP) were measured by steady state polyacrylamide
electrophoresis. The following results (means ± s.d.) were obtained
for efferent duct fluid, with serum levels in parenthesis: testo-

sterone 57.4 ± 33.4 (2.7 ± 3.6) ng/ml, 5α–dihydrotestosterone 21.3
± 9.5 (0.64 ± 0.50) ng/ml, androstenedione 5.2 ± 1.6 (0.43 ± 0.22)
ng/ml, dehydroepiandrosterone 4.2 ± 1.4 (0.48 ± 0.28) ng/ml, pregnenolone 3.3 ± 1.8 (0.53 ± 0.53) ng/ml, progesterone 1.21 ± 0.56 (0.35
± 0.21) ng/ml, estrone 0.03 ± 0.02 (0.02 ± 0.01) ng/ml, androgen
binding protein (ABP) 0.27 ± 0.12 x 10^{-6}M. Estradiol was not
measurable (< 5 pg/ml) in either efferent duct fluid or serum.
In individual rabbits, the ratios of the concentrations in efferent
duct fluid to those in serum were highest for 5α–dihydrotestosterone
(56.0) and testosterone (39.8), followed by androstenedione (12.1),
dehydroepiandrosterone (9.5) and pregnonolone (8.3). These ratios
closely parallel the relative binding affinities for androgen binding
protein (ABP). Except for two fluids with high levels of ABP, the
concentration of 5α–dihydrotestosterone was strongly correlated to
that of ABP. This, and the preferential retention of 5α–dihydrotestosterone in the fluid, indicate that ABP may be actively influencing
the "milieu interieur" of the spermatozoa.

ACKNOWLEDGEMENTS

Supported by the Swedish Medical Research Council (project 3168),
WHO (project H9/181/83) and the Ford Foundation.

REFERENCES

1. Steinberger, E. and Steinberger, A., "Handbook of Physiology." Ed.
    Ed. Greep, R. O. and Astwood, E. B. IV/2, 325, 1974.

2. Hansson, V., Ritzen, E. M., French, F. S. and Nayfeh, S. N.
    "Handbook of Physiology," Section 7: Endocrinology. Ed.
    Hamilton. D. W. and Greep, R. O. 1975, p. 173.

3. French, F. S. and Ritzen, E. M., Endocrinology. 93, 88, 1973.

4. French, F. S. and Ritzen, E. M., J. Reprod. Fertil. 32, 479, 1973.

5. Ritzen, E. M. and French, F. S., J. Steroid Biochem. 5, 151, 1974.

6. Hansson, V., Reusch, E., Trygstad, O., Torgersen, O., Ritzen,
    E. M., and French, F. S., Nature New Biol. 246, 56, 1973.

7. Vernon, R. G., Kopec, B., Fritz, B., Mol. Cell, Endocr. 1, 167,
    1974.

8. Brenner, P. F., Guerrero, R., Cekan, Z., Diczfalusy, E.,
    Steroids. 22, 775, 1973.

9. Purvis, K., Brenner, P. F., Landgren, B. M., Cekan, Z., and
    Diczfalusy. E., J. Clin. Endocr., in press 1975.

10. Ritzen, E. M., French, F. S., Weddington, S. C., Nayfeh, S. N.,
    Hansson, V., J. Biol. Chem. 249, 6597, 1974.

11. Hansson, V., Ritzen, E. M., French, F. S., Weddington, S. C.,
    and Nayfeh, S. N., Mol. Cell. Endocr., in press.

12. Ahmad, N., Holtmeyer, G. C., and Eik-Nes, K. B., Biol. Reprod.
    8, 411, 1973.

13. Clairmont, Y. and Harvey, S. C. Ciba Foundation Colloquia on
    Endocrinology, 16, 173, 1967.

14. Bartke, A., Harris, M. E., Vogelmayr, J. K. this volume, p. 197.

15. White, I. G. and Hudson, B., J. Endocr. 41, 291, 1968.

16. Ganjam, V. K. and Amann, R. P., Acta Endocr. (Kbh), 74, 186, 1973.

17. Waites, G. M. H. and Einer-Jensen, N., J. Reprod. Fertil. 41,
    505, 1974.

18. Parvinen, M., Hurme, P. and Niemi, M., Endocrinology. 87, 1082,
    1970.

19. Hagenas, L., Ritzen, E. M., Ploen, L., Hansson, V., French, F.
    S. and Nayfeh, S. N., Mol. Cell. Endocr., in press 1975.

20. Orgebin-Crist, M-C., Dyson, A. L. M. B., and Davies, J., Int.
    Congr. Series No. 273, Endocrinology, 949, Exerpta Medica,
    Amsterdam 1972.

21. Orgebin-Crist, M-C., J. Exp. Zool. 185, 301, 1973.

22. Waites, G. M. H., Jones, A. R., Main, S. J. and Cooper, T. G.,
    Adv. Biosci. 10, 101, 1973.

23. Tindall, D. J., Schrader, W. T. and Means, A. R., Hormone Binding
    and Target Cell Activation in the Testis. Eds. Dufau, M. L, and
    Means, A. R., Plenum Press, N. Y., p 167, 1974.

THE BLOOD - TESTIS BARRIER AND STEROIDS

B.P. Setchell and S.J. Main

Department of Biochemistry, A.R.C. Institute of
Animal Physiology, Babraham, Cambridge, England

Do steroids penetrate readily through the walls of the seminiferous tubules? An answer to this question is of vital importance
to anyone interested in the possible production of steroids by the
tubules or in the local action on the tubules of steroids produced
in the interstitial tissue. It is now well established (see 1 for
review) that many quite small molecules do not readily pass through
the walls of the seminiferous tubules, while for other substances,
such as glucose, there is a specific carrier system in the tubular
wall. While this "blood-testis barrier" has been reasonably well
characterized for some classes of compounds, the penetration of
steroids has not been fully investigated. The earlier experiments
involved injection of radioactively labelled steroids into the
animal and then autoradiography of the testis or separation of the
testis into tubules and interstitial tissue. The results of these
studies were rather confusing, but this may to some extent be explained by differences in the techniques used (see 1 for review).

More recently, a study has been made of the penetration of
labelled steroids from blood into rete testis fluid, by comparing
the concentrations of radioactivity in carotid blood and rete
testis fluid during intravenous infusions of labelled steroids in
rats (2). With this technique, the entry rate for a large number
of non-steroidal substances is already known (1,3,4). The label
in rete testis fluid was assumed to reflect that in the fluid inside the seminiferous tubules and the label in arterial blood was
assumed to reflect that in the blood in the testis; both assumptions,
as will appear later, may not be justified for steroids. Testosterone and dehydroepiandrosterone appeared to be readily transferred
from blood to rete testis fluid, whereas cholesterol was excluded.
Between these extremes, the appearance of radioactivity in rete

testis fluid suggested the following order of entry rates:
Progesterone > pregnenolone > 5α-reduced androgens > oestrogens >
corticosteroids.   In a ram, when [3]H- testosterone was infused into
the testicular artery, radioactivity in rete testis fluid rose to a
plateau between 2 and 3 hr, at a value about one fifth of that in
testicular venous blood. Preliminary identification of metabolites
in rete testis fluid and blood suggested that testosterone and dehydroepiandrosterone were transferred largely unchanged while androstenedione and progesterone were largely metabolised during transfer into the rete testis fluid, the former mainly to testosterone
(2).

When radioactive pregnenolone or progesterone was infused into
the testicular artery of a boar for 5 hr, comparatively little
radioactivity appeared in rete testis fluid, and most of this was
present as highly polar compounds, and not as the compounds infused
or as testosterone. However, radioactivity was also found in these
polar compounds in testicular venous blood in higher concentrations
than in rete testis fluid (Setchell, B.P. and Heap, R.B., unpublished
results) suggesting that they were formed in the interstitial tissue
and then diffused into the tubules.

However, rete testis fluid is appreciably different in ionic
composition (5) and sperm concentration (5,6,7) from fluid removed
by micropuncture from the seminiferous tubules, and the ionic composition of fluid newly secreted by the wall of the tubules is even
more distinctive (5). From these data, it was suggested that two
fluids are secreted in the testis; a potassium bicarbonate rich
fluid in the tubules themselves and a much larger quantity of a
sodium chloride rich fluid in the rete testis or in the tubuli
recti (5). Therefore, rete testis fluid cannot be taken to be truly
representative of the fluid inside the tubules. A steroid secreted
by the cells near the tubules may reach the same concentration in
the extracellular interstitial fluid and the fluid inside the tubules,
but this latter fluid could then be diluted by a steroid-poor fluid
secreted in the rete testis. Conversely, substances could enter the
rete testis fluid in the rete testis itself more quickly than they
cross the tubular wall, either with the fluid secreted in the rete
or by exchange through its walls (1). Unfortunately, the small
volumes of fluid which it has been possible to remove by micropuncture from the lumina of the seminiferous tubules have precluded direct measurements of entry rates into this fluid. However, the
fluid secreted by the rat testis can be trapped inside the tubules
and rete by ligating the efferent ducts close to the testis and
the tubular fluid recovered by dispersing and centrifuging the
cells (see Methods section).

Using this technique and collection of rete testis fluid in
the same rats, we have found that radioactive sodium enters rete

testis fluid more rapidly than tubular fluid, and potassium enters
tubular fluid more rapidly than rete testis fluid (Main and Setchell,
unpublished observations). An attempt has therefore been made to
compare the permeability to several steroids of the walls of the
seminiferous tubules and of the rete testis.

METHODS

Male albino rats, Porton Wistar strain, weighing between 280
and 430 g were used. The efferent ducts of one testis of each rat
were ligated (8) under light pentobarbitone anaesthesia and the
animal allowed to recover. Next day, the rat was anaesthetised
again and the left jugular vein was cannulated. Tritiated steroids
(testosterone, androstenedione and 5α-dihydrotestosterone from
Radiochemical Centre, Amersham, and 5α-androstane-3α, 17β-diol from
New England Nuclear Cort., Germany) in fresh plasma from normal
rats were infused (approximately 20 µl/min, 30 µCi/ml) for either
30 or 60 minutes. At the end of this time, rete testis fluid was
collected into a glass capillary tube from the ligated testis by
puncturing the rete with a needle. Approximately 100 µl was
collected in about 1 min, and this would remove most of the fluid
in the rete itself. Testicular venous blood was then collected for
about 2 min from the unligated testis by nicking some of the super-
ficial veins, the animal having been heparinised about 5 min earlier.
(500 units intraperitoneally). Both spermatic cords were then
clamped and a sample of blood removed from the aorta. The whole
sampling procedure took less than 5 min, and the infusion was continued until the sampling was complete. The testes were immediately
decapsulated and the cells dispersed by forcing the parenchyma through
a 21 SWG needle. The cell suspensions, blood and rete testis fluid
(RTF) were centrifuged (10,000 x g for 5 min). The radioactivity in
50 µl portions of plasma, sperm-free RTF and supernatant fluid from
the ligated and unligated testes was counted by liquid scintillation
spectrophotometry, and 200 µl portions were extracted with diethyl
ether (2x 1 ml). The extracts were dried under nitrogen, redissolved
in ethyl acetate (100 µl) and chromatographed on silica gel thin
layer plates, using CH_2Cl_2: diethyl ether (85: 15 v/v) and $CHCl_3$:
ethyl acetate (80 : 20) successively. Testosterone and androstendione standards were located with UV light and DHT and 5α androstane
3α-17β-diol after spraying with 35% aqueous o-phosphoric acid. One
cm bands were scraped off the plates and the radioactivity measured
by liquid scintillation. Radioactivity corresponding to metabolites
in supernatant from unligated testes was subtracted from that of the
ligated testes to obtain metabolites in "tubular fluid". Portions
of the infused plasmas were treated in the same way; in all cases,
more than 98% of the radioactivity present migrated with the
corresponding authentic steroid.

Calculation of Results

The concentration of radioactivity in tubular fluid was calculated as follows: Radioactivity / ml tubular fluid = (Total
radioactivity in supernatant fluid from the ligated testis - Total
radioactivity in supernatant fluid from the unligated testis) /
(Volume of supernatant fluid from the ligated testis - Volume of
supernatant fluid from the unligated testis).

RESULTS

Total Radioactivity

In preliminary experiments, using an exponentially decreasing
rate of infusion, constant levels of total radioactivity were
achieved in arterial plasma, but because of the accumulation of
metabolites, the levels of the steroid infused were decreasing
between 30 and 60 min. Using a constant rate intravenous infusion,
slowly rising levels of total radioactivity were achieved in
arterial blood between 15 and 60 min., but with a reasonably constant concentration of the steroid infused.

Both rete testis fluid (RTF) and calculated tubular fluid (TF)
contained appreciable amounts of radioactivity after 30 or 60 min
of infusion with either testosterone (T) or androstenedione (AD).
The final values reached were between 30% and 80% of arterial
plasma values. With 5α-dihydrotestosterone (DHT) and 5α-androstane-
3α, 17β-diol (androstanediol), there was very much less radioactivity in either RTF or TF, the values being between 5 and 30% of
the arterial levels (Table I). Previous results (Setchell, Eisenhauer
quoted in 9) which suggested that DHT did enter tubular fluid readily
were invalid because of radioactive impurities in the DHT used in
those experiments.   There were no consistent differences between
RTF and TF, or between arterial and testicular venous blood plasma,
in the levels of total radioactivity.

When cholesterol was infused, no radioactivity could be detected in tubular fluid. RTF was not collected in these experiments,
but cholesterol has previously been shown not to enter RTF (4).

Metabolites

When tritiated testosterone was infused, appreciable amounts
of radioactivity were found in plasma in a polar fraction which did
not move from the origin on TLC. The only other significant amount

TABLE I

Comparison of the Total Radioactivity in Rete Testis Fluid and Calculated Tubular Fluid Compared with that in Arterial Blood Plasma,
During Intravenous Infusions of Tritiated Steroids in Rats. Results
are Given as Mean Ratios Fluid/Plasma for Duplicate Determinations.

Steroid Infused	Rete Testis Fluid		Calculated Tubular Fluid	
	30 min	60 min	30 min	60 min
Testosterone	0.40	0.43	0.31	0.42
Androstenedione	0.33	0.69	0.39	0.51
5α-dihydrotestosterone	0.11	0.14	0.09	0.25
5α-androstane-3α, 17β-diol	0.15	0.29	0.13	0.19
Cholesterol	< 0.05*	<0.05*	<0.05	<0.05

* Data from Waites et. al., 1973 (4).

of radioactivity in the blood plasma was found in the testosterone
band. In both rete testis fluid (RTF) and calculated tubular fluid
(TF), there were comparatively few counts remaining at the origin
on the plates and the majority of the counts appeared in the
testosterone band or in the band before, which corresponded with
androstenediol. Expressed per ml of fluid, the concentration of
radioactivity in the testosterone band from RTF and TF approached
the values for aortic and testicular venous blood (Fig 1).

When 5α-dihydrotestosterone (DHT) was infused, some highly polar
compounds were found in the plasma, with very little in the testis
fluids. The largest radioactive component in both blood plasma
samples moved with authentic DHT on the TLC plates, but practically
none of that in the testis fluids behaved like DHT. In both samples,
appreciable amounts of radioactivity migrated at the same rate as
androstanediol, and a similar band of activity was found in calculated tubular fluid, but interestingly, not in rete testis fluid
(Fig 2).

When androstanediol was infused, highly polar material was
found in all samples, but apart from this, most of the activity
in blood plasma moved with authentic androstenediol on TLC. Only
a small amount of activity corresponding to the androstanediol was
found in RTF or TF, and even less in other bands. (Fig. 3).

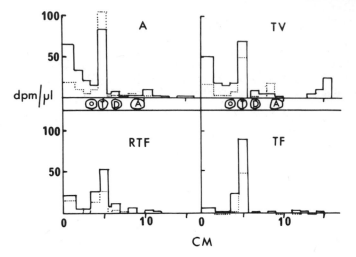

Figure 1.   The radioactivity in d.p.m./µl original fluid in Silica
gel thin layer chromatograms of aortic (A) and testicular venous
(TV) blood plasma, and in rete testis fluid (RTF) and tubular fluid
(TF) after half-hour (dotted line) and one hour (solid line) jugular infusions of ³H-testosterone.   Each line is the mean of two
rats. With this system, testosterone (T), dihydrotestosterone (D),
androstenedione (A) and 5α-androstane-3α 17β-diol (o) ran as indicated on the bar in the centre of the graph.   Because of the way
of calculating the concentration in tubular fluid, some values are
negative.

        The situation after androstenedione infusion was particularly
interesting.   Most of the radioactivity in aortic blood moved with
authentic androstenedione, but in testicular venous blood there
was more activity moving with testosterone than with androstenedione.
In the two testis fluids, there was appreciable activity moving with
testosterone, but virtually none corresponding with androstenedione.
The concentration of radioactivity migrating with testosterone was
similar in testicular venous plasma and in tubular fluid, but was
appreciably higher in rete testis fluid (Fig. 4).

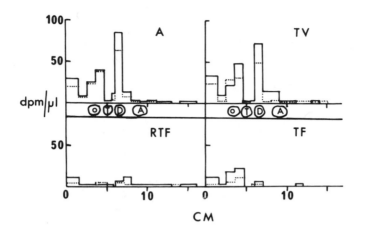

Figure 2.   The radioactivity in thin layer chromatograms of blood plasma and testicular fluids after infusion of ^{3}H-dihydrotestosterone. Details as in Fig. 1.

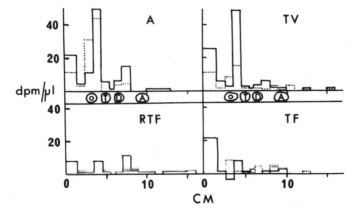

Figure 3.   The radioactivity in thin layer chromatograms of blood plasma and testicular fluids after infusion of ^{3}H-androstane-3α-17β diol.   Details as in Fig. 1.

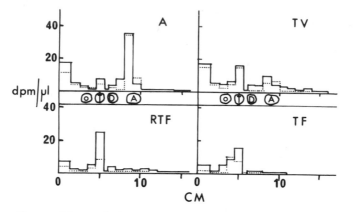

Figure 4. The radioactivity in thin layer chromatograms of blood plasma and testicular fluids after infusions of ³H-androstenedione. Details as in Fig. 1.

DISCUSSION

The results reported here are very preliminary because the metabolites have not been rigorously identified. However, they appear to confirm previous observations that different steroids penetrate into the seminiferous tubules at different rates. Testosterone enters readily but the 5α-reduced steroids enter much more slowly. The entry of testosterone would presumably be facilitated by the high concentration of androgen binding protein in the RTF (10) but this protein also binds DHT, so the differential entry of these two steroids cannot be explained on this basis. The slow entry of DHT could still be reconciled with the idea that DHT is the active form of androgen in the tubules if the steroid entered as testosterone and was transformed to DHT at the target tissue, but if this is what happens, it is perhaps strange that there were not greater amounts of radioactive DHT in the RTF or TF after infusion of elevated testosterone .

There is evidence that 5α-androstandiols are produced by the seminiferous tubules (11) as well as being important catabolites of testosterone (12). It is therefore interesting that there is radioactivity in bands corresponding with androstanediol in chromatograms of blood plasma and tubular fluid but not rete testis fluid after infusions of DHT and in TF and RTF after infusions of testosterone.

When androstenedione was infused, there were qualitative differences between aortic and testicular venous blood. Testicular venous blood is more likely to be representative of the interstitial extracellular fluid, and these results emphasise how dangerous it is to deduce what the situation is inside the testis from measurements on arterial blood.

The only clear-cut difference between the results with steroids appearing in TF and RTF was the appearance of radioactivity moving with androstanediol in TF but not in RTF following the infusion of DHT and this should be further investigated.

How physiological are the conditions of the present experiments? The pentobarbitone anaesthesia is unlikely to affect entry rates and it will be comparatively simple to repeat these experiments with the animal conscious during the infusions except during the last few minutes. More serious criticism could arise from the fact that the efferent ducts of one testis must be ligated 16 to 20 hours before the infusion. After ligation the accumulation of fluid in the testis occurs at a constant rate for about 36 hours (8) and for at least 24 hours there are no significant changes in testicular blood flow or permeability of the tubules to rubidium (5). Furthermore it has recently been shown that even 48 hours after efferent duct ligation in the mouse, when the testis was grossly distended, the structure of the junctions between adjacent pairs of Sertoli cells were unaffected (13). These junctions also appeared normal 24 hr after efferent duct ligation in rats, although at that time they appeared more "leaky" to lanthanum (14). As these junctions are probably the principal components of the blood-testis barrier (15,16) the permeability of the tubules less than 24 hours after ligation of the efferent ducts is probably normal. However, the technique used for the collection of rete testis fluid in the rat (5) also involves ligation of the efferent duct 16-24 hours earlier, so the same criticism would apply to these results also.

The collection of rete testis fluid is obviously more direct than calculation of the composition of tubular fluid by difference. However it can be calculated from measurements of tubular diameter in ligated and unligated testes, that the total fluid recovered from a ligated testis would be 76% luminal fluid, about 7% interstitial extracellular fluid and 17% from other sources, presumably from damaged cells. In the unligated testis the equivalent figures are 50%, 15% and 35%. We have assumed that the amount of interstitial fluid and fluid from damaged cells is probably similar in both ligated and unligated testes and therefore would be allowed for by subtracting the values for the unligated testis from those for the ligated testis.

"Tubular fluid" would therefore seem to be a reasonable description of the result of this calculation. The validity of the indirect method of calculation is substantiated by the demonstration that the calculated concentration in the fluid is zero for those substances which are known not to enter rete testis fluid, such as insulin, sucrose (17) and iodine-labelled albumin (18). On the other hand, 3-0-methylglucose, which is transported into the tubules by the same carrier mechanism as that which transports glucose, rapidly reaches a calculated concentration in the tubular fluid similar to that in blood. (Middleton and Setchell, unpublished results)

How does the information at present available on the penetration of steroids into the tubules relate to the questions of tubular synthesis of steroids and the role of steroids in spermatogenesis? There are suggestions of important species differences in entry rates between rat, sheep and pig, and these may be reflected in the different ratios of testosterone concentration in rete testis fluid to testicular venous blood between these species (unpublished observations). It is apparent that in the rat, testosterone penetrates into the tubules more readily than any of its precursors so far studied. It is therefore simpler to postulate that testosterone is formed outside the tubules, and, once formed, diffuses in, than to suggest production within the tubules. Most of it reaches the lumen as testosterone, but some may be present as androstanediol. so there may be important transformations inside the tubules. More rigorous identification of metabolites in the tubular and rete testis fluid is required.

Likewise, as testosterone penetrates the tubules more readily than other compounds active in maintaining spermatogenesis, and is known to be produced normally in relatively large amounts where it can easily reach the tubules, it is tempting to assume that testosterone is the normal steroid entering the tubule to regulate spermatogenesis. Once inside the tubules, it could be transformed into whatever the final active principle is. Other steroids which enter more slowly than testosterone do enter the tubules much faster than many other compounds and could also be transformed inside the tubules into active compounds.

ACKNOWLEDGEMENTS

We are grateful to Mr. A. C. Setchell for his assistance with these experiments.

REFERENCES

1. Setchell, B.P. and Waites, G.M.H., In Handbook of Physiology,
    Section 7, Endocrinology, eds. D.W. Hamilton and R.O. Greep,
    Amer. Physiol. Soc., 1975, p. 143.

2. Cooper, T. G., and Waites, G.M.H., J. Endocrin. (in press),
    1975.

3. Setchell, B.P., Voglmayr, J.K., and Waites, G.M.H., J. Physiol.
    200: 73, 1969.

4. Waites, G.M.H., Jones, A.R., Main, S.J., and Cooper, T.G., Adv.
    Biosci. 10: 101, 1973.

5. Tuck, R.R., Setchell, B.P., Waites, G.M.H., and Young, J.A.,
    Pflugers Arch. Ges. Physiol. 318: 225, 1970.

6. Levine, N., and Marsh, D.J., J. Physiol. 213: 557, 1970.

7. Howards, S.S., Johnson, A., and Miller, S., Fertil. Steril.
    (in press) 1975.

8. Setchell, B.P., J. Reprod. Fertil., 23: 79, 1970.

9. Setchell, B.P., In Male Fertility and Sterility, Mancini, R.E.,
    and Martini, L., (eds) Academic Press, London, 1974, p. 37.

10. French, F.S., and Ritzen, M., Endocrinology 93: 85, 1973.

11. Rivarola, M.A., and Podesta, E.J., Endocrinology 90: 618, 1972.

12. Baulieu, E.-E., and Robel, P., In The Androgens of the Testis,
    Eik-Nes, K.B., (ed.), 1970, p. 49.

13. Ross, M.H., Anat. Rec. 180: 565, 1974.

14. Neaves, W.B., J. Cell. Biol. 59: 559, 1973.

15. Dym, M., and Fawcett, D.W., Biol. Reprod. 3: 308, 1970.

16. Dym, M., Anat. Rec. 175: 639, 1973.

17. Setchell, B.P., and Singleton, H.M., J. Physiol. 217: 15P, 1971.

18. Setchell, B.P., and Wallace, A.L.C., J. Endocrin. 54: 67, 1972.

19. Cooper, T.G., and Waites, G.M.H., J. Endocrinol. 62: 619, 1974.

Androgen Receptors

PHYSICOCHEMICAL AND BIOLOGICAL PROPERTIES OF ANDROGEN RECEPTORS[1]

C. W. Bardin, O. Jänne, L. P. Bullock and S. T. Jacob

Departments of Medicine, Comparative Medicine and
Pharmacology

The Milton S. Hershey Medical Center of The Pennsylvania
State University, Hershey, Pennsylvania 17033

INTRODUCTION

The term "androgen receptor" has a functional connotation and
in this review will be used to designate the entity in the cell
which recognizes a specific steroid hormone and is necessary for
subsequent action. Current concepts hold that androgens initiate
their action on a wide variety of cell-types by binding to cytoplasmic proteins with high affinity. The subsequent association
of the steroid-protein complex with nuclear chromatin facilitates
RNA synthesis and eventually protein synthesis. According to this
scheme, the ultimate assay of a receptor protein would be its
ability to stimulate synthesis of specific RNA's from chromatin in
a cell-free system. Although many investigators have identified
high affinity androgen binding proteins which are believed to be
receptors, to date there are few studies which demonstrate functional capacity of these proteins other than by their ability to bind
steroids.

In the present report, we will review the physicochemical properties of proteins which are believed to be androgen receptors.
Genetic and steroid specificity studies will be presented which
substantiate the receptor function of these macromolecules.
Finally, the preliminary attempts to study the biological action
of the steroid receptor complex on chromatin will be summarized.
It should be emphasized that this is not an exhaustive review of
androgen receptors but rather a presentation of our own observations in context with selected findings of other investigators. A

[1] Supported by PHS Grant No. HD-05276

more extensive review of androgen receptors has recently been
reported by King and Mainwaring (1).

PHYSICOCHEMICAL PROPERTIES OF ANDROGEN RECEPTORS

     Androgen receptors were first studied in prostate and in other
parts of the male reproductive tract (1). More recently, these receptors have been studied in other androgen responsive tissues such
as kidney, muscle and pituitary (2-5). The similarities of these
binding proteins are illustrated by comparison of putative androgen
receptors from prostate and kidney in Table I. Both receptors are
asymmetric acidic proteins which have sedimentation coefficients
of 7-8S or 3.5-4.5S when extracted from cytoplasm or nuclei with
buffers of low or high ionic strength respectively. Receptors are
heat labile and studies with protein specific reagents suggest that
these macromolecules require cysteine and tryptophan residues for
maintenance of their binding sites. Finally, androgen receptors
as well as other steroid receptors can promote the association of
steroid with DNA. These properties serve to distinguish receptors
from extracellular androgen binding proteins such as testosterone-
estradiol binding globulin (TeBG) (7-9) (Table I) and androgen
binding protein (ABP) (10).

TABLE I

Physiocochemical Properties of the Cytoplasmic
Androgen Receptor From Rat Prostate and Mouse Kidney:
Comparison With Rabbit Testosterone-Estradiol Binding Globulin

	Receptor		TeBG
	Prostate (rat)	Kidney (mouse)	Plasma (rabbit)
Sedimentation coefficient	8	7.9	4.4
Stokes radius (Å)	84	82	44
Molecular weight (daltons)	276,000	270,000	73,000
Frictional ratio (f/fo)	1.96	1.98	1.6
Isoelectric point	5.8	4.8	5.4
Heat stable	No	No	Yes
Binds to DNA	Yes	Yes	No
References	(1)	(2,6)	(7)

It is significant that similar physicochemical properties have been found not only for androgen receptors from most tissues but for steroid receptors in general. Even though the physical properties shown in Table I may provide a means to distinguish androgen receptors from other androgen binding proteins, it is obvious that additional information is required before these macromolecules can be assigned the functional designation of "receptor." To date, the strongest arguments to suggest that these proteins are receptors are derived from genetic studies with androgen insensitive (tfm) animals, and from observations that both potentiators and inhibitors of androgen action bind to these macromolecules. These considerations are discussed in the following sections.

THE GENETICS OF THE ANDROGEN RECEPTOR

Lyon and Hawkes (11) described a mouse with testicular feminization. This disorder, like that of the rat and man (12), is transmitted by the female to half her male offspring. This pattern of inheritance, coupled with linkage studies, indicated that the tfm

TABLE II

Correlation of Androgen Responsiveness and
Androgen Receptor Activity in Normal
Male (+/y) and Female (+/+); Carrier Female (tfm/+)
and Androgen Insensitive (tfm/y) Mice

	+/+ or +/y	tfm/+	tfm/y
Androgen responsive end point[1]			
No treatment	10%	10%	10%
Androgen induced	100%	65-75%	10%
Receptor activity[2]	100%	69%	0

[1] Response expressed as percent of maximally induced normal male (+/y) or female (+/+)

[2] Receptor activity as percent of normal animals

Information summarized from references 6, 12, 14, 15.

mutation in the mouse is on the X-chromosome. Male mice with this
defect (tfm/y) are characterized by lack of androgen dependent
differentiation and by absence of a reproductive tract other than
abdominal testes. Since affected male animals have no prostate or
seminal vesicles, androgen action in these animals has been extensively studied in the kidney and submaxillary glands. Treatment
of tfm/y mice with very large doses of testosterone and other androgens produced little or no response in the parameters studied (12).
According to the Lyon hypothesis in each cell of the XX female, one
X-chromosome is inactivated, resulting in hemizygous expression of
genes on the active X-chromosome (13). Since the tfm gene is on
the X-chromosome, the androgen responsiveness of carrier females
should be variable, depending upon the percentage of normal vs.
tfm carrying X-chromosomes that are active in each target organ.
This predicted variation in androgen response was confirmed by
studies of androgen inducible proteins in kidney and submaxillary
glands of individual carrier females (14-15). Fully induced carrier
females respond only 65-75% as well as normal animals (Table II).

Several groups of investigators have demonstrated that the
androgen-receptor complex is not concentrated in nuclei of tissue
from tfm/y mice (12). These animals have been extensively studied
in our laboratory with a variety of techniques in an effort to
detect a high affinity androgen binding protein in kidney cytosol.
The assays used included dextran-coated charcoal, sucrose density
gradients, gel filtration, isoelectric focusing, and DNA-cellulose
binding. None of these techniques were able to demonstrate receptor
activity in tfm/y animals (6). By contrast, the androgen receptor
from heterozygous carrier females (tfm/+) had similar physical properties to that of normal animals (Table I). The dissociation constant (K_d) for testosterone binding to the kidney cytosol receptor
from carrier females was similar to that of normal mice: 1.3 ± 0.1
nM (mean ± S.E.M.) vs. 1.2 ± 0.1 nM for carrier and normal mice respectively. In contrast, the number of binding sites in cytosol
from carrier females was only 69% that of normal: 4.4 ± 0.2 vs.
6.4 ± 0.4 x 10^{-14} moles/mg cytosol protein. The number of binding
sites expressed as receptor activity for normal, tfm/+ and tfm/y
mice are related to the androgen responsiveness in the animals in
Table II. It is significant that the receptor content in the
carrier female is reduced to the same extent as androgen response.
These findings established an association between the tfm gene, androgen receptor activity and androgen response (6). These observations suggest that the tfm gene controls the synthesis or the
assembly of the androgen receptor. Furthermore, these studies
strongly suggest that the androgen binding protein under study in
the mouse kidney is the functional androgen receptor.

TABLE III

Androgen Metabolism in Adult Rats: Tissue Concentrations of Testosterone (T) and Dihydrotestosterone (DHT); Nuclear Androgen Uptake Following ^{3}H-Testosterone Administration; Androgen Receptor Specificity

Tissue	Tissue Androgen Concentration ng/g(a)			Nuclear Uptake Following ^{3}H-Testosterone			Androgen Receptor(b) Specificity for T vs. DHT	
	T	DHT	(Ref.)	%T	%DHT	(Ref.)		(Ref.)
Ventral prostate	2.0	2.8	(19)	15	85	(24)	T << DHT	(22)
Seminal vesicle	2.2	3.0	(19)	–	–	–	T < DHT	(73)
Epididymis	–	–	–	3	93	(25)	T << DHT	(1)
Preputial gland	–	–	–	30	70	(20)	T << DHT	(25)
Kidney	13.5	3.0	(19)	82	4	(23)	T << DHT	(12)
Hypothalamus	13.7	2.0	(19)	–	–	–	T < DHT	(26)
Pituitary	60.5	<6	(19)	63	21	(21)	T ≈ DHT	(5)
Testis	–	–	–	93	4	(c, 27)	T ≈ DHT	(5)
							T ≈ DHT	(10,28)
Levator ani muscle	7.9	<0.2	(19)	–	–	–	T < **DHT**	(4)
							T > DHT	(3)

(a) Plasma androgen levels –T– 2.5 ng/ml; DHT – <0.2 ng/ml from Reference 19.

(b) Androgen receptor – defined for the purpose of this table as a protein with the physical properties shown in Table I or as a protein extracted from isolated nuclei following androgen administration.

(c) Unpublished – G. Baker.

TABLE IV

Androgen Metabolism in Adult Mice: Nuclear Testosterone (T) and
Dihydrotestosterone (DHT) Following ^{3}H-Testosterone Administration
Compared with Steroid Specificity of the Androgen Receptor

	Nuclear Uptake Following ^{3}H-Testosterone			Androgen Receptor[a] Specificity for T vs. DHT	
	%T	%DHT	(Ref.)		(Ref.)
Seminal vesicle	13	74	(29)	T << DHT	(29)
Kidney	93	1	(30)	T ≃ DHT	(2)
Submaxillary Gland	76	9	(31)		(b)
Mammary Tumor (S115)	66	4	(32)	T ≃ DHT	(32)
	88	4	(33)		

(a)   Androgen receptor - defined for the purpose of this table as
      a protein with the physical properties shown in Table I.

(b)   An androgen binding protein has been identified which has
      many of the properties of testicular ABP (74).

STEROID SPECIFICITY OF THE ANDROGEN RECEPTOR

Binding of Dihydrotestosterone and Testosterone
to Androgen Receptors

     The classic studies of Bruchovsky and Wilson (16,17) emphasized
the important role of testosterone metabolism in androgen action on
the male reproductive tract. In prostate, testosterone is reduced
to 5α-dihydrotestosterone (DHT) and this latter steroid is believed
to be the intracellular effector of androgen action. The observations which substantiate this conclusion may be summarized as
follows: high concentrations of DHT are maintained in prostate as
a consequence of its 5α-reductase activity and the androgen receptor
which has a much higher affinity for DHT than testosterone; as a
consequence, DHT is the major androgen transferred into the nucleus
(Table III). Other tissues from the male reproductive tract and
from skin are similar to prostate with respect to these aspects of
androgen metabolism (Table III).

     Following in vivo ^{3}H-testosterone administration testosterone
(rather than DHT) is specifically concentrated in nuclei of mouse
(18) and rat (23) kidney. This observation was of particular interest

since mouse kidney has little or no 5α-reductase activity (12).
Subsequent in vitro experiments demonstrated binding of testosterone to androgen receptor from mouse kidney and further emphasized the difference in steroid specificity between prostate and
kidney. That this was primarily an organ and not a species
difference was supported by similar findings in other non-repro-
ductive tissues (Tables III and IV). These observations suggested
that testosterone was the intranuclear effector of androgen action
in some tissues. They further provided a mechanism for androgen
activation of tissues which were not able to reduce testosterone
to DHT.

The in vitro and in vivo studies of androgen metabolism and
receptor activity in mature rats and mice are summarized in Tables
III and IV. These observations suggest that androgen responsive
tissues in adult animals may be categorized according to their
5α-reductase activity and receptor specificity. Skin derivatives
and tissues of the male reproductive tract have high 5α-reductase
activity and androgen receptors which bind DHT with a higher
affinity than testosterone. In these tissues, DHT is the androgen which is transferred to the nucleus of the cell. By contrast,
many other tissues (kidney, brain, pituitary, etc.) with little or
no 5α-reductase activity have androgen receptors which bind testosterone as well as DHT. In these tissues, testosterone is usually
the dominant steroid found in the nucleus of the cell. It should
be noted, however, that not all investigators have observed these
differences in receptor specificity for testosterone and DHT between tissues (73). These findings indicate the need for a comparison of purified androgen receptors from several tissues in the
same laboratory. From the survey in Tables III and IV, we conclude
that DHT may be the major intracellular effector of androgen action
in some organs, whereas testosterone, the active androgen in others.

It is of interest to note that many of the tissues which concentrate testosterone in the nucleus respond to androgens with an
increase in RNA and protein synthesis without significant DNA synthesis. By contrast, those tissues in which the metabolite, DHT,
is concentrated in the nucleus are those in which DNA synthesis is
a component of the androgen induced response. It should be emphasized that these considerations serve only to highlight major
differences of androgen metabolism in various tissues and should
not be taken as evidence against the possibility that both testosterone and DHT can exert direct effects in a variety of tissues.

In summary, most of the above considerations suggest that the
androgen receptor in some tissues may differ from that in others.
However, in androgen insensitive tfm/y animals, all receptors are
deficient. Therefore, if the tfm gene regulates receptor activity,
then factors other than this gene must regulate individual differences in receptor steroid specificity.

Progestin - Androgen Receptor Interactions

Androgenic, Antiandrogenic, and Synandrogenic Actions of Progestins.
The ability of progestins to mimic the action of androgens has been
recognized for some time. Several studies indicate that "progestational androgenicity" is highly dependent upon the steroid as
well as the end point used. When progestins were assayed in the
adult rat, progesterone and its derivatives had only minimal androgenic effects, whereas progestins structually interrelated to 19-
nor-testosterone stimulated the male reproductive tract (34). By
contrast, both progesterone and 19-nor-testosterone derivatives
masculinize the external genitalia (35-36). In addition to their
actions on the reproductive system, a variety of progestins can
also simulate androgen action on mouse kidney (37), liver (38),
preputial glands (39), and submaxillary gland (40).

While there are numerous studies showing that progestins
stimulate androgen responsive tissue, there are few experiments
to indicate the mechanism by which this activity is initiated.
Observations of the effect of progestin in androgen insensitive
(tfm/y) mice and rats indicate that these animals also have an end
organ resistance to this class of steroids. These studies suggest
that progestin action on some androgen sensitive tissues is similar
to that of testosterone. Since the tfm animals lack an androgen
receptor, it is possible that in some tissues, progestin activation
of the cell is mediated by way of the androgen receptor (12,37).

Several progestins such as cyproterone acetate have antiandrogenic effects on the male reproductive tract (41). Inhibition of
androgen action by these steroids is related to their ability to
compete with testosterone and DHT for binding sites on intracellular
androgen receptors (42). Recent studies have also demonstrated
that cyproterone acetate will inhibit androgen action on kidney
and preputial glands. In mouse kidney, the suppression of androgen action correlates with cyproterone acetate induced inhibition
of testosterone uptake by androgen receptors and nuclei (12).
Similar observations have been reported concerning DHT displacement
from preputial gland androgen receptors (12).

In addition to the androgenic and antiandrogenic actions of
progestins, several investigators recently reported unexpected
potentiation of androgen action following administrations of
several synthetic progestins. One of the most striking examples
of this progestin-androgen interaction is produced by testosterone
and cyproterone acetate on mouse kidney (Fig. 1). When the dose
of cyproterone acetate was the same or up to 2-3 times higher than
the dose of testosterone, cyproterone acetate potentiated androgen
action. However, with increasing amounts of cyproterone acetate,
the expected antiandrogenic effect was observed (Fig. 1). The
potentiating effect of medroxyprogesterone acetate (MPA) on testo-

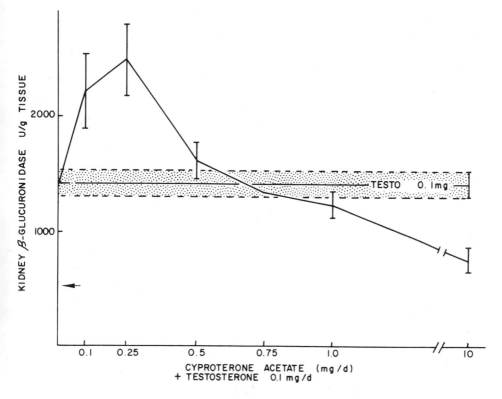

Figure 1. Syn- and antiandrogenic actions of cyproterone acetate
on kidney β- glucuronidase of female mice. Testosterone alone
(0.1 mg/d) increased β-glucuronidase 2-fold (horizontal shaded bar :
mean ± SEM). When combined with various doses of cyproterone acetate (0.1-10 mg/day), this response was first potentiated and then
inhibited (solid line - mean ± SEM). Cyproterone acetate alone
(0.1-10 mg) produced no effect in this experiment. Mice were
treated for 6 days. The arrow indicates the enzyme activity in
oil-treated control animals. Mowszowicz, et al., 1974 (37).

sterone action is shown in Fig. 2. This latter steroid also was
mildly androgenic but had no antiandrogenic properties. The potentiating effects of progestins has been termed synandrogenic and
this action has been shown to be a general property of several
progestational agents (37). To determine whether the synandrogenic
action was a function of the progestational or the antiandrogenic
activity of the steroid, 3 non-progestational antiandrogens were
tested and found to have no synandrogenic activity. From these
studies, it would appear that in vivo synandrogenic activity is
associated with progestational structure-function relationships whereas antiandrogenic activity is not (37).

There is an extensive body of information on the biologic activity of progestins from which one can formulate mechanisms for both
androgenic and antiandrogenic actions of these steroids. However,
relatively little is known about how these agents synergize with
androgens. Although it is possible that different molecular mechanisms may be involved in each of the individual actions, it would
be of interest to account for all actions by a common mechanism.
Since many progestins are known to bind to the androgen receptors
and since the androgenic and antiandrogenic actions of these compounds may be explained by direct interaction with this protein,
it is possible that the synandrogenic actions may also be mediated
in a similar manner. In this regard, allosteric models have been
proposed to explain the kinetics of an enzyme whose activity is both
potentiated and inhibited by the same ligand (43,44). A similar
system may account for the differential effects of various steroids
on tyrosine amino-transferase in hepatoma cells (45,46). If an
allosteric model is to explain both the syn- and antiandrogenic
actions of progestins, then these steroids should be able to : (a)
bind to the androgen receptor; (b) potentiate androgen binding
at low concentrations; and (c) inhibit androgen binding at high
concentrations. Studies designed to investigate these possibilities
are reviewed in the next section.

Progestin Binding to the Androgen Receptor. The fact that androgen insensitive mice do not respond to MPA suggested that androgens
and progestins may share a common receptor. To test this possibility,
$3H$-MPA was synthesized as follows : MPA was refluxed in benzene solution with 2,3,-dichloro-5,6-dicyaro-1, 4-benzoquinone to yield 6α-
methyl-17α-hydroxy-1,4-pregnandiene-3,20-dione acetate. This latter
compound was selectively reduced with tritium to yield $(1,2-{}^{3}H)$-6α-
methyl-17α-hydroxy-4-pregnene-3,20-dione acetate $({}^{3}H$-MPA$)$.

Medroxyprogesterone acetate binding to the androgen receptor
was then evaluated by incubating kidney cytosol with ^{3}H-testosterone
or ^{3}H-MPA in the presence and absence of cold steroids. Samples
were sedimented on sucrose gradients and the results are summarized
in Fig. 3. ^{3}H-testosterone and ^{3}H-MPA labeled macromolecules sedimented in the 7.9S region of the gradient. Cold testosterone and
MPA competed with both ^{3}H-ligands for their respective binding sites.
Furthermore, neither ^{3}H-testosterone nor ^{3}H-MPA was bound by kidney
cytosol from tfm/y mice. These observations are consistent with the
hypothesis that progestins bind to the androgen receptor.

In a similar set of experiments, the ability of progestins to
inhibit testosterone binding to the kidney receptor were tested.
Cyproterone acetate, MPA, megestrol acetate were all shown to be
effective inhibitors of testosterone binding. Preliminary studies
indicate that low concentrations of cyproterone acetate and MPA can
also potentiate testosterone binding to this receptor. These observations, along with studies reported above, are consistent with

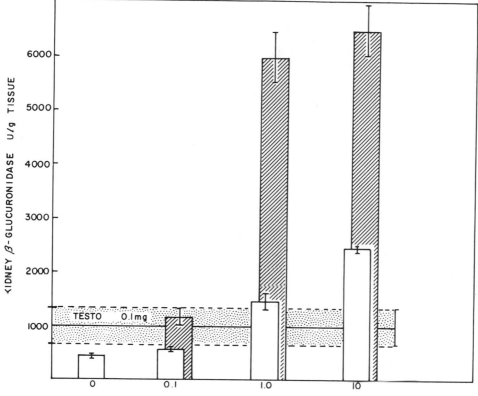

Figure 2. Effect of testosterone (0.1 mg) (horizontal bar – mean ± SEM), various doses of medroxyprogesterone acetate (open bars) and the combination of 0.1 mg testosterone plus various doses of medroxyprogesterone acetate (hashed bars) on female mouse kidney β-glucuronidase. The synandrogenic effect is obtained with 1 and 10 mg of medroxyprogesterone acetate. Mice were treated daily for 6 days. Mean ± SEM. Mowszowicz et al. 1974 (37).

the hypothesis that the androgenic, antiandrogenic and synandrogenic actions of progestins all may be mediated by way of the androgen receptor. Although the antiandrogenic effects of progestins have been demonstrated for many androgen receptors, to date, the synandrogenic action has been most extensively studied in mouse kidney. Whether this latter effect is a property of all or selected androgen receptors remains to be established. It is nonetheless important to emphasize that androgen receptors, in general, bind progestins, a property which may be used to distinguish receptors from other androgen binding proteins such as TeBG and ABP.

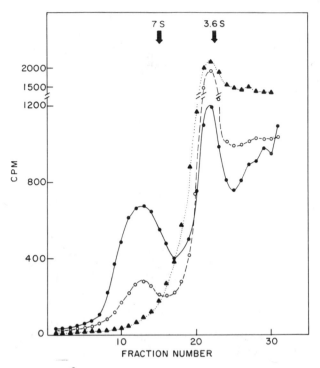

Figure 3. In vitro ^{3}H-testosterone (closed circles) and ^{3}H-medro-
xyprogesterone acetate (open circles) binding in kidney cytosol.
^{3}H-steroids were incubated with kidney cytosol from castrate mice
and analyzed on sucrose gradients. Cold medroxyprogesterone acetate
competed for ^{3}H-testosterone (closed triangles) and cold testosterone
competed for ^{3}H-medroxyprogesterone acetate (not shown). No specific
binding of ^{3}H-testosterone or ^{3}H-medroxyprogesterone acetate was
demonstrated in kidney cytoplasm of androgen insensitive (tfm/y)
mice (not shown).

BIOLOGICAL ACTIVITY OF THE STEROID RECEPTOR COMPLEX

As noted in the above sections, the physical properties and the
steroid specificity of androgen receptors have been studied extensively. Even though numerous lines of investigation indicate that
the steroid-receptor complex exerts a regulatory role on gene
transcription, there are relatively few studies which have attempted
to measure the biological activity of any steroid receptor. The
techniques used to assay steroid-receptor in cell-free systems are
summarized in Table V. Since the experiments with estrogen and glucocorticoid receptors illustrate some of the problems and technical
difficulties with this approach, these studies are reviewed along with
a critique of the experiments with the androgen receptor complex.

TABLE V

Methods Used to Study the Influence of
Steroid-Receptor Complex on In Vitro Transcriptional Events

Template/Enzyme	Description of Technique	References
Isolated nuclei	Preincubation of nuclei with hormone-labeled receptor; separation of nuclei by centrifugation and assay of nuclear RNA polymerase activities or actinomycin-D binding to nuclei	(47-51,54, 55,58-60)
Chromatin	Incubation of isolated chromatin with steroid-receptor complex and subsequent measurement of chromatin template activity with crude or partially purified mammalian and/ or bacterial RNA polymerases	(56-62)
DNA	Influence of steroid-receptor complexes on the in vitro transcription of native DNA by mammalian RNA polymerases	(52, 57, 58)

Most of the studies with the estrogen receptor complex utilized
isolated nuclei (Table V). In these experiments, uterine cytosol
fractions or nuclear extract labeled with estradiol stimulated an
increase RNA synthesis which was specific to uterine nuclei (47-50).
These studies were performed under conditions favoring nucleolar RNA
polymerase activity and the newly formed RNA was GC-rich in its
base composition (50). A salt and temperature dependent activation
of the cytosol receptor was necessary for the stimulation of RNA
synthesis (50). A major disadvantage with these studies in isolated
nuclei was that they did not allow the investigators to determine
with certainty the site of action of receptor complex (i.e., chromatin template, RNA polymerases, newly formed RNA) and this information,
if available, was derived indirectly from other studies. For example,
estrogen receptor appeared to stimulate chromatin activity when
actinomycin-D binding was used as an index for this process (51).
In addition, Jensen et al. (48,50) and Arnaud et al. (52) suggested
an estrogen receptor mediated activation of the nucleolar RNA polymerase. The recent observation that estrogen receptor bound to
RNA polymerase I of quail oviduct is compatible with this postulate; however, the molecular weight for oviduct polymerase-re-

ceptor complex was only 130,000 daltons as opposed to 500,000 daltons reported for other eukaryotic RNA polymerases. This latter observation suggests that the estrogen receptor was associated with a factor other than intact RNA polymerase I (53).

In accord with the results obtained with estrogen-receptor complexes, glucocorticoid receptor from liver cytosol has been shown to enhance RNA formation in isolated nuclei (54,55). Furthermore, recent studies by Sekeris and van der Meulen indicated that the ability of liver cortisol-receptor to activate nucleoplasmic RNA polymerase and/or chromatin persisted through a number of receptor purification steps (56). Similarly, studies from our own laboratory demonstrated that partially purified rat liver dexamethasone-receptor complex could activate liver chromatin in vitro making it a more efficient template for partially purified liver RNA polymerases I and II. In these studies, part of the stimulatory effect of the receptor on RNA synthesis remained when native DNA was substituted for chromatin as the template of RNA polymerase II (57).

The androgen receptor complex was studied by Davies and Griffiths (58-60). These investigators indicated that prostatic 5α-dihydrotestosterone-receptor complexes (cytosol 8S and 3S and nuclear 4.5S receptors) facilitated a tissue specific increase in RNA synthesis in either an isolated nuclear incubation or reconstituted chromatin-RNA polymerase assay system (Table V). In these studies, androgen receptor complex increased the RNA synthesis catalyzed by both RNA polymerase I and II. Removal of histones and the bulk of the non-histone proteins from the chromatin did not change the template activation by dihydrotestosterone-receptor complexes. However, when DNA was used instead of chromatin as the template, much smaller stimulation of RNA synthesis was observed in response to the prostatic androgen receptor complexes (58). These observations were recently confirmed and extended by Mainwaring (61) who showed that prostatic 5α-dihydrotestosterone-receptor complex preferentially stimulated elongation during the in vitro transcription of chromatin by partially purified homologous RNA polymerase II.

Our own studies examined the ability of mouse kidney testosterone-receptor complex to enhance chromatin and DNA transcription. For these studies, mammalian RNA polymerases I and II were purified from mouse, rat or pig kidney nuclei (62,63). Chromatin was prepared as previously described (63) and testosterone receptor was obtained by ammonium sulfate precipitation (33% fractional saturation) of the renal cytosol. The results of these studies are summarized in Fig. 4. Kidney testosterone receptor was able to increase kidney chromatin transcription in a concentration dependent manner in the case of both mammalian RNA polymerase I and II.

By contrast, no increase (but a slight decrease) was seen in E.
coli RNA polymerase transcription. The stimulation of chromatin
transcription by androgen receptor seemed to exhibit some tissue
specificity, since transcription of spleen chromatin was increased
to a much smaller extent (Fig. 4). Moreover, spleen cytosol "androgen receptor fraction" (prepared identically with the renal receptor)
did not bring about any significant enhancement in the transcription
of renal chromatin by any of the polymerases investigated (unpublished observations). These results provide preliminary evidence which
suggests that steroid receptor complexes can stimulate RNA synthesis
in vitro. It should be stressed, however, that all of the studies
conducted thus far have utilized relatively crude components, thus
limiting the interpretation of results. Before the role of steroid-
receptor complexes in the regulation of the transcription can be
assessed, an assay system with purified components must be devised.
Of crucial importance is the exclusion (from both receptor and RNA
polymerase preparations) of all nonreceptor factors known to stimulate transcription by nucleolar and nucleoplasmic RNA polymerases
(64-72). Moreover, the specificity of the stimulation of RNA synthesis brought about by steroid hormone-receptors remains to be
established. Finally, to our knowledge, no information is available
to exclude the possibility that steroid hormone-receptors function
in the in vitro reconstituted systems through product (RNA) stabili-
zation.

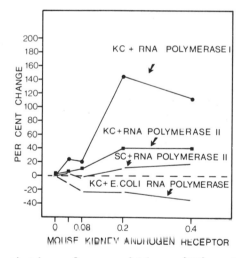

Figure 4. Transcription of mouse kidney (KC) and spleen chromatin
(SC) by renal RNA polymerases I and II as well as by E. coli RNA
polymerase in the presence of various concentrations of mouse kidney
androgen receptor (nM) expressed as testosterone bound at the beginning of the incubation. Chromatins and androgen receptor were
pre-incubated in 0.1 M KCl at 0°C for 60 min prior to the template
activity assays with various RNA polymerases. Each point represents
a mean of two separate experiments performed in triplicate.

REFERENCES

1. King, R.J.B., and Mainwaring, W.I.P., Steroid-Cell Inter-
    actions, University Park Press, Baltimore, 1974, pp. 41-101.

2. Bullock, L.P. and Bardin, C.W., Endocrinology 94: 746, 1974.

3. Jung, I., Baulieu, E.E., Nature New Biology 237: 24, 1972.

4. Krieg, M., Szalay, R., and Voigt, K.D., J. Steroid Biochem. 5:
    453, 1974.

5. Naess, O., Attramadal, A., and Aakvaag, A., Endocrinology 96:
    1, 1975.

6. Bullock, L.P., Mainwaring, W.I.P., Bardin, C.W., Endocrinol.
    Res. Comm., In press, 1975.

7. Hansson, V, Ritzen, E.M., Weddington, S.C., McLean, W.S.,
    Tindall, D.J., Nayfeh, S.N., and French, F.S., Endocrinology
    95: 690, 1974.

8. Mercier-Bodard, C., Alfsen, A., and Baulieu, E.-E, Karolinska
    Symposia on Research Methods in Reproductive Endocrinology,
    2nd Symposium, March 23-25, 1970.

9. Corvol, P.L., Chrambach, A., Rodbard, D., and Bardin, C.W.,
    J. Biol. Chem. 246: 3435, 1971.

10. Hansson, V. Trygstad, O., French, F.S., McLean, W.S., Smith, A.A.,
    Tindall, D.J., Weddington, S.C., Petrusz, P., Nayfeh, S.N., and
    Ritzen, E.M., Nature 250: 387, 1974.

11. Lyon, M.F., and Hawkes, S.G., Nature (London) 227: 1217, 1970.

12. Bardin, C.W., Bullock, L.P., Sherins, R.J., Mowszowicz, I., and
    Blackburn, W.R., Rec. Progr. Horm. Res. 29: 65, 1973.

13. Lyon, M.F., Biol. Rev. 47: 1, 1972.

14. Ohno, S., and Lyon, M.F., Clin. Genetics 1: 121, 1970.

15. Lyon, M.F., Hendry, I., and Short, R.V., J. Endocr. 58: 357, 1973.

16. Bruchovsky, N., and Wilson, J.D., J. Biol. Chem. 243: 2012, 1968.

17. Bruchovsky, N., and Wilson, J.D., J. Biol. Chem. 243: 5853, 1968.

18. Bullock, L.P., Bardin, C.W., and Ohno, S., Biochem. Biophys.
     Res. Commun. 44: 1537, 1971.

19. Robel, P., Corpechot, C., and Baulieu, E.-E., FEBS Letters 33:
     218, 1973.

20. Bullock, L.P. and Bardin, C.W., J. Steroid Biochem. 4: 139,
     1973.

21. Thieulant, M.L., Samperez, S., and Jouan, P., J. Steroid
     Biochem. 4: 677, 1973.

22. Liao, S., Liang, T., Fang, S., Castaneda, E., and Shao, T.C.,
     J. Biol. Chem. 248: 6154, 1973.

23. Ritzen, E.M., Nayfeh, S.N., French, F.S., and Aronin, P.A.,
     Endocrinology 91: 116, 1972.

24. Anderson, K.M., and Liao, S., Nature 219: 277, 1968.

25. Blaquier, J.A., Biochem. Biophys. Res. Commun. 45: 1076, 1971.

26. Suzuki, K., and Tamaoki, B., Steroids Lipids Res. 4: 266, 1973.

27. Mulder, E., Peters, M.J., van Beurden, W.M.O., and van der Molen,
     H.J., FEBS Letters 47: 209, 1974.

28. Mulder, E., Peters, M.J., DeVries, J., van der Molen, H.J.,
     Molecular and Cellular Endocrin. 2: 171, 1975.

29. Mainwaring, W.I.P., and Mangan, F.R., J. Endocr. 59: 121, 1973.

30. Bullock, L.P. and Bardin, C.W., Steroids 25: 107, 1975.

31. Goldstein, J.L. and Wilson, J.D., J. Clin. Invest. 51: 1647, 1972.

32. Gordon, J., Smith, J.A., and King, R.J.B., Molecular and Cellu-
     lar Endocrin. 1: 259, 1974.

33. Bruchovsky, N., Biochem. J. 127: 561, 1972.

34. Edgren, R.A., Jones, R.C., and Peterson, D.L., Fertil. Steril.
     18: 238, 1967.

35. Suchowsky, G.K., and Junkmann, K., Endocrinology 68: 341, 1961.

36. Revesz, C., Chappel, C.I., and Gaudry, R., Endocrinology 66:
     140, 1960.

37. Mowszowica, I., Bieber, D.E., Chung, K.W., Bullock L.P. and
     Bardin, C.W., Endocrinology 95: 1589, 1974.

38. Fahim, M.S., and Hall, D.G., Amer. J. Obstet. Gynecol. 106: 124, 1970.

39. Huggins, C., Parsons, F.M., and Jensen, E.V., Endocrinology 57: 25, 1955.

40. Desclin, J. Jr., CR Acad. Sci. (Paris) 264: 1494, 1967.

41. Neumann, F., von Berswordt-Wallrabe, R., Elger, W., Steinbeck, H., Hahn, J.D., and Kramer, M., Rec. Progr. Horm. Res. 26: 337, 1970.

42. Fang, S., Anderson, K.M., and Liao, S., J. Biol. Chem. 244: 6584, 1969.

43. Monod, J., Wyman, J., and Changeux, J.-P., J. Mol. Biol. 12: 88, 1965.

44. Rubin, M.M., and Changeux, J.-P., J. Mol. Biol. 21: 265, 1966.

45. Samuels, H.H., and Tomkins, G.M., J. Mol. Biol. 52: 57, 1970.

46. Rousseau, G.G., Baxter, J.D., and Tomkins, G.M., J. Mol. Biol. 67: 99, 1972.

47. Raynaud-Jammett, C., and Baulieu, E.-E., CR Acad. Sci. (Paris) 268: 3211, 1969.

48. Mohla, S., DeSombre, E.R., and Jensen, E.V., Biochem. Biophys. Res. Commun. 46: 661, 1972.

49. DeSombre, E.R., Mohla, S., and Jensen, E.V., Biochem. Biophys. Res. Commun. 48: 1601, 1972.

50. Jensen, E.V., Brecher, P.I., Mohla, S., and DeSombre, E.R., Acta Endocr. 177: Suppl. 191, 159, 1974.

51. Leclercq, G. Hulin, N., and Heuson, J.C., Europ. J. Cancer 9: 681, 1973.

52. Arnaud, M., Beziat, Y., Borgna, J.L., Guilleux, J.C., and Mousseron-Canet, M., Biochim. Biophy. Acta 254: 241, 1971.

53. Muller, W.E.G., Totsuka, A., and Zahn, R.K., Biochim. Biophys. Acta 366: 224, 1974.

54. Bottoms, G.D., Stith, R.D., and Roesel, O.F., Proc. Soc. Exptl. Biol. Med. 140: 946, 1972.

55. Ribarac-Stepnic, N., Trajkovic, D., and Kanazir, D., Steroids 22: 155, 1973.

56. Sekeris, C.E., and van der Meulen, N., Acta Endocr. 177: Suppl.
     191, 1973, 1974.

57. Jacob, S.T., Janne, O., and Rose, K.M., In Regulation of Growth
     and Differentiated Function in Eukaryote Cells, Talwar, G.P.
     (ed.), Raven Press, New York, In press, 1975.

58. Davies, P., and Griffiths, K., Biochem. J. 136: 611, 1973.

59. Davies, P., and Griffiths, K., Biochem. J. 140: 565, 1974.

60. Davies, P., and Griffiths, K., J. Endocr. 62: 385, 1974.

61. Mainwaring, W.I.P., J. Steroid Biochem., In press, 1975.

62. Jacob, S.T., Janne, O., and Sajdel-Sulkowska, E.M., In
     Isozymes, Vol. 3: Developmental Biology, Markert, C.L. (ed.),
     Academic Press, New York, In press, 1975.

63. Janne, O., Bardin, C.W., and Jacob, S.T., Submitted for publi-
     cation, 1975.

64. Stein, H., and Hausen, P., Europ. J. Biochem. 14: 270, 1970.

65. Lentfer, D., and Lezius, A.G., Europ. J. Biochem. 30: 278, 1972.

66. Higashinakagawa, T., Oniski, T., and Muramatsa, M., Biochem.
     Biophys. Res. Commun. 48: 937, 1972.

67. Froehner, S.C., and Bonner, J., Biochem. 12: 3064, 1973.

68. Sugden, B., and Keller, W., J. Biol. Chem. 248: 3777, 1973.

69. Lee, S.-C., and Dahmus, M.E., Proc. Nat. Acad. Sci. 70: 1383,
     1973.

70. Seifart, K.H., Juhasz, P.P., and Benecke, B.J., Europ. J.
     Biochem. 33: 181, 1973.

71. Banks, S.P., Gilbert, B.E., and Johnson, T.C., Life Sci. 14:
     303, 1974.

72. Chuang, R. Chuang, L., and Laszlo, J., Biochem. Biophys. Res.
     Commun. 57: 1231, 1974.

73. Krieg, M., Steins, P., Szalay, R., and Voigt, K.D., J. Steroid
     Biochem. 5: 87, 1974.

74. Dunn, J.F., Goldstein, J.L., and Wilson, J.D., J. Biol. Chem.
     248: 7819, 1973.

ANDROGEN RECEPTOR IN RAT TESTIS

A.A. Smith, W.S. McLean, S.N. Nayfeh, and F.S. French

Departments of Pediatrics, Biochemistry, and The
Laboratories for Reproductive Biology, University of
North Carolina, School of Medicine, Chapel Hill,
North Carolina 27514 U.S.A.;

Vidar Hansson, Institute of Pathology, Rikshospitalet,
Oslo, Norway;

Martin Ritzen, Karolinska Institutet, Stockholm, Sweden

Testosterone, in large doses, maintains spermatogenesis following hypophysectomy (1,2), suggesting a direct effect on the
testis. Androgen target cells in other organs such as prostate
(3-8), epididymis (9-14), and seminal vesicles (15) have been shown
to contain receptor proteins for 5α-dihydrotestosterone (DHT) and
testosterone (T). It is believed that androgenic stimuli to target
cells are mediated through such receptor proteins.

The androgen-receptor complexes formed in cytoplasm have been
reported to be translocated into nuclei (16-18), where they bind to
chromatin (17,19) and stimulate the synthesis of RNA (20,21). We
have recently demonstrated the presence of such receptor proteins
for T and DHT in the rat testis (22-24). This receptor is shown to
have properties similar to cytoplasmic receptors in prostate and
epididymis, but different from the androgen binding protein, ABP,
a secretory product of the seminiferous tubule, presumed to be
formed in the Sertoli cell (25-31).

MATERIALS AND METHODS

Materials

1,2,6,7-^{3}H-testosterone (91 Ci/mMole, ^{3}H-T) and 1,2-^{3}H-5α-

dihydrotestosterone (44 Ci/mMole, 1,2-^{3}H-DHT) were obtained from New
England Nuclear Corporation (Footnote 1). 1,2,4,5,6,7-^{3}H-dihydro-
testosterone (100 Ci/mMole, ^{3}H-DHT) was obtained from Amersham-Searle.
Radiochemical purity was checked by thin layer chromatography on
Brinkman precoated sheets of silica gel GF-254 in methylene
chloride:diethyl ether (4:1, v/v). Aluminum oxide gel (E. Merck)
was obtained from Brinkman. Cyproterone acetate was obtained from
Schering A.G., Berlin. Acrylamide, N,N,N',N'-tetramethyl-
ethylenediamine (TEMED) and N,N'-methylene-bis-acrylamide (Bis) were
obtained from Mann Research Laboratories. P-chloromercuriphenylsulfonate (PCMPS) was obtained from Sigma Chemical Co. PCMPS was
dissolved in water as a 10 mM solution immediately before mixing with
the supernatant. Dry charcoal (Norit-A) was obtained from Matheson,
Coleman and Bell. Ribonuclease-A (RNase) and bovine serum albumin
(BSA) were obtained from Sigma Chemical Co., neuroaminidase from
Worthington Biochemical Corporation, Deoxyribonuclease I (DNase)
1430 Kunitz Units/mg protein and Pronase from Calbiochem. Medium
199 was obtained from Grand Island Biological Company. Ampholyte
solution (pH 3-10) was obtained from LKB. Insta-Gel was from Packard
Instruments Company. Stanley-Gumbreck androgen insensitive rats
were obtained from Introgene Lab., Oklahoma City. All rats were
hypophysectomized by Hormone Assay Laboratories, Chicago, Ill.

Preparation of animals and labeling tissues

Sprague-Dawley rats were hypophysectomized at 25, 35, 40, 50
or 60 days of age. After various postoperative periods (3-60 days),
the animals were eviscerated and functionally hepatectomized (32,33),
and ^{3}H-testosterone (50 μCi) in 0.25 ml of 15% EtOH in normal saline
was injected via the femoral vein. After 3 hr, the animals were
sacrificed by decapitation. Blood was collected and immediately
chilled in ice. Organs were removed, trimmed of excess fat, and
placed in saline at 0-2 C.

To separate seminiferous tubules from the interstitial tissue
of immature rats, the testicular capsule was removed and the tubules
gently teased apart and washed repeatedly with Hank's salts (total
of 100 ml/testis). The initial washings, containing interstitial
cells, were collected on ice. Seminiferous tubules from rats hypophysectomized at 50 days of age were purified by the manual
dissection method of Christensen and Mason (34).

Preparation of labeled supernatants and nuclei

In vivo labeled tissue was minced and homogenized in 3 or 4
volumes of 50 mM Tris-HCl buffer, pH 7.4 at 4 C, containing 3 mM
MgCl$_2$ and 0.32 M sucrose (TSM) using either a Teflon-glass Potter-
Elvehjem or an all-glass Duall homogenizer. Nuclei were sedimented
at 600 g for 10 minutes. Crude nuclear pellets were resuspended

in TSM buffer containing 0.2% Triton X-100 and resedimented as above. Pellets were resuspended in 10 volumes of 2.0 M sucrose in TSM buffer and centrifuged at 20,000 RPM for 1 hr in a Spinco SW-27 rotor. The pellets were washed repeatedly by suspending in 10 volumes of TSM until a constant amount of radioactivity was removed in successive washes.

Androgen-receptor complexes were extracted from purified nuclei by homogenizing in TKE buffer (20 mM Tris, pH 7.6 at 4°, containing 1.0 M KCl, 1.5 mM EDTA, 1 μM, T, and 1 μM DHT) and allowing to stand 2 hr at 0°. Extracts were centrifuged at 30,000 g for 45 min to obtain the supernatant containing receptor protein. In later experiments, a lower concentration of KCl (0.5 M) was used in TKE buffer since it was equally effective, extracted less DNA and caused less background interference with measurement of radioactivity.

Postnuclear supernatants were centrifuged at 105,000 x g at 0-2 C. Protein concentration in the 105,000 x g supernatants was determined by the method of Lowry et al. (35).

In vitro labeling of testis was carried out in two ways: (a) Decapsulated testes were incubated in 5 vol of medium 199 containing ^{3}H-T and/or ^{3}H-DHT (50 nM) for 2 hr at 0 C. (b) Testes were homogenized in 50 mM Tris-HCl buffer, pH 7.4 at 4 C, containing 1 mM EDTA, 0.5 mM 2-mercaptoethanol and 10% glycerol (TEMG), and 105,000 g supernatants were equilibrated with ^{3}H-T at 0 C.

Sucrose gradient centrifugation

Gradient analysis was performed according to Martin and Ames (36) using BSA as reference standard. Samples of supernatants (250 μl) were layered over 5-20% (w/v) sucrose gradients (4.4 ml) prepared in 50 mM Tris-HCl, containing 3 mM $MgCl_2$ and 10% glycerol, pH 7.4 at 4 C. Centrifugation and collection of fractions was as described previously (9).

Gel filtration

All chromatographic procedures were performed at 4 C. Columns of Sephadex G-200 were packed using hydrostatic pressure, 1 cm H_2O cm^2, increasing to 4 cm H_2O cm^2 over a 40 hr period. The columns were eluted with 0.1 M Tris-HCl buffer, pH 7.5 at 4 C, containing 0.02% NaN_3, as described in Figure 2.

Bound and unbound radioactivity were separated by chromatography on columns of Sephadex G-25. Nuclear extracts in TKE buffer were layered on 1.6 x 30 cm columns preequilibrated with TKE buffer containing a concentration of KCl equal to that of the nuclear extract. Columns were eluted at a flow rate of 1.0 ml per min.

Eighty fractions of 40 drops each (1.8 ml) were collected.

Polyacrylamide gel electrophoresis (PAGE)

Gels containing 3.25% acrylamide and 0.5% agarose were prepared by a modification of the method of Dingman _et al._ (37,10).

Isoelectric focusing

Isoelectric focusing was performed in polyacrylamide gels containing 3.5% acrylamide and 0.5% agarose as described previously
(10) with the modifications of Naess et al. (38).

Identification of labeled androgens

(a) Homogenates, 105,000 g supernatants and serum: Aliquots
of homogenates and supernatants were placed in tubes containing
carrier 5α-androstanediol, testosterone, 5α-dihydrotestosterone,
androsterone, androstenedione, and 5α-androstanedione (100 µg of
each). Steroids were extracted by the method of Folch et al. (39).
Extracts were chromatographed on silica gel GF-254 in methylene
chloride:diethyl ether (4:1). After detection of carrier steroids by
short wave ultraviolet light and iodine vapor, the area corresponding
to each carrier steroid was eluted in ethyl acetate and the radioactivity was measured by liquid scintillation counting. DHT was
further separated from androsterone by thin-layer chromatography
on highly activated aluminum oxide gel in diethyl ether.

Sera from each animal were placed in tubes containing carrier
steroids and extracted with 4 vol of methylene chloride. The extracts were dried and chromatographed on silica gel.

(b) Nuclei: Carrier androgens indicated above were added to
each pellet of purified nuclei. Steroids were extracted 3 times
with 5 ml of acetone at 45 C. Extracts were dried under nitrogen,
dissolved in diethyl ether, and washed with 0.1 vol water. The
ether was dried under nitrogen and the residues dissolved in
ethanol. Aliquots were taken for measurement of radioactivity and
for chromatography on silica gel in methylene chloride:ether
(4:1, v/v).

(c) Protein bound androgens: Polyacrylamide gel slices were
eluted in 1 ml toluene overnight at room temperature. Aliquots were
taken for measurement of radioactivity. The toluene extracts from
slices containing the receptor were pooled and carrier androgens
added. Toluene was evaporated under nitrogen at 50 C, and the
samples chromatographed on silica gel in methylene chloride:diethyl
ether (4:1, v/v).

Fractions corresponding to the peak of bound radioactivity from Sephadex G-200 supernatants or G-25 (nuclear extracts) were pooled and extracted twice with 4 vol of diethyl ether. The extracts were dried under nitrogen and chromatographed on silica gel as above. DHT was further separated from androsterone as described above.

(d) <u>Crystallization of androgens</u>: Radioactive metabolites corresponding to carrier T and DHT were recrystallized from cyclohexane:acetone and methanol:water to constant $^3H/^{14}C$ ratios after addition of ^{14}C-testosterone or ^{14}C-dihydrotestosterone.

Measurement of radioactivity

Radioactivity was measured in a Packard Tri-Carb liquid scintillation spectrometer in scintillation fluid containing 0.4%, 2,5-diphenyl-oxazole and 0.01%, 1,2-bis-2-(4-methyl-5-phenyloxyzolyl)-benzene in toluene. The radioactivity in aqueous samples was measured using Insta-Gel (Packard):toluene (1:1).

RESULTS AND DISCUSSION

THE ANDROGEN RECEPTOR IN 105,000 g SUPERNATANT (CYTOPLASMIC RECEPTOR)

Sucrose Gradient Centrifugation

Testis supernatant labeled <u>in vivo</u> with ^3H-testosterone and analyzed by sucrose gradient centrifugation formed a single peak of bound radioactivity migrating at about 7S in buffer of low ionic strength. The labeled 7S complex was destroyed by heating at 50 C for 30 min, but remained intact in the presence of an excess of unlabeled DHT after equilibration for 1 hr at 0 C.

The androgen-receptor complex in testis is similar to the epididymis and ventral prostate receptors in its sedimentation behavior (7,14) and different from rat ABP which consistently sediments as a 4.5S complex (26,27).

Gel Filtration

Chromatography of <u>in vivo</u> labeled supernatant on Sephadex G-200 in buffer of low ionic strength yielded a single peak of bound radioactivity in or close to the void volume of the column (Figure 1A). This androgen-protein complex was identical to the 7S complex with respect to temperature stability and dissociation. Binding was destroyed by heating at 50 C for 30 min prior to chromatography, and there was little or no decrease in bound

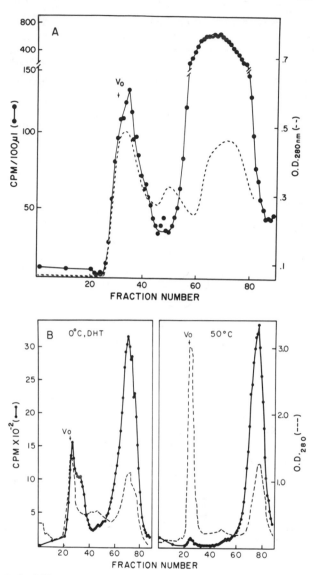

Figure 1. Gel filtration chromatography of _in vivo_ labeled testis
105,000 x g supernatant. Testicular supernatants were labeled and
prepared as in Methods. Separate 2 ml aliquots of supernatant were
(A) untreated, or (B) incubated at 0 C with a 1000 fold excess of
unlabeled DHT and heated at 50 C for 1 hr prior to chromatography
on a column of Sephadex G-200 (1.6 x 30.8 cm). The column was
eluted with 0.1 M Tris-HCl buffer, pH 7.5, 4 C, at a flow rate of
7.5 ml/hr, and fractions of 40 drops were collected. Optical density
of each fraction was measured at 280 nM and the radioactivity was
counted in Insta-Gel:toluene (1:1). ------ (OD 280). ●-----●,
radioactivity (CPM). From McLean _et al_. (24).

radioactivity after equilibration with a thousand fold excess of
unlabeled DHT for 1 hr at 0 C (Figure 1B). The elution volume
of the androgen-receptor complex from Sephadex G-200 columns suggests
a molecular radius of greater than 80 A which is similar in size
to the large forms of the cytoplasmic receptors in epididymis and
ventral prostate (5-7, 14) and different from the Stokes radius
of ABP (47 A) (14,40).

Polyacrylamide Gel Electrophoresis (PAGE)

The androgen-receptor protein in testis supernatants from
immature hypophysectomized rats had an electrophoretic mobility
identical to the cytoplasmic androgen receptors (CR) in rat
epididymis and ventral prostate (R_f = 0.4-0.5 relative to bro-
mophenol blue) and different from ABP (Figure 2). The slower moving
androgen-protein complexes (CR), like the complexes described by
sucrose gradient centrifugation and gel chromatography, were heat
sensitive (as shown below) and did not dissociate in the presence
of excess unlabeled DHT at 0 C for 1 hr.

Isoelectric Focusing

In several experiments with in vivo labeled testicular supernatants of immature hypophysectomized rats, a major peak of radioactivity focused between pH 5.5-6.0 (mean 5.8) and a minor peak
focused at pH 3.5 (Figure 3). The peak at pH 5.8 was identified as
the cytoplasmic androgen receptor by its heat sensitivity and slow
rate of dissociation at 0 C. Major peaks focusing at pH 5.8 were
also observed in labeled supernatants of prostate and epididymis (not
shown) as reported previously for the androgen receptors in these
target organs (10,44) and for a binding protein in rat testis,
presumed to be the cytoplasmic androgen receptor (42). The small
peak focusing at pH 3.5 was observed in all organs. It was not
destroyed by heating to 50 C but was not characterized further.
No peak of bound radioactivity was observed when rat serum was
focused after equilibration with ^{3}H-T or ^{3}H-DHT.

Radioactive Androgens in Serum, Testicular Homogenates and 105,000 g Supernatants

In serum, the major radioactive androgens present 3 hr after
injection of ^{3}H-T were polar metabolites remaining at the origin
of the chromatoplate (31%), androstanediol (9%), testosterone
(12%), dihydrotestosterone (11%), and androsterone (27%).
Testicular homogenates contained metabolites at origin (20%),

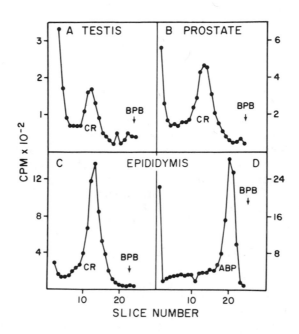

Figure 2.   Polyacrylamide gel electrophoresis of 105,000 x g supernatants of testis (a), prostate (B), epididymis (C) labeled in vivo, and epididymis (D) labeled in vitro.   Twenty-five day old rats were hypophysectomized and 8 days later were eviscerated, functionally hepatectomized and injected with 1,2,6,7-^{3}H-testosterone i.v.   The rats were killed 3 hr after the injection.   ABP was labeled in vitro by equilibrating 10 nM 1,2-^{3}H-DHT in charcoal (1 mg/mg protein) extracted epididymal supernatants.   Aliquots (100 μl) of in vivo and in vitro labeled supernatants were run in 3.5% acrylamid gels containing 0.5% agarose using Tris-glycine buffer, pH 8.6 at 0-2 C.   Bromphenol blue (BPB) was used as marker and allowed to migrate to the end of the gels.   Gels were sliced in 2.3 mm segments, and the radioactivity extracted overnight at room temperature in toluene counting solution.   From McLean et al. (24).

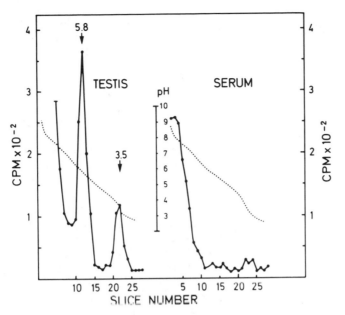

Figure 3. Isoelectric focusing of 105,000 x g supernatant from testis of hypophysectomized rats and serum in 3.5% acrylamide gels containing 0.5% agarose and 2% ampholines. Testes were homogenized in 4 vol TEMG buffer. Rat serum was diluted 1:10 in TEMG buffer. Testis supernatant containing 8 mg/ml protein and serum were equilibrated with 1 nM ^{3}H-T for 16 hr at 0 C and 0.1 ml aliquots of each were focused on 5 x 70 mm gels as described under Methods. From McLean et al. (24).

Table 1

Radioactive Androgens in Rat Testicular 105,000 g Supernatants[*] 3 hr After Injection of 1,2,6,7-^{3}H-Testosterone, I.V.

Percentage of Total Radioactivity Recovered from the Chromatoplates

Metabolites at origin	Experiment #			
	1	2	3	4
5α-androstanediol	12	16	25	17
Testosterone	58	56	45	54
Dihydrotestosterone	3	9	12	9
Androsterone	5	6	12	5
Androstenedione	3	3	2	4
5α-androstanedione	2	2	1	1

[*]Rats hypophysectomized at 25-30 days of age, 10 days prior to the experiments.

androstanediol (28%); and testosterone (36%), as the major fractions of the total radioactivity (Footnote 1). In 105,000 g super-natants, the distribution of radioactivity among carrier androgens was similar, as shown in Table 1.

Androgen Specificity of the Cytoplasmic Receptor

Studies in vivo: Bound and free radioactive androgens in testicular supernatants were separated by chromatography on Sephadex G-200 or G-25 or by PAGE (Table 2). Radioactive androgens were identified by thin layer chromatography and crystallization to constant specific activity. Only ^{3}H-T and ^{3}H-DHT were bound to the receptor even though the free fractions contained substantial amounts of radioactivity chromatographing at the origin or with carrier androstanediol and androsterone. More ^{3}H-T than ^{3}H-DHT was found; however, the amounts of ^{3}H-T in total supernatant (Table 1) and in unbound fractions (Table 2) were greater than ^{3}H-DHT, indicating that more ^{3}H-T might be available for binding. In these same experiments the relative amounts of ^{3}H-T and ^{3}H-DHT bound and un-bound in epididymis supernatant were in striking contrast with testis. Radioactivity bound to the receptor was 98% ^{3}H-DHT and on-ly 2% ^{3}H-T. Moreover, ^{3}H-DHT was the major metabolite present in extracts of total radioactivity in epididymal supernatants. These finding are in agreeement with previous in vivo studies in rat epi-didymis (9) and prostate (8) showing that ^{3}H-DHT is a major metabo-lite in supernatant after injection of ^{3}H-T and that ^{3}H-DHT is also the major androgen bound by the cytoplasmic receptors in these or-gans (4-9, 14).

Studies in vitro: The metabolism and binding of ^{3}H-T and ^{3}H-DHT were examined further in vitro. Testes from immature hypo-physectomized rats were decapsulated and incubated for 1 hr at 0 C in a medium containing equimolar amounts of ^{3}H-T and ^{3}H-DHT. Fol-lowing the incubation, tubules were washed and homogenized. 105,000 g supernatant fractions were prepared and binding was analyzed by chromatography on Sephadex G-25. Bound radioactivity was 80% ^{3}H-T and 20% ^{3}H-DHT (Table 3); however, relatively little ^{3}H-DHT remained in the free fraction at the termination of the incubation, indicating that it was metabolized rapidly at 0 C. In subsequent experiments, we have shown that ^{3}H-DHT is rapidly converted to andro-stanediol when incubated with 105,000 g supernatant of immature rat testis at 0 C. The apparent lower affinity of the testis receptor for ^{3}H-DHT might, therefore, result from its conversion to an androgen which is not bound by the receptor.

Table 2

Bound and Unbound Radioactive Androgens in Testicular 105,000 g Supernatant 3 h

After Injection of 1,2,6,7-³H-Testosterone I.V.

Experiment No.	Hypophysectomy Age*	Post-op period days	Percentage of total radioactivity recovered from the chromatoplates						
			Polar	5α-Androstanediol	Testosterone	Dihydrotestosterone	Androsterone	Androstenedione	5α-Androstanedione
			Bound						
1	25	8			60	40			
2	25	8			81	19			
3	45	3			61	38			
4	25	15			80	20			
			Unbound						
2	25	8	12	29	44	10**	3	2	1
3	40	3	26	6	50	11**		4	3
4	25	15	12	34	46	5		2	1

*Refers to age at hypophysectomy and postoperative days until experiment.
**Dihydrotestosterone and Androsterone not separated.

From McLean et al. (24).

Table 3

Binding to the Androgen Receptor In Vitro[*]

	% of total radioactivity recovered from chromatoplates	
	Bound to Receptor	Free
Metabolites at origin		1
5α-androstanediol		35
Testosterone	80	55
Dihydrotestosterone	20	4
Androsterone		1
Androstenedione		2
5α-androstanedione		2

[*]Relative amounts of bound and free androgens in 105,000 g supernatant after incubation of rat testis with equimolar concentrations (50 nM) of ^{3}H-testosterone and ^{3}H-dihydrotestosterone.
Bound radioactivity was analyzed after Sephadex G-25 chromatography on two columns in succession.

Saturability of the Cytoplasmic Receptor

Studies in vivo: A limited binding capacity characteristic
of steroid receptors was demonstrated by injection of nonlabeled
testosterone 5 min prior to the injection of ^{3}H-testosterone (100
μCi/rat). Animals were sacrificed after 3 hr and binding was
analyzed by PAGE. Accumulation of radioactivity in testis supernatant was not influenced by unlabeled testosterone (60 times the
weight of ^{3}H-T); however, binding of labeled androgen to the cytoplasmic androgen receptor was abolished. Complete inhibition of
labeled androgen binding was also noted after prior injection of the
anti-androgen, cyproterone acetate (1000 times the weight of ^{3}H-T).

Studies in vitro: Saturation of androgen receptor sites in
testicular supernatants was demonstrated in vitro after equilibration at 0 C with ^{3}H-T. Binding sites were almost saturated
at a concentration of 3 nM (Figure 4). A single class of high
affinity sites with an apparent K_D of 7×10^{-10} M was indicated
by Scatchard analysis. From the intercept with the x-axis, the
testicular supernatant was estimated to contain about 10 fmoles of
available receptor sites per mg of supernatant protein (assuming
one binding site per molecule of binding protein).

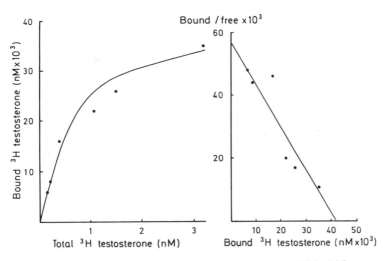

Figure 4. Saturation of androgen receptors in 105,000 g supernatants of testicular homogenates. Rats were hypophysectomized
at 60 days of age and studied 60 days later. ^{3}H-T in several
concentrations up to 3 nM was equilibrated in 0.5 ml supernatant
(4.9 mg protein/ml) for 16 hr at 0 C, and receptor binding was
analyzed in 0.2 ml aliquots by PAGE as described in Methods.
Left: Plot of bound radioactivity versus concentration of total
testosterone. Right: Scatchard plot of bound/free versus concentration of bound testosterone. The equilibrium constant of
dissociation (K_D), 7×10^{-10} M, was calculated from the x and y
intercepts of the regression line which are equal to n (the number
of binding sites) and n/K_D, respectively. From McLean et al. (24).

Susceptibility of Receptor to Heat, Degradative
Enzymes, and Sulfhydryl Reagent

The temperature stability of the testicular androgen receptor
(CR) was similar to the cytoplasmic receptors (CR) in epididymis
and prostate. Cytosol fractions labeled in vivo with ^{3}H-testo-
sterone were incubated at various temperatures prior to measurement
of binding by PAGE. Binding to CR in prostate, epididymis, and
testis was unaffected by 25 C but destroyed completely by heating
at 50 C for 30 min. In contrast to the receptors, binding to
ABP was not influenced by heating at 50 C, but was destroyed at
60 C for 30 min.

Binding to the androgen receptor in testis supernatant
labeled in vivo was destroyed by incubation at 0 C for 10 min with

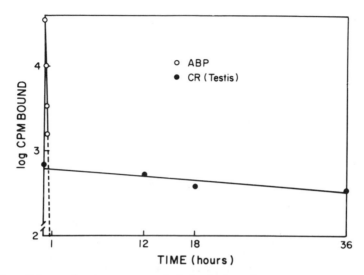

Figure 5.   Dissociation rate of labeled androgen-receptor complexes
in testis supernatant in comparison with ^{3}H-DHT-ABP complexes.
Twenty-five day old rats were hypophysectomized and sacrificed 8
days later.   Testis supernatant was equilibrated with 2 nM ^{3}H-DHT
and chromatographed on Sephadex G-200.   The peak fractions of bound
radioactivity were pooled and aliquoted.   Unlabeled DHT (1000 nM)
was added to separate aliquots at time 0 and specific binding was
assayed on Sephadex G-25 columns at 12, 18, and 36 hr after the
addition of the unlabeled DHT.   ABP was labeled in charcoal adsorbed
epididymal supernatants from intact rats by equilibration with
10 nM 1,2-^{3}H-DHT.   Unlabeled DHT (3000 nM) was added to separate
aliquots at time 0 and specific binding was assayed by Sephadex G-25
after 1, 5, 10, and 20 min.   The Sephadex G-25 columns were equilibrated and eluted with 0.1 M Tris-HCl (pH 7.4) containing 0.02%
NaN$_3$.   From McLean et al. (24).

Pronase (100 µg/ml), but not with neuraminidase (500 µg/ml), RNase (100 µg/ml), or DNase (100 µg/ml). Androgen receptors in epididymis and prostate, as well as the androgen binding protein (ABP), responded similarly to these enzymes (10,14). Exposure to the sulfhydryl reagent, p-chloromercuriphenylsulfonate (PCMPS) 1 mM for 1 hr at 0 C decreased receptor binding by more than 50% but did not eliminate it completely. Binding to ABP, on the other hand, was unaffected by a similar concentration of PCMPS.

Dissociation Rate of Androgen-Receptor Complexes

A characteristic feature of androgen-receptor complexes in epididymis and prostate is their slow rate of dissociation at 0 C (10). The labeled androgen-receptor complex in testicular supernatant was shown to have a similar slow dissociation rate (Figure 5). In these experiments, testicular supernatants were prepared from immature hypophysectomized rats after labeling in vivo with ^{3}H-T. A large excess of unlabeled dihydrotesterone or testosterone (1000 x amount of radioactive androgen) was added to prevent re association of labeled androgen, and binding was measured by chromatography on Sephadex G-25. The slow dissociation rate of labeled androgen-receptor complexes was in striking contrast to the very rapid dissociation of ^{3}H-DHT-ABP complexes.

The Nuclear Receptor

Nuclear accumulation of radioactive androgens in testis of immature hypophysectomized rats was compared with other tissues after injection of ^{3}H-T I.V. as shown in Figure 6. Accumulation of androgen in testis nuclei was less than in epididymal nuclei but greater than in kidney or submandibular gland. In the androgen insensitive rat, only negligible amounts of radioactivity were present in nuclei of testis as well as kidney.

The radioactivity remaining in testis nuclei after purification through 2.0 M sucrose and extensive washing was extracted completely in buffer containing 0.5-1.0 M KCl (TKE buffer). Chromatography of the nuclear KCl extracts on columns of Sephadex G-25 yielded a peak of bound radioactive androgens in the void volume of the column well separated from free radioactive androgens (Figure 7). This salt extractable androgen-receptor complex in testis nuclei had a sedimentation coefficient of 3-4S as determined by centrifugation on 5-20% sucrose gradients (22).

When bound and unbound steroids in testicular supernatants were separated on Sephadex G-25 or G-200 columns, ^{3}H-T and ^{3}H-DHT were shown to be bound selectively by the cytoplasmic receptor (Table 4).

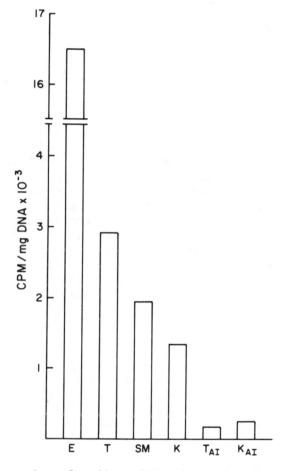

Figure 6. Retention of radioactivity by nuclei from various tissues of immature hypophysectomized rats 3 hr following injection of ^{3}H-T I.V. Nuclei were purified, and the radioactivity extracted in acetone. DNA was measured in the residues as described under Methods. Epididymis (E), Testis (T), Submandibular gland (SM), Kidney (K), testis of androgen insensitive rat (T_{AI}), Kidney of androgen insensitive rat (K_{AI}). From Smith et al. (23).

Table 4

Radioactive Androgens in 105,000 g Supernatants and Nuclei of Immature* Rat Testis 3 hr After Injection of ³H-T I.V.

	Experiment 1			Experiment 2			Experiment 3		
	Supernatant		Nuclei	Supernatant		Nuclei	Supernatant		Nuclei
	Unbound	Bound	Bound	Unbound	Bound	Total	Unbound	Bound	Total
Metabolites at origin	26			30			10		4
Androstanediol	6	61	56	41			29	84	5
T	50			16	27	30	42		85
Androsterone	**			**			3	1	
DHT	11	38	44	13	73	70	13	11	5
Δ⁴-androstenedione	4			1			2	2	1
5α-androstanedione	3			1			1	2	
Nonpolar†	1			1			1		

*Rats hypophysectomized at 25-35 days of age and experiments performed 7-14 days later.

**Not separated from DHT.

†Nonpolar = radioactive steroids at or near the solvent front.

From Smith et al. (23).

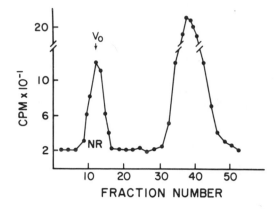

Figure 7. Gel filtration chromatography of 0.5 M KCl extract of purified testis nuclei. Eight rats were hypophysectomized at 30 days of age and studied 10 days later. They were eviscerated, hepatectomized and injected with 50 µCi ^{3}H-T I.V. as described in Methods. Crude nuclear pellets from 3.6 g of testis were washed in 0.2% Triton X-100 in TSM buffer and sedimented through 2.0 M sucrose. The pellets were washed 5 times by suspending in TSM buffer and extracted in TKE buffer. The extract was chromatographed on Sephadex G-25 as described in Methods. From Smith et al. (23).

Likewise, ^{3}H-T and ^{3}H-DHT were the only labeled androgens bound in TKE extracts of purified nuclei. The ratio of bound ^{3}H-T to bound ^{3}H-DHT was similar in supernatant and nuclear fractions as shown in Table 4.

Saturability of the nuclear androgen binding protein was examined by injecting a 60-fold greater amount of unlabeled T 5 min before ^{3}H-T. Accumulation of radioactivity in 105,000 g supernatant was reduced by only 17%; however, nuclear accumulation of radioactivity was decreased by 85%, and receptor binding in supernatant and nuclei was abolished (Table 5). Injection of a 1000 fold greater amount of cyproterone acetate 5 min before ^{3}H-T did not influence total radioactivity in supernatant but reduced total nuclear radioactivity by 83%. The reduction in nuclear accumulation of radioactive androgens was again associated with total elimination of binding of radioactive androgens to receptors in cytoplasm and nuclei.

The nuclear androgen binding component, like the cytoplasmic androgen receptor, was found to be a heat labile protein. Binding was destroyed completely by heating nuclei to 50 C for 30 min or by treatment with the proteolytic enzyme, Pronase. Binding was unaffected by DNase.

Table 5

Inhibition of Radioactive Androgen Accumulation in Testis Nuclei In Vivo

	Supernatant Radioactivity cpm/ml		Nuclear Radioactivity cpm/mg DNA	
	Total[†]	Bound[1]	Total[††]	Bound[2]
Control *[3]H-T (0.308 µg/rat)	5.2×10^4	6.5×10^3	1.3×10^4	0.26×10^4
Testosterone *[3]H-T (0.308 µg/rat) **T (18.5 µg/rat)	4.3×10^4	-0-	0.2×10^4	-0-
Control *[3]H-T (0.154 µg/rat)	9.4×10^4	3.8×10^3	1.8×10^3	0.7×10^3
Cyproterone Acetate (CA) *[3]H-T (0.154 µg/rat) **CA (250 µg/rat)	9.5×10^4	-0-	0.3×10^3	-0-

* Rats were sacrificed 3 hr after injection of $1,2,6,7-^3$H-testosterone I.V.

** Injected I.V. 5 min before ^{3}H-T.

† Total radioactivity in 105,000 g supernatant.

†† Total radioactivity extracted from purified nuclei.

(1) Binding measured by polyacrylamide gel electrophoresis.

(2) Binding measured by chromatography on Sephadex G-25 column.

The rate of dissociation of androgen-protein complexes in testis nuclei was similar to that of the androgen-receptor complexes in testis cytoplasm. When salt extracts of in vivo labeled testis nuclei were incubated at 0 C in the presence of a large excess of unlabeled T and DHT to prevent reassociation of labeled androgens, there was only a small decrease in bound radioactivity after a period of several hours.

The nuclear androgen receptor in rat testis therefore has certain properties similar to the cytoplasmic androgen receptor. It binds T and DHT in ratios similar to the ratios bound to the cytoplasmic receptor. Its androgen binding sites are saturable and can be inhibited by the anti-androgen, cyproterone acetate. It is heat sensitive, and forms complexes with androgen which dissociate very slowly at 0°.

Androgen receptor complexes in testis nuclei resist extraction in low ionic strength buffers but are extractable in 0.5 M KCl, suggesting an interaction with chromatin. Conditions required to extract these receptor complexes from testis nuclei are similar to those used for extraction of androgen receptors from nuclei of prostate and epididymis (3,6,9).

The finding that androgen receptors in rat testis bind ^{3}H-T as well as ^{3}H-DHT after labeling in vivo is in agreement with the recent reports by Mulder et al. (43,44). Under similar conditions of labeling in vivo, androgen receptors in epididymis and prostate (8) bind ^{3}H-DHT to a much greater extent than T. In testis, it appears likely that the androgen receptor has a similar affinity for T and DHT. The relative amounts of T and DHT bound are probably determined by the concentrations of unbound T and DHT available to receptor sites, this being controlled by the rates of T and DHT metabolism. In rat ventral prostate, ^{3}H-T is rapidly converted to ^{3}H-DHT, thus less ^{3}H-T is available for binding (45,46). When binding to the prostate receptor was measured after short periods of labeling with ^{3}H-T in vivo, however, Rennie and Bruchovsky found nearly as much ^{3}H-T as ^{3}H-DHT bound to the receptor (47). These same authors have pointed out that competition studies in vitro may not accurately reflect the in vivo affinity of the prostate receptor for T relative to DHT (8).

Unbound radioactivity in TKE extracts of purified testis nuclei was almost exclusively ^{3}H-T and ^{3}H-DHT indicating that these androgens accumulated via a selective mechanism. Although much of this fraction may have resulted from receptor degradation during extraction it is equally possible that it might represent a physiological pool resulting from the intranuclear dissociation of androgen-receptor complexes during the process of metabolic turnover (47).

ANDROGEN RECEPTORS IN CYTOPLASM (CR) AND NUCLEI (NR)

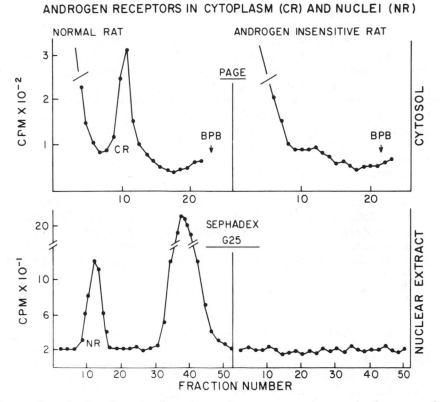

Figure 8. Lack of cytoplasmic androgen receptor and absence of nuclear accumulation of radioactivity in the Stanley–Gumbreck androgen–insensitive rat. Rats were hypophysectomized at 30 days of age and studied 10 days later. Testes were labeled by injection of ³H-testosterone I.V. 50 µCi/rat and supernatants analyzed by gel electrophoresis as in Figure 2. Nuclei were purified, extracted with TKE buffer and chromatographed on Sephadex G-25 as described in Figure 7.

Evidence that the cytoplasmic receptor has an essential role in the nuclear accumulation of androgen has been obtained from studies on the androgen insensitive (Stanley–Gumbreck) rat. This rat, with a congenital defect in target cell response to androgen has been shown to lack the ability to accumulate androgen in target cell nuclei of such tissues as kidney and preputial gland (48,49). The lack of androgen accumulation in nuclei is associated with a total absence of cytoplasmic androgen receptors (49). Similar results are obtained in testis of the androgen insensitive rat (Figure 8). Hypophysectomized androgen insensitive rats were injected with tritiated testosterone, and binding in supernatant and nuclei was examined. The presence of the cytoplasmic androgen receptor was demonstrated in the normal male littermate by gel electrophoresis, but there was a conspicuous absence of receptor in the androgen insensitive rat testis. In normal male littermates nuclear radioactivity extracted with 0.4 M KCl was bound to receptor as shown by chromatography on Sephadex G-25. In the androgen insensitive rat, however, nuclear accumulation was negligible (Figure 6) and no bound radioactivity could be extracted (Figure 8). Studies of this genetic defect support the concept that nuclear accumulation of androgen is dependent on androgen binding to cytoplasmic receptors and subsequent transport into the nucleus as androgen-receptor complexes.

The results presented here are in support of earlier evidence that the seminiferous tubule is androgen dependent. Intracellular receptors for androgens very likely mediate the androgen stimulus to spermatogenesis. The androgens bound selectively by the receptor (T and DHT) are both capable of maintaining spermatogenesis.

ACKNOWLEDGMENTS

Supported by National Institutes of Health, U.S.A. (research grant HD04466 and training grant AMO5330), World Health Organization (grant H9/181/83), The Rockefeller Foundation, the University of North Carolina Research Council, the Norwegian Research Council for Sciences and Humanities, and the Swedish Medical Research Council.

REFERENCES

1. Ludwig, D.J., Endocrinology 46: 453, 1950.
2. Desjardins, C., Ewing, C.L., and Irby, D.C., Endocrinology 93: 450, 1973.
3. Bruchovsky, N., and Wilson, J.D., J. Biol. Chem. 243:5953, 1968.
4. Unhjem, O., Tveter, K.J., and Aakvaag, A., Acta Endocrinol., 62:153, 1969.
5. Fang, S., Anderson, K.M., and Liao, S., J. Biol. Chem. 244: 6584, 1969.
6. Mainwaring, W.I.P., J. Endocrinol., 45:531, 1969.
7. Baulieu, E.E., and Jung, I., Biochem. Biophys. Res. Commun., 38:59, 1970.
8. Rennie, P., and Bruchovsky, N., J. Biol. Chem., 247:1546, 1972.
9. Tindall, D.J., French, F.S., and Nayfeh, S.N., Biochem. Biophys. Res. Commun., 49:1391, 1972.
10. Tindall, D.J., Hansson, V., McLean, W.S., Ritzen, E.M., Nayfeh, S.N., and French, F.S., Molec. Cell. Endocrinol., 1975, in press.

11. Tindall, D.J., Hansson, V., Sar, M., Stumpf, W.E., French,
     F.S., and Nayfeh, S.N., Endocrinology 95:1119, 1974.
12. Blaquier, J.A., Biochem. Biophys. Res. Commun. 45:1076, 1971.
13. Blaquier, J.A., and Calandra, R.S., Endocrinology 93:51, 1973.
14. Hansson, V., Djoseland, O., Reusch, E., Attramadal, A., and
     Torgersen, O., Steroids 22:19, 1973.
15. Stern, J.D., and Eisenfeld, A.J., Science 166:233, 1969.
16. Blaquier, J.A., and Calandra, R.S., Endocrinology 93:51, 1973.
17. Liao, S., and Fang, S., J. Biol. Chem. 246:16, 1971.
18. Mainwaring, W.I.P., In: Some Aspects of the Aetiology and
     Biochemistry of Prostatic Cancer, K. Griffiths, and C.G.
     Pierrepoint (Eds.), p. 109.
19. Mainwaring, W.I.P., and Peterken, B.M., Biochem. J. 125:285,
     1971.
20. Davies, P., and Griffiths, K., Biochem. Biophys. Res. Communc.
     53:373, 1973.
21. Davies, P., and Griffiths, K., J. Endocrinol. 62:385, 1974.
22. Hansson, V., McLean, W.S., Smith, A.A., Tindall, D.J.,
     Weddington, S.C., Nayfeh, S.N., French, F.S., and Ritzen, E.M.,
     Steroids 23:823, 1974.
23. Smith, A.A., McLean, W.S., Hansson, V., Nayfeh, S.N., and
     French, F.S., Steroids 25:569, 1975.
24. McLean, W.S., Smith, A.A., Hansson, V., Naess, O., Nayfeh,
     S.N., and French, F.S., Molec. Cell Endocrinol., in press.
25. French, F.S., and Ritzen, E.M., Endocrinology 93:88, 1973.
26. Hansson, V., Djoseland, O., Reusch, E., Attramadal, A., and
     Torgersen, O., Steroids, 21:457, 1973.
27. Ritzen, E.M., Dobbins, M.C., Tindall, D.J., French, F.S., and
     Nayfeh, S.N., Steroids 21:593, 1973.
28. Hansson, V., Reusch, E., Trygstad, O., Torgersen, O., Ritzen,
     E.M., and French, F.S., Nature New Biol. 246:56, 1973.
29. Vernon, R.G., Kopec, B., and Fritz, I.B., Molec. Cell
     Endocrinol. 1:167, 1974.
30. Hansson, V., Trygstad, O., French, F.S., McLean, W.S., Smith,
     A.A., Tindall, D.J., Weddington, S.C., Petrusz, P., Nayfeh,
     S.N., and Ritzen, E.M., Nature 250:387, 1974.
31. Sanborn, B.M., Elkington, J.S.H., and Steinberger, E., In:
     Hormone Binding and Target Cell Activation in the Testis,
     M. Dufau, and A. Means (Eds.), Plenum Press: New York,
     1974, p. 291.
32. Ingle, D.J., Exper. Med. Surg. 7:34, 1949.
33. Hotta, S., and Chaikoff, I.C., Arch. Biochem. Biophys. 56:
     28, 1955.
34. Christensen, A.K., and Mason, N.R., Endocrinology 84:488, 1969.
35. Lowry, O.H., Rosebrough, N.S., Farr, A.L., and Randall, A.J.,
     J. Biol. Chem. 193:265, 1951.
36. Martin, R.G., and Ames, B.N., J. Biol. Chem. 236:1372, 1961.
37. Dingman, C.W. and Peacock, A.C., Biochemistry 7:659, 1968.
38. Naess, O., Hansson, V., and Attramadal, A., Endocrinology,
     1975, in press.

39. Folch, J., Leese, M., and Stanley, G.H.S., J. Biol. Chem.
     226:499, 1957.
40. Hansson, V., Steroids 20:475, 1972.
41. Mainwaring, W.I.P., and Irving, R., Biochem. J. 134:113, 1973.
42. Mainwaring, W.I.P., Mangan, F.R., Wilce, P.A., and Milroy,
     E.G.P., In: Receptors for Reproductive Hormones, B.W. O'Malley
     and A.R. Means (Eds.), Plenum Press: New York, 1973.
43. Mulder, E., Peters, M.J., DeVries, I., and van der Molen,
     H.J., Molec. Cell. Endocrinol. 2:171, 1975.
44. Mulder, E., Van Beurden-Lamers, W.M.O., DeBoer, W.,
     Mechzelsen, M.J., and van der Molen, H.J., F.E.B.S. Letters
     47:209, 1974.
45. Bruchovsky, N., and Wilson, J.D., J. Biol. Chem. 243:2012, 1968,
46. Mainwaring, W.I.P., and Mangan, F.P., J. Endocrinol.59:121,1973.
47. Rennie, P., and Bruchovsky, N.J., J. Biol. Chem. 248:3288,
     1973.
48. Ritzen, E.M., Nayfeh, S.N., French, F.S., and Aronin, P.A.,
     Endocrinology 91:116, 1972.
49. Bardin, C.W., Bullock, L.P., Sherins, R.J., Mowszowicz, I.,
     and Blackburn, W.R., Rec. Prog. Hormone Res. 29:65, 1973.

FOOTNOTE 1

The following trivial names are used:

dihydrotestosterone = 17β-hydroxy-5α-androstan-3-one

5α-androstanediol = 5α-androstane-3α-17β-diol.

5α-androstanedione = 5α-androstane-3-17-dione

androsterone = 5α-androstan-3α-01-17-one

The following abbreviations are used:

PAGE = polyacrylamide gel electrophoresis

TSM = 50 mM Tris-HCl buffer, pH 7.4 at 4 C, containing 3 mM $MgCl_2$
      and 0.32 M sucrose.

TEMG = 50 mM Tris-HCl buffer, pH 7.4 at 4 C, containing 1 mM EDTA,
       0.5 mM β-mercaptoethanol and 10% glycerol

BSA = bovine serum albumin.

LOCALIZATION OF ANDROGEN RECEPTORS IN RAT TESTIS: BIOCHEMICAL STUDIES

Elizabeth M. Wilson and Albert A. Smith

Departments of Pediatrics and Biochemistry

University of North Carolina, School of Medicine
Chapel Hill, North Carolina 27514 U.S.A.

Rat testis has been shown to contain an intracellular receptor protein for testosterone and 5α-dihydrotestosterone (1-5) which is thought to mediate the androgenic stimulus to spermatogenesis. Further identification of the androgen receptor within specific testicular cell types has proved difficult due to their hetero-geneity. Localization of receptors in germ cells and/or supporting cells would help establish the mechanism of androgen action in spermatogenesis. In this report, we have measured receptor con-centrations in isolated tubules, in a germ cell-free testis obtained from prenatally irradiated rats, and in nonirradiated controls. The data suggest that the androgen receptor is present both in germ cells, interstitial and Sertoli cells.

Sprague-Dawley rats were hypophysectomized at 50 or 70 days of age (Hormone Assay Laboratory, Chicago, Ill.). In the in vivo studies, rats were eviscerated, functionally hepatectomized (5) and injected with 80 µCi of 1,2,6,7-^{3}H-testosterone (91 Ci/mmole) in 0.25 ml 15% ethanol in saline via the femoral vein 1 hr prior to sacrifice. The seminiferous tubules of the decapsulated testes were manually teased apart in saline at 4°C according to the method of Christensen and Mason (6). This laborious procedure yields a rather pure preparation of seminiferous tubules and a residual fraction containing interstitial cells and tubules. Both fractions were homogenized in a teflon pestle-glass homogenizer in 2 volumes of 0.32 M sucrose, 3 mM $MgCl_2$ and 50 mM Tris-HCl, pH 7.5 at 4°C. Androgen receptor binding activity was measured in the 105,000 x g supernatants by polyacrylamide gel electrophoresis (cf. article #18 by Smith et al.). For in vitro binding studies, decapsulated

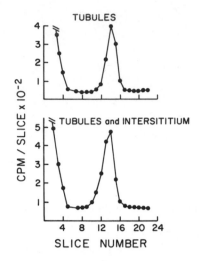

Figure 1.   Androgen receptor binding by subfractions of the testis
from hypophysectomized rats.   Receptor binding was analyzed in the
105,000 x g supernatant fractions of seminiferous tubules and a
residual fraction (cf. text) using polyacrylamide gel electrophoresis.

testes from rats irradiated in utero and nonirradiated controls were
homogenized in 4 volumes of 10% glycerol, 1 mM EDTA, 0.5 mM 2-mer-
captoethanol, and 0.05 M Tris-HCl, pH 7.5   Various concentrations
from 0.2 to 20 nM ^{3}H-testosterone were incubated for 20 hours at
0°C with the 105,000 x g supernatants.   Binding activity was measured
by polyacrylamide gel electrophoresis and by a charcoal adsorption
assay.

Androgen receptor binding in the 105,000 x g supernatant of
in vivo labeled seminiferous tubules was found to be similar to that
in the residual fraction containing interstitial cells and tubules
(Figure 1).   It appears likely that interstitial cells contain
receptor as do tubular cells.   Further, it was found that nuclei
prepared and analyzed as previously described (4) from the in vivo

labeled seminiferous tubules retained both testosterone and dihydrotestosterone (not shown). These observations are in agreement with the autoradiographic studies of Sar et al. showing nuclear accumulation of labeled androgen in seminiferous tubular epithelium and interstitial cells (cf. article # 22).

In an attempt to further localize the receptor within seminiferous tubular cells, we have utilized the technique of irradiation of the fetal rat. Prenatal rat testis has previously been shown to be sensitive to irradiation (150 rads from a ^{60}Co source) on the 18th-19th days of gestation. The primary radiation effect is a loss of germ cells from the tubule (7). Figure 2 shows a comparison of light microscope cross sections of germ cell-free (Fig. 2a) and non-irradiated (Fig. 2b) seminiferous tubules. The seminiferous epithelium of the nonirradiated hypophysectomized rat contains spermatogonia, spermatocytes, and Sertoli cells, while the epithelium of the prenatally irradiated rat consists only of Sertoli cells.

The 105,000 x g supernatants of germ cell-free testes and non-irradiated controls were found to contain similar concentrations of receptor when analyzed by gel electrophoresis or by charcoal adsorption (Fig. 3). The average amounts of total supernatant protein per testis in the germ cell-free and nonirradiated testes were 5 and 12 mg, respectively. In the germ cell-free testis, total numbers of receptors per testis were therefore reduced by about one-half. Since this loss of receptors was concomitant with a loss of germ cells, it would appear that germ cells contain androgen receptors. A possibility remains, however, that the loss of receptors in the germ cell-free testis might have resulted from a loss of receptors in Sertoli cells, perhaps by contraction of Sertoli cell cytoplasmic volume. The relatively high concentration of receptors in the germ cell-free testis suggests that Sertoli cells contain androgen receptors, since this is a predominant cell type in this preparation. The presence of androgen receptors in Sertoli cells would suggest that androgen stimulation of ABP production results from a direct action of the steroid on its target cell.

In summary, androgen receptors have been demonstrated in seminiferous tubules from testes of hypophysectomized rats. Comparison of receptor concentrations in germ cell-free and non-irradiated control testes suggests the presence of receptors in germ cells, i.e., spermatogonia and/or spermatocytes, and in Sertoli cells. From these studies, it also appears that receptors are present in interstitial cells.

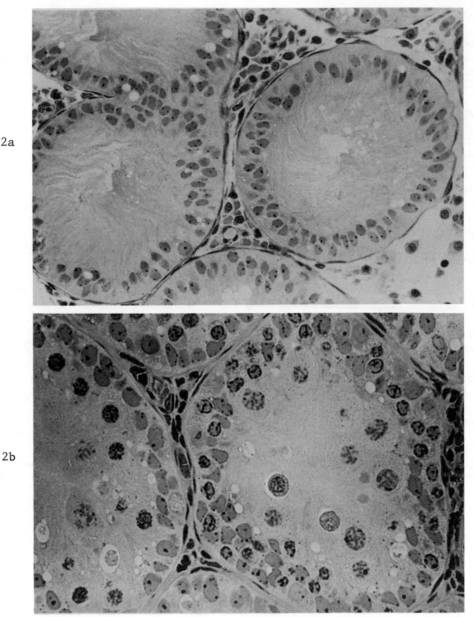

Figure 2. Light micrographs of cross-sections of testis from
irradiated germ cell-free hypophysectomized rats (2a) and non-
irradiated hypophysectomized controls (2b). Slices of testis were
fixed in 3% glutaraldehyde and infiltrated with glycol methacrylate.
Sections of about 2 μm thickness were stained with toluidine blue
(2a) and Noct's buffered azure-eosin (2b).

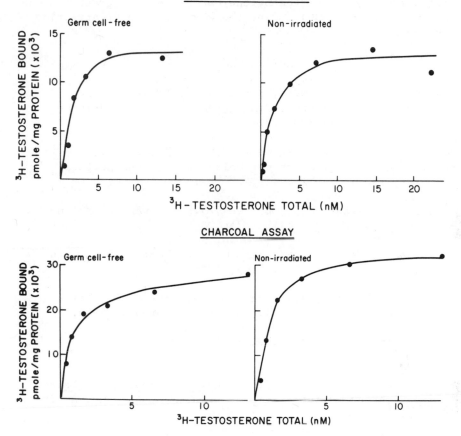

Figure 3.   Androgen receptor binding in 105,000 x g supernatants of irradiated germ cell-free testis and nonirradiated controls. Rats were hypophysectomized at 70 days of age and studied 30 days later.   Analysis of receptor binding by gel electrophoresis has been described previously (cf. article # 18).   Details for analysis of receptor binding using charcoal will be published elsewhere (Wilson, E.M. et al.).   Briefly, a 1% charcoal solution containing 0.1% dextran-80 and 0.1% gelatin was added to the labeled supernatant and incubated for 20 min with intermittent shaking.   Centrifugation for 15 min at 2000 x g separated free from bound radioactivity.   Nonspecific binding was accounted for by including samples containing a 100 fold excess of unlabeled steroid for each concentration of labeled steroid.

ACKNOWLEDGEMENTS

We would like to thank Dr. Frank French for his encouragement and helpful advice. Supported by the USPHS research grant HD04466 and training grant AM05330) and by the World Health Organization (grant H9/181/83).

REFERENCES

1. Hansson, V., McLean, W.S., Smith, A.A., Tindall, D.J., Weddington, S.C., Nayfeh, S.N., .French, F.S., and Ritzen, E.M., Steroids 23: 823, 1974.

2. Mulder, E., Van Beurden-Lamers, W.M.O., DeBoer, W., Mechzelsen, M.J., and van der Molen, H.J., FEBS Letters 47: 209, 1974.

3. Mulder, E., Peters, M.J., DeVries, J., and van der Molen, H.J., Mol. Cell. Endocr. 2: 171, 1975.

4. Smith, A.A., McLean, W.S., Hansson, V., Nayfeh, S.N., and French, F.S., Steroids 25: 569, 1975.

5. McLean, N.S., Smith, A.A., Hansson, V., Naess, O., Nayfeh, S.N., and French, F.S., Mol. Cell. Endocr. (in press), 1975.

6. Christensen, A.K., and Mason, N.R., Endocrinology 84: 488, 1969.

7. Means, A.R., and Huckins, C., in Hormone Binding and Target Cell Activation in the Testis. Dufau, M. and Means, A. (Eds.), 1974, p. 145.

ANDROGEN RECEPTORS IN TESTIS TISSUE ENRICHED IN SERTOLI CELLS

Eppo Mulder, Marjan J. Peters and Henk J. van der Molen

Department of Biochemistry (Division of Chemical Endocrinology

Medical Faculty
Erasmus University Rotterdam, Rotterdam, The Netherlands

A specific receptor for androgens is present in the tubular
compartment of the testis. In contrast to androgen binding protein (ABP) this receptor protein is located intracellularly, and
can be demonstrated both in cytoplasmic and nuclear fractions (1-3).
In mature rats the steroid bound by this receptor is mainly
testosterone (1,2) and in immature rats both dihydrotestosterone
and testosterone are bound (3).

Re-initiation of spermatogenesis can be obtained in hypophysectomized rats by injections of large doses of testosterone (4).
Despite the degeneration of the testes in hypophysectomized animals
the Sertoli cells are retained and these cells might be the prime
target for the action of testosterone during the re-initiation of
spermatogenesis. In order to obtain information on the possible
relationship between androgen receptor content of tubular tissues
and the presence of Sertoli cells we have tried to compare the
receptor content of normal rat testes and of testes which contain
a relatively large fraction of Sertoli cells. At different time
intervals after hypophysectomy of mature rats the amount of receptor in the nuclear fraction was estimated in an in vitro assay.
In testes of the male offspring of X-irradiated pregnant female
rats (5) spermatogenesis is almost completely absent and the Sertoli
cells are the quantitatively dominant cell types in the seminiferous
tubules. Therefore, we have also analysed testes of prenatally
irradiated rats for androgen receptors in the nuclear fraction after
in vitro incubatin with testosterone.

287

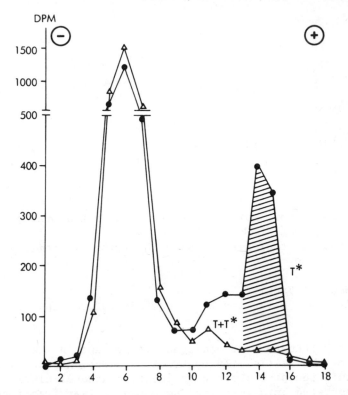

Figure 1.   Agar-gel electrophoresis of androgen binding proteins obtained from nuclear extracts of testis tissue incubated in vitro. Testis was obtained from 27 day old, prenatally irradiated rats which were hypophysectomized 3 days before the experiment.   The decapsulated testes were incubated for 45 min at 32°C with 2×10^{-8} M ^{3}H-testosterone (T*) or with 2×10^{-6} M unlabeled testosterone and 2×10^{-8}M ^{3}H-testosterone (T + T*).   The shaded area reflects specific binding of steroid to the nuclear receptor.

        The in vitro method for estimation of nuclear binding was used as described in detail previously (2).   In brief, decapsulated testis tissue was incubated in Eagle's Medium, containing 2×10^{-8}M ^{3}H-testosterone for 45 min at 32°C and subsequently the tissue was homogenized and a nuclear fraction was prepared.   The 0.4 M KCl extract of this fraction was subjected to agar gel electrophoresis.

As illustrated in Fig. 1, free steroid moves to the cathode as a
result of the electro-endosmotic effect, while receptor bound
steroid moves to the anode. A control sample containing a large
excess of non-radioactive steroid was run in parallel and the
difference in binding obtained in the receptor region was calculated.

Table I shows the results obtained for the hypophysectomized
mature rats. The amount of exogenous testosterone that could be
bound per mg of testis tissue increases gradually after hypophysectomy. Thin-layer chromatography of the radioactivity present
in the anodic peak on the agar-gel showed that 95% of the ^{3}H-
labeled compound was associated with testosterone. The increase
of the binding of exogenous steroid during the first days after
hypophysectomy may reflect the lower level of exogenous testosterone.
Testosterone production was completely absent within 1-2 days after
hypophysectomy. The still increasing binding capacity at 19 days
after hypophysectomy might reflect a predominant localization of
the receptor in the Sertoli cells because at that time most spermatogenic cell types had disappeared and interstitial Leydig cells
and Sertoli cells were the main cell types present. It has been
shown that receptor binding of androgen by testis tissue occurs
mainly in the seminiferous tubules (2,3).

TABLE I

Effect of Time After Hypophysectomy
on Binding of Testosterone by Extracts of Testicular Nuclei

Days after hypophysectomy	Weight of the testicle (g)	Bound testosterone (fmole/mg protein)
0	1.2	2.7 ± 0.5
2-3	1.0 - 0.9	6.3 ± 1.9
5-7	1.0 - 0.8	7.4 ± 2.4
8-10	0.8 - 0.7	14.4 ± 4.5
14-16	0.6 - 0.4	16.3 ± 4.7
19	0.3	31.7 ± 4.4

TABLE II

Effect of Prenatal Irradiation on Binding of
Testosterone Extracts of Testicular Nuclei Obtained from
Hypophysectomized 27 d. Old Rats

Pretreatment	n	Testis weight (mg)	Bound testosterone (fmole/mg protein)
Hypox. 3 days	11	175 ± 25	29 ± 9
Hypox 3 days 150 Rad 2-4 days before birth	9	50 ± 20	55 ± 16

n = Number of different experiments.

Table II shows the results obtained for 27 day old rats prenatally irradiated with 150 r between day 17 and 19 of embryonic
life (5). Both the irradiated and control animals were hypophysectomized 3 days before the experiment in order to decrease
endogenous levels of androgens and in order to prevent the possible
occupation of receptor sites by endogenous steroid. Sections of
the testicular tissue of the hypophysectomized irradiated rats
fixed in Bouin's solution and stained with periodic acid-Schiff-
hematoxylin showed mainly Sertoli cells and only a few germinal
elements. In the testes of the irradiated rats the concentrations of receptor when expressed per mg protein were higher than
in testes of normal rats. For the irradiated rats the radioactivity present in the receptor peak on the agar gel was analysed by
thin-layer chromatography and consisted for approximately 60% of
testosterone, 20% of androstanediol and 20% of dihydrotestosterone.
The relative amounts of testosterone, androstanediol and dihydrotestosterone in the remaining free radioactivity isolated after agar
gel electrophoresis were in the order of 40%, 55% and 5% respectively. This may reflect that the affinity of the receptor for androstanediol is lower than for DHT and T. When testis tissue was incubated with a three-fold excess of unlabeled estradiol together
with the ^{3}H-testosterone no significant depression of testosterone
binding was observed. Binding of androgens to the estradiol receptor in the interstitial cells (6) might therefore be excluded.

The present findings suggest that the intercellular androgen receptor is localized mainly in Sertoli cells. It is tempting to speculate that the effect of androgens on the germinal cells is mediated by the Sertoli cell.

REFERENCES

1. Mulder, E., Peters, M.J., Van Beurden, W.M.O. and van der Molen, H.J.; FEBS letters $\underline{47}$: 209, 1974.

2. Mulder, E., Peters, M.J., de Vries, J. and van der Molen, H.J.; Mol. Cell. Endocr. $\underline{2}$: 171, 1975.

3. Hansson, V., McLean, W.S., Smith, A.A., Tindall, D.J., Weddington, S.C., Nayfeh, S.N., French, F.S. and Ritzen, E.M.; Steroids $\underline{23}$: 823, 1974.

4. Vonberswordt-Wallrabe, R. and Mehing, M.; J. Steroid Biochem. $\underline{5}$: 380, 1974.

5. Means, A.R. and Huckins, C.; in Hormone Binding and Target Cell Activation in the Testis, Dufau, M.L. and Means, A.R. (eds), Plenum Press, p. 145-165.

6. Mulder, E., van Beurden, W.M.O., de Boer, W., Brinkmann, A.O. and van der Molen, H.J.: in Hormone Binding and Target Cell Activation in the Testis, Dufau, M.L. and Means, A.R. (eds), Plenum Press, p. 343-355.

ANDROGEN BINDING IN THE TESTIS: IN VITRO PRODUCTION OF ANDROGEN
BINDING PROTEIN (ABP) BY SERTOLI CELL CULTURES AND MEASUREMENT OF
NUCLEAR BOUND ANDROGEN BY A NUCLEAR EXCHANGE ASSAY

B. M. Sanborn, J. S. H. Elkington, A. Steinberger, and
E. Steinberger

Department of Reproductive Biology and Endocrinology,
University of Texas Medical School
Houston, Texas 77025

L. Meistrich

Section of Experimental Radiotherapy, The University
of Texas Cancer Center, M. D. Anderson Hospital and
Tumor Institute
Houston, Texas 77025

Until three years ago, little was known about macromolecules
which bound androgens in the testis, although physiologists and reproductive biologists had been investigating the androgen-dependent
aspects of spermatogenesis for some time +, see (1) for review.
Since that time it has become clear that there are two types of an-
drophilic macromolecules in the testis. The first to be described,
termed androgen binding protein or ABP, was found in high concentration in rete testis fluid and was transported from the testis into the epididymis (2-6). The ABP-androgen complex was found to
have a rapid dissociation rate with a $t\frac{1}{2}$ of 3 min_3(7). The second
androphile, demonstrated by in vivo injection of ^{3}H-testosterone,
had the characteristics of an intracellular receptor - a slow complex dissociation rate, heat instability, and a 6-8S sedimentation
coefficient (8).

IN VITRO PRODUCTION OF ANDROGEN BINDING PROTEIN
BY SERTOLI CELL CULTURES

ABP levels in the testis decline following hypophysectomy, rapidly in the immature animal (9,10) and more gradually in the adult

(6,7,11,12). FSH administration <u>in</u> <u>vivo</u> has been shown by these
same investigators to maintain testicular ABP levels after hypophysectomy and to restore them following their decline. In the mature
animal, testosterone propionate (13) or LH (6) can also achieve this
effect. While testosterone treatment markedly enhances the response
of the immature testis to FSH (14), this synergism has not been observed in the adult (15).

The restoration of ABP in post-hypophysectomy regressed testes
suggested, along with several other lines of evidence, that Sertoli
cells were the source of this protein. The demonstration that Sertoli cells which had been freshly isolated from rat testis or cultured for 11 days respond to FSH with increased levels of cAMP (16,
17) prompted us to assess the <u>in</u> <u>vitro</u> responsiveness of the Sertoli cell to FSH with respect to ABP secretion. Sertoli cells have
been reported to secrete ABP in response to FSH after 1-2 days of
culture by Fritz <u>et</u> <u>al</u> (12).

Sertoli cells were isolated from rat testes and cultured as described elsewhere (17, 18). After a 2-3 day preincubation period,
the culture medium was replaced with serum-free medium and the cells
were kept in culture for additional intervals. In this system, Sertoli cells isolated from 41 day old rats continued to secrete ABP
into the medium in the absence of any exogenously added hormones
(Rf 4.1, Fig. 1A). Unlabeled dihydrotestosterone in 50 fold molar
excess successfully competed for the ABP binding activity (Fig. 1B),
demonstrating that the binding activity was saturable in this concentration range.

The effect of FSH on ABP production was also tested in cultures
of Sertoli cells isolated from adult rats (Fig. 2). In untreated
cultures, there was still an appreciable amount of ABP produced after a total of 9 days of culture. The addition of NIH-FSH-S1 to the
medium 10 or 100 µg/ml, with or without 0.1mM methyl-isobutylxanthine (MIX) increased ABP levels above those found in comparable control cultures. There seemed to be little effect of MIX in the first
medium samples (4 day collection) but after an additional 3 days of
treatment, the amounts of ABP in the media from cultures treated
with FSH plus MIX were elevated when contrasted with those receiving
FSH alone. The amounts of ABP per day per culture found in the second media collections (a total of 9 days in culture) were lower
than those found in the first collection period (6 days in culture)
and may reflect a decreasing responsiveness of the Sertoli cells to
FSH. Certain FSH preparations (NIH-FSH-P2, for example) were found
to contain material toxic to the cultured cells. The enhancing effect of MIX on FSH-stimulated ABP production is most likely due to
its inhibitory action of cAMP phosphodiesterase. This effect appeared to be more pronounced in the older cultures.

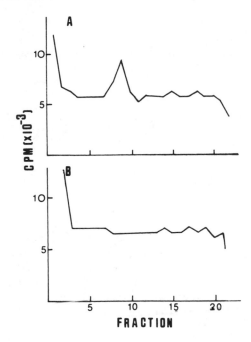

Figure 1. The secretion of ABP by Sertoli cell cultures. Sertoli
cells were isolated from rats (41 days old) and cultured for 3 days
in petri dishes. After this time the culture dishes were rinsed with
Hank's balanced salt solution and fresh serum-free medium was applied to the cultures. After a further 4 days of culture, the medium was assayed for ABP by the PAGE method of Ritzen et al (34).
Aliquots of medium were electrophoresed on 7.5% polyacrylamide gels
containing (A) ^{3}H-DHT (2nM) or (B) ^{3}H-DHT (2nM) + unlabeled DHT
(100nM) (11).

    This culture system should serve as a useful in vitro model for
defining the mechanisms by which hormones exert controls on ABP
levels and for measuring this specific parameter of Sertoli cell responsiveness under altered experimental conditions.

MEASUREMENT OF NUCLEAR BOUND ANDROGEN BY A NUCLEAR EXCHANGE ASSAY

    The measurement of androgen receptors in the testis is compli-
cated by the high local endogenous testosterone levels. Carbon extraction has been reported to destroy the receptors labeled by in
vivo injection (8). Reduction of local testosterone levels by hypophysectomy could conceivably cause degeneration of receptors themselves or of the cell types which possess them.

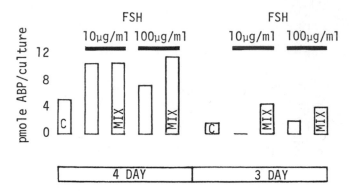

Figure 2. The effect of FSH and FSH plus methyl-isobutylxanthine
(MIX) on ABP production in Sertoli cell cultures. Sertoli cells
were isolated from adult rats (100 day old), cultured for 2 days,
washed with Hank's balanced salt solution and incubated ± NIH-FSH-
S1 or FSH + MIX for 4 days. The medium was then collected and replaced with fresh medium plus additives for an additional 3 days.
ABP was measured in the medium as described in the legend to Fig. 1.
Each bar represents the determination on medium pooled from 2 dishes
and assayed at 2 dose levels.

Hansson et al (8) reported that the intracellular androgen receptors were of tubular origin and persisted for up to 24 days following hypophysectomy in immature rats. Mulder et al (19) found
testicular nuclear uptake into 0.4M KCl extractable material 3-20
days after hypophysectomy in adult animals. These data are consistent with the hypothesis that the receptors are located in the Sertoli cells or young germ cells. Galena et al (20), on the other
hand, reported macromolecules which bound androgens in non-flagellate
germ cells from intact adult rats. They also found androgen binding
in epididymal sperm, a finding not corroborated by others (21,22).

The nuclear exchange method developed by Anderson et al (23) to
study nuclear-bound uterine estrogen receptor seemed particularly
suited for the study of testicular androgen receptors. The principle of this method is represented schematically in Fig. 3. Activated
steroid-receptor complexes migrate to the nucleus and bind to acceptor sites. The nuclei are then isolated and labeled hormone is exchanged for unlabeled hormone under conditions where the nuclear-
bound receptor complex is stable.

An attempt was made to apply this methodology in the testis.
Preliminary studies in this laboratory using in vitro labeling of
testicular minces had shown significant incorporation into nuclear
0.4 M KCl-extractable material by 15 min, with increasing uptake for
60-90 min at 33 C. Therefore, for nuclear exchange, in vitro preincubations with testosterone were carried out for 1 hr at 33°C.

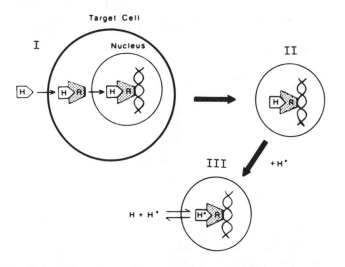

Figure 3.   The principle of the nuclear exchange method to measure
nuclear bound steroid hormone receptor as described by Anderson et
al (23).   Step I: (A)   The hormone, H endogenous or exogenous, enters the target cell and binds to specific cytoplasmic H, receptor.
(B)   The hormone-receptor complex migrates to the nucleus and binds
to an acceptor site depicted on the chromatin.   Step II: The crude
nuclear pellet (contaminated with membrane fragments) is isolated
and washed free of exogenous hormone.   Step III: The unlabeled
hormone in the nuclear-bound complex is exchanged by labeled hormone at intact receptor sites.   The nuclei are then washed, and the
radioactivity extracted and counted.   The assumptions behind this
method are listed by Anderson et al (23).

This procedure was found to be more reproducible from experiment to
experiment and to result in higher specific nuclear exchange levels
than in vivo injection (subcutaneous, intraperitoneal, or intrascro-
tal).

     The nuclear exchange activity was relatively stable for the in-
cubation interval employed (45 min, 26°C) but was less stable at
extended intervals (Fig. 4). ^{3}H-testosterone was chosen as the
labeled ligand instead of   5α-dihydrotestosterone because it was
more stable under the incubation conditions employed (Sanborn, B
and Tcholakian, R., unpublished observations), and was found to give
more consistent results.   In support of this approach, Hansson et
al (8) had found about equal quantities of labeled testosterone and
5α-dihydrotestosterone in testicular nuclei after in vivo injection
of ^{3}H-testosterone while Mulder et al (19) found predominantly testosterone.   In addition, androgen receptors in other tissues bind
both of these androgens (24-26).   Once the exchange system has been

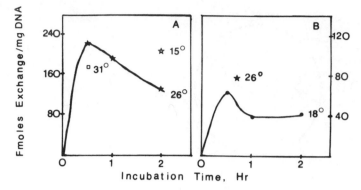

Figure 4. Nuclear exchange activity as a function of exchange incubation time. A. Exchange using the nuclear pellet obtained from the testes of a 119 day old, 19 day hypophysectomized rat. B. Exchange using the nuclear pellets obtained from the testes of three 55 day old, 20 day hypophysectomized rats. The perfused testes were decapsulated, minced and placed in the incubation medium (0.85% NaCl, 0.1% glucose, 0.01 M Tris Cl pH 7.4 containing 200 µg/ml testosterone in 4% dimethylsulfoxide), and incubated at $33°C$ for 1 hr. The tissue was then washed three times with Tris-saline, homogenized in 0.32 M sucrose, 3 mM $MgCl_2$, 0.01 M TrisCl pH 7.4, filtered through cotton gauze, centrifuged (15 min, 800x g), and washed three times by resuspension and centrifugation. The resulting crude nuclear pellet was resuspended by gentle homogenization in the homogenization buffer, pipetted in 0.5 ml aliquots (containing ∿40 µg DNA) into tubes containing 0.1 ml ^{3}H-testosterone (50 Ci/mmole, 22nM final concentration) with or without unlabeled testosterone (11 µM) and incubated for 45 min at $26°C$. The reaction mixtures were diluted with cold 3mM $MgCl_2$, 0.01M Tris Cl pH 7.4. The tubes centrifuged (10 min, 800x g chloroform 4:1 counted), and the resulting pellets washed three times. Radioactivity was extracted with 2 x 1.5 ml ether:chloroform: 4:1, evaporated to dryness, and counting in Scinti Prep 1/ toluene (Fisher). Each point represents the difference between total and nonspecific counts determined in triplicate or quadriplicate. The nuclear suspension contained predominantly intact nuclei with little clumping, cytoplasmic membrane fragments, or cellular debris. The DNA content/tube (33) varied by less than 12%.

refined, it will be important to reexamine differences between exchange using labeled testosterone and 5α-dihydrotestosterone.

Specific exchange was defined as the difference between total counts associated with the crude nuclear fraction and counts measured in the presence of 100–500 fold molar excess unlabeled hormone. Specific binding ranged from 30–50% of total binding in nuclear fractions prepared from homogenates of whole testes from intact and hypophysectomized rats. In some subfractions of the testis (vide infra) specific binding approached 70%. The proportion of specific binding was neither improved nor adversely affected by washing the nuclear pellet with 0.1% Triton-X 100 prior to exchange. This degree of specific binding was comparable to the 30% observed by Hsueh for progesterone exchange in the uterus (27). Estradiol-17β and cortisol did not compete for ³H-testosterone in the exchange assay in a concentration-dependent manner at 100-500 molar excess (Fig. 5). Somewhat surprisingly, progesterone was as effective as testosterone. The specificity using ³H-dihydrotestosterone was si-milar. There is evidence that progesterone and synthetic progestins are reasonably potent inhibitors of androgen uptake by prostate (25, 28). More recently, Mowszowicz et al (29) have postulated that cer-tain progestins exert "synandrogenic" effects by interacting with kidney androgen receptors but found no effect of progesterone itself.

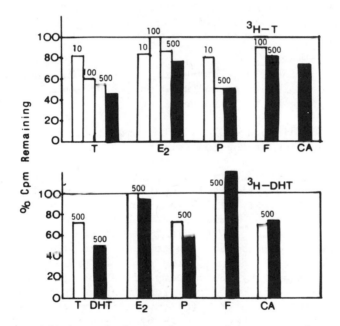

Figure 5. Specificity of the nuclear exchange reaction. Nuclear sus-pensions were incubated with ³H-androgen with or without the excess by weight of unlabeled hormone indicated as described in the legend to Fig. 4. The ³H-testosterone data represent a composite from three experiments using 7, 18, and 22 day hypophysectomized, adult rat tes-tes obtained 50 min after a 1 mg s.c. injection of testosterone (open bars) or a germ cell fraction (30) from two 63 day old rat testes af-ter in vitro preincubation (solid bars). The ³H-dihydrotestosterone data were obtained using the testes from a 19 day hypophysectomized rat (open bars) or the germ cell fraction described above (closed bars), both after preincubation in vitro. T: testosterone; DHT: dihydrotestosterone; E₂: estradiol-17β; P: progesterone; F: cortisol; CA: cyproterone acetate.

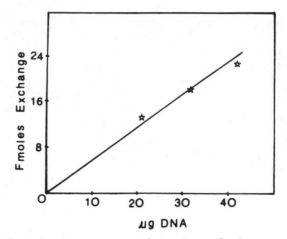

Figure 6. Nuclear exchange as a function of the amount of nuclei added. The exchange reaction was performed on a germ cell fraction (30) from the testes of a 104 day old rat.

Galena et al (20) found more uptake of progesterone than of androgens in their germ cell fractions and also observed competition for ^{3}H-progesterone uptake by testosterone.

Under the conditions employed, the amount of nuclear exchange was a linear function of the concentration of nuclei (Fig. 6).

The following evidence is consistent with the hypothesis that some nuclear exchange activity is located in the Sertoli cells of the seminiferous tubules: (1) Significant but reduced exchange/mg DNA remains in testes and seminiferous tubules from adult rats hypophysectomized for 6-42 days (Table I). The binding is 2-10 fold greater in tissue preincubated with testosterone than in that incubated without hormone (Table I). The exchange specificity does not change with duration of hypophysectomy (data not shown). (b) Significant exchange occurs in testes from immature rats hypophysectomized for 20-28 days (Table I). (c) Specific exchange is still present in tubules freed of Leydig cells by extensive washing and minced to remove the bulk of the germinal cells (Table II). Sertoli cells isolated from rat testes (17, 18) show specific exchange, calculated per testis or per mg of DNA, equal to or greater than that in corresponding intact testes from 42 day hypophysectomized rats (Fig. 7).

Nuclear exchange activity appears also to be present in the germ cells. Significant exchange activity with the same specificity as observed for whole testis was found in germ cells isolated from intact adult rat testes (Fig. 5). With one exception, the concentra-

Table I

Exchangeable Nuclear Sites in Intact and Hypophysectomized Rats

Days After Hypophysectomy		Pretreatment		Fmoles Exchange/ mg DNA
		In Vitro	In Vivo	
Mature	0	− T		99,88
		+ T		200
	6	+ T		680
	7	+ T		130,310
	8	+ T		400
	15		+ T	130
	18		+ T	230,280
	19	− T		27
		+ T		260,190,180
	20	+ T		150
	21		+ T	130
	42	− T		17
		+ T		28,30
Immature	0		+ T	99
	20	+ T		78,62
	28	− T		26
		+ T		70

Exchange reactions were executed as described in the legend to Fig. 4. Adult animals were 100 days of age at hypophysectomy; immature animals were 35 days old at surgery. In vitro preincubations utilized 100-200 μg/ml testosterone in 2-4% dimethylsulfoxide; pretreatment in vivo involved a s. c. injection (1 mg testosterone in 25% ethanol in 0.85% saline) 1 hr prior to sacrifice. Data represent specific binding with individual points measured in triplicate or quadruplicate. Multiple values represent determinations on separate preparations.

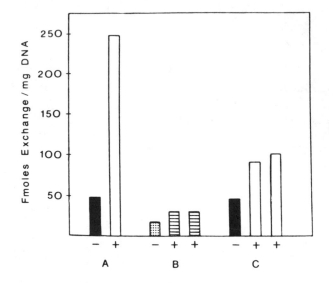

Figure 7. Nuclear exchange activity in intact testes and Sertoli cell fractions. Preincubations were performed in vitro in 4% dimethylsulfoxide (-) or 200 μg/ml testosterone in 4% dimethylsulfoxide (+). Sertoli cell fractions (17, 18) were used immediately after enzyme treatment. A: Exchange in Sertoli cell fractions from the testes of a 132 day old rat, and hypophysectomized for 32 days. B: Exchange in individual intact testes from rats 142 days old, and hypophysectomized for 42 days. C: Exchange in Sertoli cell fractions from testes of rats comparable to B.

tion of exchangeable sites per mg DNA was greater in the germ cell fraction than in the remaining tubule fraction (Table II).

Germinal elements were separated into enriched fractions in a Beckman Elutriator rotor (31). The results of one such experiment are summarized in Table III. The exchange sites were reasonably stable throughout the separation procedure subsequent to preincubation with the unlabeled hormone (4 hr) as judged by the recovery of exchange sites in the eluted fractions (82% of the activity in the initial suspension); cell recovery from the rotor was quantitative. The fractions obtained were enriched in (a) pachytene spermatocytes; (b) round spermatids and early elongating spermatids; (c) late spermatids and residual bodies; and (d) intact spermatozoa and sperm heads according to the criteria of Meistrich et al (32). Cytological examinations of the fractions were performed and the results are presented in Table IV. As can be see in Table III, the bulk of the exchangeable sites expressed as per cent of the total was found to be located in the most mature cell types. Expressed per nucleus or per DNA, the concentration of exchangeable sites exhibited striking cell specificity and represents an enrichment compared to the total

Table II

Nuclear Exchange in Washed Tubule and Germ Cell Fractions

Age of Animal, Days Hypox	Fraction	Pmoles Exchange per mg DNA
107d, 7d hypox	Tubules Germ Cells	0.25 0.80
108d, 8d hypox	Tubules Germ Cells	0.17 0.73
111d, 11d hypox	Tubules Germ Cells	0.73 0.35
84d, intact	Tubules Germ Cells	0.22 0.54
104d, intact	Germ Cells	0.54
22d, intact	Germ Cells	0.32

Testes were primed as described in the legend to Fig. 4 except that after the capsules were removed, the tubules were only gently teased apart. After preincubation, the testes were washed copiously on a 125 μ stainless steel grid with a forceful stream of 0.85% NaCl in 0.01 M Tris pH 7.4 to dislodge the interstitial cells (30). The tubules were then finely minced and the freed germ cells washed through the grid with buffer. The washed tubules (obviously depleted but still significantly contaminated with germ cells) and the germ cell fractions (containing primarily spermatocytes, spermatids, and occasional interstitial cells and Sertoli cells) were processed according to the procedure described in the legend to Fig. 4.

cell suspension. These results have been consistently obtained in two separate experiments, indicating that the exchange sites are located in the nuclei of the spermatozoa or are associated with contaminating structures such as sperm tails or residual bodies. Preliminary experiments show marked exchange activity in epididymal sperm, a finding which is consistent with the pattern in Table III.

At this point, it is not possible to equate nuclear exchange activity in the testis with the presence of nuclear-bound receptor.

Table III

Nuclear Exchange in Enriched Germ Cell Fractions

Fraction	Nuclei/Cells % Recovery	μg DNA/ 10^6 Nuclei	Pmoles Exchange per		
			mg DNA	10^9 Nuclei	Total Fraction
Initial germ cell fraction	52	8.1	0.38	3.0	3.3
Cells loaded on elutriator	47	3.7	0.92	3.3	3.9
Pachytene spermatocytes	75	9.6	0.25	2.4	0.14
Round spermatids	47	4.0	0.21	0.8	0.48 82%
Late spermatids	37	1.6	0.98	1.5	0.69
Sperm, sperm heads	31	3.3	2.8	9.3	1.9

Testes (8) from 100 day old Sprague-Dawley rats were perfused, decapsulated, gently spread, and incubated as described in the legend to Fig. 4 (20ml) except that 50 mg trypsin (Difco) was added during the final 20 min. The tubules were then washed, minced finely, and the liberated germ cells washed thoroughly with Dulbecco's phosphate-buffered saline plus 0.1% glucose (30). The germ cells were then treated with trypsin and deoxyribonuclease and spun through the elutriator rotor (Beckman) as described by Grabske et al (31). The resulting fractions were used to prepare nuclear pellets which were subjected to the exchange procedure. Cell and nuclei counts were determined using a hemocytometer and phase contrast microscopy. Nuclei were also counted after staining with methylene blue. Total exchange values are corrected for the recovery of nuclei. Counts may include cytoplasmic fragments detached from late spermatids (residual bodies) contributing to the low DNA recoveries in the late spermatid fraction. The DNA content of the sample saved for assay prior to loading onto the rotor may be low due to residual deoxyribonuclease activity. Note that the total number of sites in this sample is essentially the same as in the initial fraction.

Table IV

Cellular Composition of Fractions of Rat Testicular Cells
Separated by Centrifugal Elutriation

Cell Type	Elutriator Fraction				
	Pachytene Spermato- cytes	Spermatids Round	Late	Sperma- tozoa	Cells Loaded
Spermatogonia & spermatocytes (a)	2(m)	1	<1	0	<1
Spermatocytes (b)	34	<1	0	0	3
Early spermatids (c)	39(m)	51	11	0	29
Elongating spermatids (d)	10(m)	34	21	0	18
Sperm heads (e)	2	4	15	32	12
Spermatozoa (f)	<1	<1	12	68	25
Residual bodies	2	7	38	<1	9
Sertoli cells	10	0	0	0	2
Leydig cells	0	<1	0	0	<1
Unknowns (g)	<1	2	3	0	2

Numbers represent the per cent of each cell type based on differential counts of 500-750 cells on PAS-hematoxylin stained smears. (m)
refers to a predominance of multinucleate cells which most likely
arise by coalescence of cells through cytoplasmic bridges during
cell suspension preparation.   Residual bodies (cytoplasmic fragments containing ribonuclear protein aggregates) detached from late
stage spermatids are found in the nuclear fraction as isolated and
are included in the cell counts (35).

(a) To zygotene
(b) Pachytenes, some in meiotic division and some secondary spermat-
     ocytes
(c) Steps 1-11
(d) Steps 12-15, with cytoplasm but no flagella.
(e) Nucleus of step 12-19 spermatids
(f) Spermatids with flagella, steps 16-19, some 12-15.
(g) Macrophages, fibroblasts and degenerating cells.

The fact that preincubation with exogenous steroid results in significantly greater exchange levels under conditions where the uptake of 0.4M KCl extractable labeled androgen is increased is certainly consistent with this interpretation. The present attempts
also cannot be considered as quantitative estimates of exchange
activity since experimental aspects such as the stability of receptors during preincubation and exchange are still being evaluated.
The data do, however, give useful information, on a relative scale,
about the ability of testes components to exchange nuclear bound
androgen.

The data presented suggest that androgen receptors might exist
in both Sertoli cells and in components of the germ cell fraction.
Since the androgen dependent processes in germ cell maturation include the meiotic division (1), one might expect to find receptors
in the spermatocytes. The contamination of the pachytene fraction
with spermatids was sufficiently high as to preclude any statements
about the existence of nuclear exchange in the spermatocytes. The
role of the exchange activity in spermatid maturation remains to
be investigated. The study of the control of androgen responsiveness, i.e. androgen receptor concentration, will be of great importance in understanding hormonal influences in the testis.

SUMMARY

Androgen binding activity in the testis has two components.
One component, ABP, has been shown to be produced by Sertoli cell
cultures for at least 9 days in the absence of exogenously added
hormones. FSH (10-100 μg/ml) markedly enhances the secretion of
ABP. MIX has a potentiating effect after long treatment intervals
(7 days).

In order to study the second component, intracellular androgen receptor, a nuclear exchange assay was developed. Competition
for exchange activity using ^{3}H-dihydrotestosterone was significant
for a 500 fold excess of testosterone, dihydrotestosterone, progesterone, and cyproterone acetate. The exchange activity was increased 2-10 fold by prior treatment in vitro or in vivo with testosterone. Significant exchange activity was found in long-term hypophysectomized adult and immature animals and in tubule and germ
cell fractions. In isolated germ cell fractions, the highest concentration of exchange activity was associated with the most mature
elements. These data suggest that androgen exchange activity may
exist in both Sertoli cell and germ cell fractions and suggest that
the mechanism of action of androgens in the testis is quite complex.

ACKNOWLEDGEMENTS

The authors gratefully acknowledge the assistance of Dr. A. K. Chowdhury in the morphological examination of the germ cell nuclei and for helpful discussion. They thank Ms. H. Kuo, C. Williamson, R. Rodriguez and P. Trostle for valuable assistance in various aspects of this work. The FSH was a gift from the Pituitary Distribution Program, NIAMD. This work was supported by Contract NO1-HD3-2782, NICHHD (BMS) and grants from the Population Council and NCI, Grant CA06294 (MLM).

REFERENCES

1. Steinberger, E., Physiol. Rev. 51: 1, 1971.

2. Hansson, V., Djoseland, O., Reusch, E., Attramadal, A. and Torgersen, O., Steroids 21: 457, 1973.

3. Ritzen, E., Dobbins, M., Tindall, D., French, F. and Nayfeh, S., Steriods 21: 593, 1973.

4. French, F. and Ritzen, E., J. Reprod. Fert. 32: 479, 1973.

5. French, F. and Ritzen, E., Endocrinology 93: 88, 1973.

6. Vernon, R., Kopec, B. and Fritz, I., Molecular and Cellular Endocrinology 1: 167, 1974.

7. Sanborn, B., Elkington, J. and Steinberger, E., In Hormone Binding and Target Cell Activation in the Testis, ed. Dufau, M. L. and Means, A. R., Plenum Press, New York, 1974, p. 291.

8. Hansson, V., McLean, W., Smith, A., Tindall, D., Weddington, S., Nayfeh, S. and French, F., Steroids 23: 823, 1974.

9. Hansson, V., Reusch, E., Trygstad, O., Torgersen, O., Ritzen, E. and French, F., Nature New Biology 246: 56, 1973.

10. French, F., McLean, W., Smith, A., Tindall, D., Weddington, S., Petrusz, P., Sar, M., Stumpf, W., Nayfeh, S., Hansson, V., Trygstad, O. and Ritzen, E., In Hormone Binding and Target Cell Activation in the Testis, ed. Dufau, M. L. and Means, A. R., Plenum Press, New York, 1974, p. 265.

11. Sanborn, B., Elkington, J., Tcholakian, R., Chowdhury, M. and Steinberger, E., Endocrinology 96: 326, 1975.

12. Fritz, I., Kopec, B., Lam, K. and Vernon, R., In Hormone Binding and Target Cell Activation in the Testis, ed. Dufau, M. L. and Means, A. R., Plenum Press, New York, 1974, p. 311.

13. Elkington, J., Sanborn, B., and Steinberger, E., Molecular and Cellular Endocrinology 2: 157, 1975.

14. Hansson, V., French, F., Weddington, S., Nayfeh, S. and Ritzen, E., In Hormone Binding and Target Cell Activation on the Testis, ed. Dufau, M. L. and Means, A. R., Plenum Press, New York, 1974, p. 287.

15. Elkington, J., Society for the Study of Reproduction, Ottawa, Canada, Abstr/ 22, 1974.

16. Heindel, J., Rothenberg, R., Robison, G. and Steinberger, A., J. Cyclic Nucleotide Research, 1975 (in press).

17. Steinberger, A., Heindel, J., Lindsey, J., Elkington, J., Sanborn, B. and Steinberger, E., Endocrine Research Communications, 1975 (submitted).

18. Steinberger, A., Heindel, J., Lindsey, J., Elkington, J., Sanborn, B. and Steinberger, E., 1975, this volume p.

19. Mulder, E., Peters, M., van Beurden, W. and van der Molen, H., FEBS Letters 47: 209, 1974.

20. Galena, H., Pillai, A. and Terner, C., Endocr. 63: 223, 1974.

21. Blaquier, J., Biochem. Biophys. Res. Commun. 45: 1076, 1971.

22. Tindall, D., French, F. and Nayfeh, S., Biochem. Biophys. Res. Commun. 49: 1391, 1972.

23. Anderson, J., Clark, J. and Peck, E., Jr., Biochem. J. 126: 561, 1972.

24. Jung, I and Baulieu, E., Biochimie 53: 807, 1971.

25. Fang, S., Anderson, K. and Liao, S., J. Biol. Chem. 244: 6584, 1969.

26. Krieg, M., Steins, P., Szalay, R., and Voigt, K. D., J. Steroid Biochem. 5: 87, 1974.

27. Hsueh, A., Peck, E., Jr., and Clark, J., Steroids 24: 599, 1974.

28. Mangan, F. and Mainwaring, W., Gynec. Invest. 2: 300, 1971/72.

29. Mowszowicz, I., Bieber, D., Chung, K., Bullock L. and Bardin, C., Endocrinology 95: 1589, 1974.

30. Steinberger, A., In Methods in Enzymology, Vol. 39, Part D, ed. O'Malley, B. O. and Hardman, J. G., Academic Press, New York, 1975 (in press).

31. Grabske, R., Lake, S., Gledhill, B. and Meistrich, M., J. Cell. Physiol., 1975 (in press).

32. Meistrich, M., Bruce, W. and Clermont, Y., Exp. Cell. Res. 79: 213, 1973.

33. Burton, K., Methods Enzymol. XII, Part B, 163, 1968.

34. Ritzen, E., French, F., Weddington, S., Nayfeh, S. and Hansson, V., J. Biol. Chem. 249: 6597, 1974.

35. Platz, R., Grimes, S., Meistrich, M. and Hnilica, L., Biol. Chem., 1975 (in press).

LOCALIZATION OF ANDROGEN TARGET CELLS IN THE RAT TESTIS:

AUTORADIOGRAPHIC STUDIES

M. Sar, W.E. Stumpf, W.S. McLean, A.A. Smith, V. Hansson, S.N. Nayfeh, and F.S. French

Departments of Anatomy, Pediatrics, Biochemistry, and The Laboratories for Reproductive Biology, University of North Carolina, School of Medicine, Chapel Hill, North Carolina 27514 U.S.A.

Testosterone and 5α-reduced androgens maintain spermatogenesis in hypophysectomized rats (1,2). A specific receptor protein for testosterone and dihydrotestosterone has been demonstrated in testis (3-6), however, the androgen target cells containing these receptors have not yet been identified. In the present study, we used an autoradiographic technique (7), which avoids translocation and diffusion artifacts during tissue preparation. Experiments were carried out to determine whether the accumulation of androgen can be localized to specific types of cells within the testis.

MATERIALS AND METHODS

Immature male Sprague-Dawley rats from Hormone Assay Labs., Chicago, were hypophysectomized at 35 days of age. Androgen in-sensitive (Stanley-Gumbreck) rats were obtained from Introgene Labs., Oklahoma City, and hypophysectomized by Hormone Assay Labs. Ten days after hypophysectomy, the rats were eviscerated and functionally hepatectomized. 1,2,6,7-^{3}H-testosterone (New England Nuclear Corp.) with a specific activity of 91 Ci/mmole was injected intravenously at a dose of 50 μCi per 100 g body weight of the animal. Rats were killed either at 1 or 3 h after the injection of labeled hormone. Testes were removed and pieces were frozen at -180°C in liquified propane. The remaining portions of testis were utilized for receptor binding studies (c.f., Smith et al., article #18). Four μm frozen sections were cut in a Wide Range Cryostat (Harris Mfg. Co., North Billerica, Mass.) and freeze-dried with a Cryopump (Thermovac Industries, Copiague, N.Y.). The

311

freeze-dried sections were dry-mounted on desiccated emulsion (Kodak NTB-3) coated slides. After autoradiographic exposure for 7-9 months, the slides were photographically processed and stained with either H & E or methylgreen pyronin.

In order to show the specificity of androgen localization in testis, hypophysectomized rats were injected simultaneously with ^{3}H-testosterone and the anti-androgen, cyproterone acetate, in 150 fold excess of labeled testosterone. To examine the distribution of estrogen target cells in relation to androgens, rats were injected with 2,4,6,7-^{3}H-estradiol (90 Ci/mmole) in a dose similar to that of ^{3}H-testosterone. Rats were also injected with 1,2-^{3}H-5α-dihydrotestosterone (44 Ci/mmole), a nonaromatizable androgen, to exclude that the localization of labeled androgen might result from its conversion to estrogen.

RESULTS

Autoradiograms of testis prepared 3 h after the injection of ^{3}H-testosterone showed nuclear concentration of radioactivity in certain cells within the seminiferous tubule and the interstitium (Figs. 1 and 2). In some seminiferous tubules, cells of the basal layer concentrated little radioactivity when compared with the second and third layers of cells. In other tubules, however, distinct nuclear concentration of radioactivity was present in basilar cells. On the whole, nuclear concentration of radioactivity in basilar cells was weaker than in the second layer of cells. In hypophysectomized rats, Sertoli cell nuclei may appear in the second layer and in the innermost layer of cells; however, in these freeze-dried sections, it was not possible to distinguish between Sertoli cells and germ cells.

Peritubular myoid cells and interstitial cells concentrated radioactivity in their nuclei (Figures 1 and 2). In addition, cells in tunica albuginea showed nuclear labeling (Figure 3). The intensity of nuclear concentration of radioactivity in tubular cells was weaker than the heavy nuclear concentration in epithelial cells of the caput epididymis (Figure 3).

Nuclear accumulation of radioactivity (Figure 4) was abolished when the anti-androgen cyproterone acetate was administered in 150-fold excess of labeled testosterone (Figure 5). In testes of the immature androgen insensitive (Stanley-Gumbreck) rat, an animal lacking in androgen receptors, radioactivity did not accumulate in nuclei of seminiferous tubular epithelial cells, peritubular cells or interstitial cells (Figure 6).

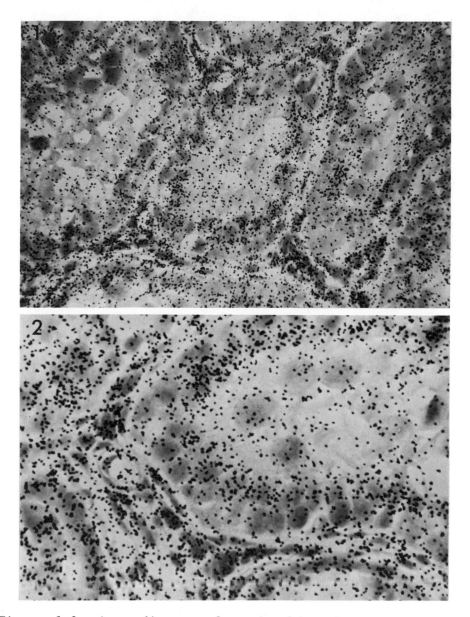

Figures 1-2. Autoradiograms of testis of hypophysectomized rats, 3 hrs after injection of ^{3}H-testosterone, showing nuclear concentration of radioactivity in tubular, peritubular and interstitial cells. Exposure time 200 days, 4 μm section x 540 (Figure 1); x 880 (Figure 2). Stained with methylgreen pyronin.

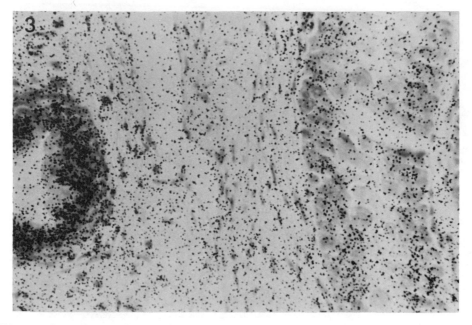

Figure 3.   Autoradiograms of testis of hypophysectomized rats, 3 hrs after injection of ^{3}H–testosterone, showing nuclear concentration of radioactivity in cells of tunica albuginea and seminiferous tubules as well as in epithelial cells of epididymis.   Note the stronger labeling of cells in caput epididymis as compared with labeling of cells in the seminiferous tubules.   Exposure time 200 days, 4 μm sections x 540.   Stained with methylgreen pyronin.

After the injection of ^{3}H–estradiol, nuclear concentration of radioactivity was seen only in interstitial cells (Figure 7) and not in tubular cells.   Nuclear concentration of radioactivity after the injection of ^{3}H–dihydrotestosterone was seen both in interstitial cells and tubular epithelial cells (Figure 8).

DISCUSSION

In these autoradiograms, selective accumulation of radioactivity in nuclei of seminiferous epithelial cells and peritubular myoid cells has been observed 3 hr after injection of ^{3}H–testosterone. Similar results were obtained at 1 hr after ^{3}H–testosterone injection (8).   These observations suggest the existence of several different types of androgen target cells in the testis.   The localization appears specific for androgen since the anti–androgen cyproterone acetate inhibits nuclear concentration of radioactivity.   After injection of ^{3}H–estradiol, nuclear accumulation of radioactivity

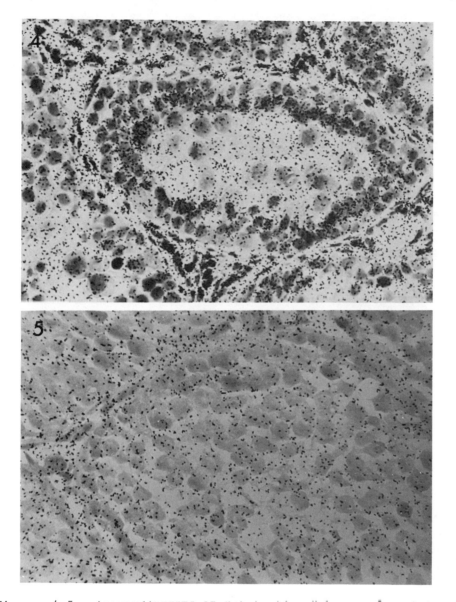

Figures 4-5. Autoradiograms of rat testis, 3 hours after injection
of ³H-testosterone into hypophysectomized rats, showing nuclear concentration of radioactivity in tubular and peritubular cells in
control animals without cyproterone acetate treatment (Figure 4) and
lack of nuclear concentration in cells of seminiferous tubules after
cyproterone acetate treatment(Figure 5). Exposure time 190 days,
4 μm sections x 540 stained with H & E (Figure 4) and methylgreen
pyronin (Figure 5).

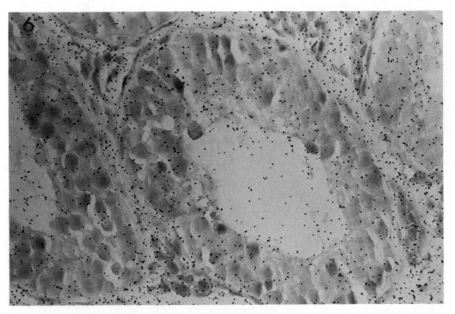

Figure 6. Lack of nuclear concentration of radioactivity in cells
of seminiferous tubules from hypophysectomized pseudohermaptro-
dite rats 3 hrs after injection of ^{3}H-testosterone. Exposure
time 190 days 4 μm sections x 540. Stained with methylgreen
pyronin.

is confined to the interstitial compartment and there is no
localization in cells of the seminiferous tubules.

The autoradiographic results agree with results from biochemical
studies in which a specific receptor protein in the seminiferous
tubules has been demonstrated to bind testosterone and dihydrotestosterone (c.f., Wilson, E.M., and Smith, A.A., article # 19 ;
and Mulder et al., article # 20). The lack of nuclear accumulation
of radioactive androgens in testes of androgen insensitive rats is
also consistent with the absence of intracellular androgen receptors
in testis of these rats (c.f., Smith et al., article # 18).

Stumpf (9) earlier demonstrated nuclear concentration of ^{3}H-
estradiol in interstitial cells of immature rat testis. In the
present studies we have observed nuclear concentration of radioactivity in interstitial cells of hypophysectomized rats after
injection of ^{3}H-estradiol as well as ^{3}H-testosterone or ^{3}H-dihydro-
testosterone. This suggests that there are different receptors for
estrogen and androgen in interstitial cells, or that one receptor
binds both estrogen and androgen. Mulder et al. have shown,
however, that the estradiol receptor in interstitial cells has a very
low affinity for androgens (10). Nuclear accumulation in interstitial

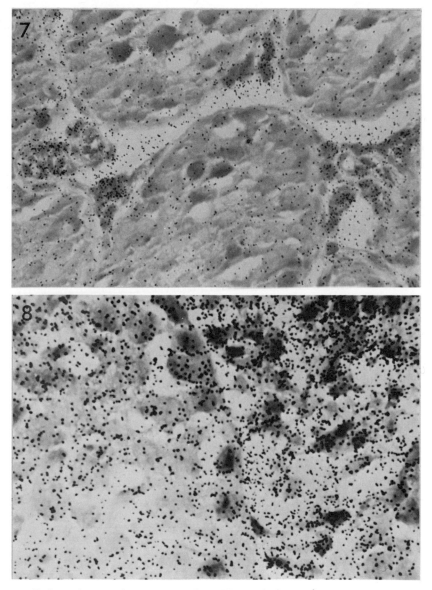

Figures 7 8. Autoradiograms of testis of hypophysectomized rats 1 hr after injection of ^{3}H-estradiol (Figure 7), or ^{3}H-dihydrotestosterone (Figure 8) showing nuclear concentration of radioactivity in interstitial cells. Exposure time 330 days, 4 μm sections x 540 (Figure 7); x 820 (Figure 8). Stained with methylgreen pyronin.

cells after injection of radioactive androgens probably does not result entirely from conversion to estrogen, since dihydrotestosterone is not aromatized to estradiol.

In the present study, the seminiferous tubular epithelium of these immature hypophysectomized rats consisted of 2-3 cell layers containing primarily Sertoli cells, spermatogonia and primary spermatocytes. Although there is an indication that Sertoli cells and spermatogonia as well as spermatocytes accumulate androgens, further studies are needed to clearly identify the androgen target cells. Nuclear accumulation of radioactivity in interstitial cells and myoid cells also suggests a direct action of androgen on these extratubular cells. This observation is supported by the findings that maturation and function of the myoid cells is dependent on androgen stimulation (11). The functional significance of androgen action on interstitial cells remains to be clarified.

ACKNOWLEDGEMENTS

Supported by Research grant HS09914, HD04466 and Training Grant AMO5330 from the National Institutes of Health, Grant P4B0873 from the National Science Foundation, the World Health Organization (Grant H9/181/135) and by the Rockefeller Foundation. V.H. was a Fogarty International Fellow. We thank Ms. Gerda Michalsky and Ms. C. Moussalli for their technical assistance.

REFERENCES

1.   Albert, A. The Mammalian Testis. In Sex and Internal Secretion, W.C. Young (Ed.), Vol. I, Williams and Wilkins Co., Baltimore, pp. 305-365, 1961.

2.   Steinberger, E., and Steinberger, A. The Testis: Growth Versus Function. In Regulation of Organ and Tissue Growth, R.J. Goss (Ed.), Academic Press, New York, pp. 299-314, 1972.

3.   Hansson, V., McLean, W.S., Smith, A.A., Tindall, D.J., Weddington, S.C., Nayfeh, S.N., French, F.S., and Ritzen, E.M., Steroids 23: 823-832, 1974.

4.   McLean, W.S., Smith, A.A., Hansson, V., Naess, O., Nayfeh, S.N., and French, F.S., Mole. Cell. Endocr. (in press), 1975.

5.   Smith, A.A., McLean, W.S., Hansson, V., Nayfeh, S.N., and French, F.S. Steroids 25: 569, 1975.

6.   Mulder, E., Peters, M.J., deVries, J., and van der Molen,
      H.J., Mol. Cell. Endocr. 2:   171, 1975.

7.   Stumpf, W.E., and Sar, M. Autoradiographic Techniques for
      Localizing Steroid Hormones. In Methods in Enzymology,
      O'Malley, B.W., and Hardman, J.G. (Eds.), Vol. 36,
      Academic Press, N.Y., pp. 135-156, 1975.

8.   Stumpf, W.E., and Sar, M. Autoradiographic Localization of
      Estrogen, Androgen, Progestin and Glucocorticosteroid in "target
      tissues" and "non-target tissues." In Receptors and Mechanism
      of Action of Steroid Hormones, Pasqualini, J. (Ed.),
      Marcel Dekker, N.Y., in press, 1975.

9.   Stumpf, W.E. Endocrinology 85:   31-37, 1969.

10.   Mulder, E., van Buerden-Lamers, W.M.O., DeBoer, W., Brinkman,
      A.O., and van der Molen, H.J. In Hormone Binding and Target
      Cell Activation in the Testis, Dufau, M., and Means, A. (Eds.),
      Plenum Press, p. 343, 1974.

11.   Hovatta, O. Z. Zellforsch. 131:   299-308, 1972.

Hormonal Regulation
of
Sertoli Cell Function

TESTICULAR ANDROGEN BINDING PROTEIN (ABP) - A PARAMETER OF SERTOLI CELL SECRETORY FUNCTION

V. Hansson, S.C. Weddington, O. Naess and
A. Attramadal

Institute of Pathology, Rikshospitalet, Oslo, Norway

F.S. French, N. Kotite and S.N. Nayfeh

Departments of Pediatrics, Biochemistry and The
Laboratories for Reproductive Biology, University
of North Carolina, School of Medicine, Chapel
Hill, North Carolina, USA

E.M. Ritzen and L. Hagenäs

Pediatric Endocrinology Unit, Clinical Research
Laboratory, Karolinska Sjukhuset, Stockholm, Sweden

It has become increasingly evident that many factors affecting spermatogenesis are mediated by the Sertoli cells that carry the developing germ cells in a close embracement during the most critical periods of spermatogenesis. Due to the vital importance of the Sertoli cells, increasing interest has been devoted to finding a biochemical index of Sertoli cell function. Testicular androgen binding protein is so far the only known specific product of Sertoli cells.

Paradoxically, the testicular androgen binding protein (ABP) was first demonstrated in the rat epididymis (1,2). It was later found that it was produced in the testis and then transported with the testicular fluid into the caput epididymidis where it seems to be absorbed by the lining epithelium or destroyed in the lumen (see reference 3 for review). The concentration of ABP in the efferent duct fluid of rat (4-8×10^{-8}M) and rabbits (2×10^{-7}M) is sufficient to explain the very high concentrations of testosterone and DHT in these fluids (3,5).

Evidence obtained in rats conclusively shows that ABP is produced by the Sertoli cells: ABP is present in high concentrations
in the testicular efferent duct fluid but not in the intertubular
lymph (6,7). Testes whose germinal epithelia have been destroyed
often contain increased concentrations of ABP (4,6,7,21) and finally,
androgen binding protein is produced by Sertoli cell cultures in
vitro (8,10).

The precise function of ABP in the germinal epithelium and its
relationship to spermatogenesis is not finally established. We
have proposed (3,4) that ABP might be important in order to concentrate sufficient amounts (increased uptake and/or decreased
metabolic inactivation) of active androgens in close proximity to
target cells within the tubules (Fig. 1). ABP also has the potential

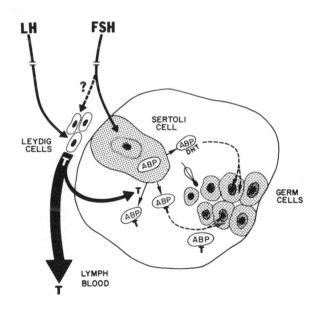

Figure 1. Schematic drawing of our concept how FSH and androgens
are acting synergistically on spermatogenesis. Testosterone (T)
is secreted from the Leydig cells due to LH stimulation. Most of
the testosterone is transported away from the testes by blood and
lymph. ABP is produced by the Sertoli cells in response to FSH
stimulation and secreted into the tubular fluid. ABP within the
seminiferous tubules causes increased accumulation of active androgens in close proximity to androgen dependent cells in this compartment. ABP also has the potential of selectively localizing
the androgenic stimulus within the germinal epithelium. From
Hansson et. al., 1973 (4).

of selectively concentrating the active androgens around some cells
and keeping them away from others.   Such selective localization of
ABP in the germinal epithelium has still to be proven.

The fact that ABP is produced by the Sertoli cell provides a
well characterized secretory product of these cells that is of
great value as a parameter of Sertoli cell function.   A high rate
of ABP production indicates optimal secretory function of the Sertoli cells, and a low rate of ABP production indicates failure of
Sertoli cell function.   The rate of ABP production is determined
from the accumulation of ABP in a testis where the efferent ducts
have been ligated for a defined period of time.   Measurements of
ABP in the caput epididymidis also give an indication of ABP production rate (Fig. 2).

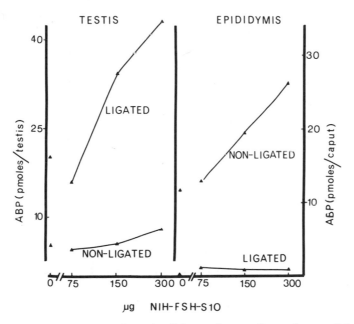

Figure 2. ABP concentration in ligated testis and non-ligated caput
epididymidis after injection of different doses of NIH-FSH-S10 (75,
150 and 300 µg of total doses).   Twenty eight days old intact rats
in groups of 4 were injected with FSH immediately after unilateral
ligation of efferent ducts.   Animals were killed 24 hours later and
ABP measured in testis and caput epididymidis of the ligated and non-
ligated side.   ABP was measured by steady state polyacrylamide gel
electrophoresis (SS-PAGE)   (18) with 2 nM ^{3}H-DHT in the gels.   Note
dose response effect to FSH in the ligated testis and, in the non-
ligated caput epididymidis.   Each point is duplicate measurements
from pool of 4 rats.

Having a good parameter of Sertoli cell secretory function, several critical questions can be asked:

How does treatment with different hormones or drugs affect the secretory function of the Sertoli cells? Increased testicular temperature is known to inhibit spermatogenesis. Is the gradual loss of germ cells in the cryptorchid testis exclusively an effect of elevated temperature on these cells, or does cryptorchidism influence the secretory activity of the Sertoli cells?

The following examples show how ABP can be used as a tool to investigate Sertoli cell function in health and disease. It will be shown that the secretory function of the Sertoli cell is dramatically influenced both by FSH and androgens. FSH stimulates ABP production at all times after hypophysectomy. Androgens alone can completely maintain (hormone given immediately after hypophysectomy) but not reinitiate (androgen given after posthypophysectomy regression) the secretory function of the Sertoli cell. There is a serious impairment of Sertoli cell secretory function in secondary cryptorchidism which might explain the gradual loss of germinal cells occurring in the cryptorchid testis. Drugs like nitrofurazone and ethionine, as well as x-irradiation, also have a slight inhibitory effect on the secretory function of the Sertoli cell; however, this is not likely the only reason for the dramatic failure in the proliferation of germinal cells after such treatments.

HYPOPHYSECTOMY AND FSH

ABP disappears both from the testis and the epididymis after hypophysectomy and reappears after treatment with pituitary gonadotrophins (3,4,9--13). In the immature rat (28 days) ABP in caput epididymidis decreases to undetectable levels within 5 days after hypophysectomy, while in the mature rat a somewhat slower decline has been found. Within 24 hours after injection of FSH to immature hypophysectomized rats, ABP accumulation can be measured both in the testis and caput epididymidis. The levels in the epididymis reach a plateau within 2-4 days, and further treatment does not give a proportional increase in ABP content (13). When hypophysectomized rats are injected with different doses of FSH, a dose-response effect is seen (13). The sensitivity of this ABP response is comparable to that of the ovarian weight augmentation assay (Steelman-Pohley assay) (19). The ABP response to FSH administration was found to be specific, since other pituitary hormones, and androgens

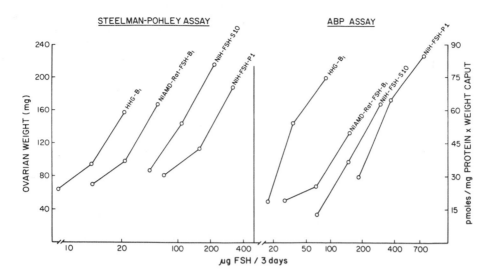

Figure 3. Comparison of ovarian weight and ABP levels in caput
epididymidis after administration of different FSH preparations
for 3 days. Steelman Pohley assays (19) were performed on
immature, intact, female rats weighing 50–60 g. In the ABP "assays",
animals were hypophysectomized at 28 days of age, and treatment was
started 2 days later. Note, various FSH preparations show the same
order of potency in the two assays. From Hansson et al., 1975 (13).

(2 mg/3 days) had no effect when administered for the same time
periods (3,12,13). The ability of different FSH preparations to in-
duce ABP secretion from the Sertoli cells and the ability of the
same preparations to increase ovarian weight are depicted in Fig. 3.
The preparation with the highest potency in the Steelman-Pohley assay
(HHG-B$_1$) is also the most potent preparation in inducing ABP, and
different preparations show the same relative potencies in the two
systems. These findings provided evidence that FSH is the hormone
stimulating Sertoli cell production of ABP. Recent studies by Means
and Tindall (24) have convincingly shown ABP response to FSH a very
short time (1 hr) after hormone administration to prenatally x-
irridated rats (Sertoli cell only (SCO) rats). However, the turnover

of ABP is very rapid. Four hours after i.v. FSH administration,
ABP concentrations are back to normal. Such a rapid effect of FSH
on ABP levels in immature rat testis has recently been confirmed in
our laboratories (Kotite et al., unpublished). In our previous
studies, ABP was measured after 1-3 days of hormone administration
and always at least 12 hr after the last hormone injection. Thus,
whereas these rapid effects of FSH on ABP most probably are reflecting the FSH induced synthesis and breakdown of ABP, we have in
our previous studies examined the overall process of synthesis and
secretion. All these studies on FSH effects on ABP show that the
Sertoli cell must be a target cell for FSH. This assumption is
supported fully by work on FSH stimulation of cyclic AMP and FSH
binding. Dorrington et al. (22) have shown that FSH stimulates
the formation of cyclic AMP by isolated Sertoli cells in culture.
Means and Huckins (23) demonstrated specific binding of ^{3}H-
labeled FSH to membrane receptors of seminiferous tubules devoid of
germ cells. FSH is also capable of stimulating ABP production in
vitro, both in organ culture (14) and in cell culture (10,15).
Thus, independent studies in several laboratories now strongly
suggest that the Sertoli cell is the main and perhaps the only
target cell for FSH in the testis.

                          EFFECT OF ANDROGENS

     The sensitivity of the Sertoli cell to FSH, as measured by
ABP response, decreases dramatically following hypophysectomy
(12,16) but can be restored by pretreatment with testosterone
propionate. When hypophysectomized immature rats are treated with
2 mg testosterone daily beginning at day 1 after hypophysectomy,
Sertoli cell sensitivity is not only maintained but even increased
compared to that seen in the two-day-hypophysectomized "controls".
Thus, in prepubertal animals androgens appear to dramatically influence the sensitivity of the Sertoli cell for FSH. The secretory
function of the Sertoli cell during this time period is not only
dependent on FSH but also on androgens (12,16).

     Also in the ten-day-old rat testis the FSH and androgen act
synergistically in stimulating ABP secretion (Kotite et al.,
unpublished).

     How androgens are affecting these processes is still not known;
it might affect either synthesis or secretion as well as the
destruction of ABP in the testis.

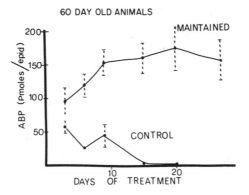

Figure 4. Maintenance of ABP production in adult hypophysectomized rats by testosterone propionate (TP). Sixty day old rats were injected in groups of 6 with 10 mg TP for 3 to 27 days starting immediately after hypophysectomy. ABP was measured in individual animals by SS-PAGE with 2 nM ^{3}H-DHT in the gels. Note, complete maintenance of ABP in TP treated animals. Mean ± S.D.

Sertoli Cell Secretory Function at Different Time Intervals After Hypophysectomy

It is known that spermatogenesis can be maintained with androgens alone in the absence of pituitary hormones if treatment is started immediately after hypophysectomy. However, if the testis is allowed to regress completely after hypophysectomy, it is much more difficult to re-initiate spermatogenesis (17). An important question was therefore: Is androgen capable of maintaining and/or re-initiating the secretory function of the Sertoli cell after hypophysectomy? As illustrated in Fig. 5, there is a complete quantitative maintenance of ABP in hypophysectomized adult rats when androgen treatment is started immediately after hypophysectomy. Animals in groups of 6 were treated with 10 mg testosterone propionate daily from 1 to 27 days after hypophysectomy and ABP measured in the epididymis. In the hypophysectomized controls ABP levels in the epididymis declined rapidly, and reached undetectable levels 14 days following hypophysectomy. Androgen does not seem to be able to restore the secretory activity of the Sertoli cell when the testis is allowed to regress after hypophysectomy.

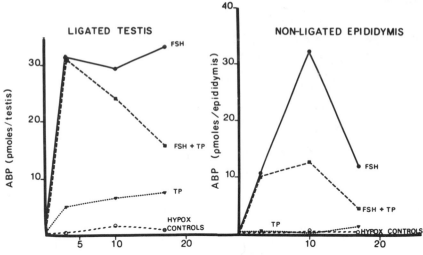

Figure 5. Effect of testosterone propionate (TP) and FSH on the
production of ABP in the fully regressed, adult, hypophysectomized
testis. "Ligated" indicates unilateral ligation of efferent ducts
18 hr before the rats were killed, to prevent the outflow of ABP.
The rats were hypophysectomized at 60 days of age, and treatments
were started 60 days later as follows. ABP was measured in pooled
tissue from 4 rats by SS-PAGE (18).

Note: FSH but not TP was capable of re-initiating Sertoli cell secretion of ABP. TP did not fully maintain ABP secretion after having
been "started" by 5 days of FSH treatment.

TP: TP 10 mg/day
FSH: NIH-FSH-S10 500 µg/day
FSH + TP: Combined treatment with FSH (500 µg/day) and TP
(10 µg/day) for 5 days, after which only TP was given.
Hypox: Non-treated hypophysectomized rats.

As shown in Figure 5, 10 mg of testosterone propionate daily for
as long as 17 days did not cause any secretion of ABP into the
epididymis. A small increase in ABP levels was found in the testis
supernatant, but there was very little or no difference between
the ligated and the non-ligated side. The small but significant
increase in ABP levels in the completely regressed testis might be
explained by some increase in the intracellular content of ABP within the Sertoli cells, and that other hormonal factors (FSH) are
needed to get ABP out of the Sertoli cell and into the testicular
fluid and epididymis. As shown in the same figure, FSH is capable
of immediate stimulation of the secretory activity of the Sertoli
cells even after two months of posthypophysectomy regression. The
finding that androgen alone is less effective in

re-initiating than maintaining the secretory function of the Sertoli
cell is possibly one explanation why androgen alone is less capable
of re-initiating than maintaining spermatogenesis. Similar results
are reported for immature rats hypophysectomized at 28 days of age
(25). These studies emphasize the importance of the Sertoli cell for
spermatogenesis and clearly show that spermatogenesis requires
functioning Sertoli cells as well as androgen. Thus, it looks like
after a long time of hypophysectomy the Sertoli cell is transformed
into a state of relative "androgen insensitivity" with respect to
ABP production. It is not known what factor or factors from the
pituitary are needed to restore androgen sensitivity of the Sertoli
cell.

In another set of experiments (Fig. 6) we tried to treat adult
animals after 60 days of post-hypophysectomy regression with FSH
for 5 days in order to obtain a maximum ABP secretion before continuing the treatment with testosterone propionate alone. The
question was: at a time when the secretory function of the Sertoli
cell is already established by FSH after post-hypophysectomy
regression, will the testosterone then be capable of "taking over"
and maintaining the secretory function of the Sertoli cells? From
our studies this does not seem to be the case. After stopping FSH
treatment there was a gradual decrease in ABP content both in the
testis and epididymis in spite of continued testosterone treatment,
indicating that testosterone propionate alone is not capable of
maintaining the secretory function of the Sertoli cells under these
experimental conditions. This could be due to the fact that 5 days
of FSH treatment is too short a time for restoring the components
which are necessary for optimal androgen sensitivity. However,
the possibility that factors other than FSH might be needed to
normalize Sertoli Cell response to androgens cannot be excluded.

The above findings and the relationship to earlier studies on
spermatogenesis can be summarized as follows: FSH alone in rats
maintains Sertoli cell secretory function at all times after hypophysectomy, but cannot effectively stimulate spermatogenesis in
the absence of androgen. On the other hand, when androgen maintains
the Sertoli cell secretory function it is also capable of maintaining
spermatogenesis. When androgen fails to re-initiate the secretory
function of the Sertoli cell, it also fails in re-initiating spermatogenesis. Androgen plus FSH stimulates Sertoli cell function and
spermatogenesis under conditions of maintenance as well as re-
initiation.

Androgen Insensitivity Syndrome (Testicular Feminization, Tfm)

Since androgens have such marked effects on ABP production,
both in immature and mature rats, it was of great interest to
examine if ABP was present in the androgen insensitive (Stanley-
Gumbreck) rat with testicular feminization (Tfm). As illustrated

TABLE I

Content and Concentration of Testicular Androgen Binding Protein
(ABP) in Testis of Rats with Testicular Feminization (Tfm) and
in Normal Littermates.

Animal	ABP pmol/mg prot. (mean ± S.D.)	ABP pmol/testis (mean ± S.D.)	n
Control	0.41 ± 0.07	34.3 ± 6.7	(6)
Tfm	2.90 ± 0.51	63.7 ± 14.8	(6)

Testes were homogenized in 4 volumes of 50 mM Tris-HCl buffer, pH 7.4
containing 1 mM EDTA (TE buffer) and 105,000 x g supernatants were
prepared. The cytosols were diluted with equal volumes of TE-buffer
containing 20% (v/v) glycerol and 10 mM ^{3}H-DHT (44 Ci/nM). Binding
was measured by steady state electrophoresis with 2 mM ^{3}H-DHT in the
gels (18).
(n); number of individual animals per group.

in Table I, the Tfm rat testis contained almost 10 times as much
ABP as the normal littermates, calculated per mg of protein. Also
when calculated as ABP per testis, the Tfm rats contained more ABP
than the normal rats. This clearly shows that ABP is formed even
in the absence of androgen stimulation. To what extent the ABP
production in the Tfm testis is higher or lower than that in the
normal littermates remains to be determined. The very high levels
of ABP in the testes of the Tfm rats could be due to impaired flow
of testicular fluid from the testis.

EFFECT OF CRYPTORCHIDISM

Cryptorchidism is an important condition in clinical medicine
with a complete failure of the seminiferous tubular epithelium. It
is also well known that in most experimental animals spermatogenesis
is arrested if the testicles are located intra-abdominally. Since
the viability of Sertoli cells has previously been assessed mainly
by morphological means, Sertoli cells have been thought to remain
intact, even in the cryptorchid state. However, this does not seem
to be the case. Sertoli cell secretory function was studied experimentally by making rats cryptorchid either unilaterally or bi-
laterally, and the rate of ABP production was measured both in the
abdominal and in the scrotal testis (20). Surprisingly, the abdominal testis was shown to produce much less ABP than the scrotal
one, and after 4 weeks of cryptorchidism there was an almost complete arrest in ABP production in the abdominal testis. In the

contralateral (scrotal) testis, the rate of ABP production was not reduced. This strongly suggests that serious impairment of Sertoli cell secretory function might be the explanation for the gradual loss of germ cells in the cryptorchid testis.

IONIZING RADIATION

X-irradiation of adult rats as well as of the fetuses is known to cause a more or less complete destruction of the germ cells in the seminiferous tubules. The high rate of formation of ABP by the Sertoli cells after X-irradiation indicates that relatively little damage is done to these cells by such treatment. (6,7) Adult rats were irradiated with 600 r locally towards the lower part of the abdomen and ABP was measured in the testis and epididymis at different time intervals after the X-ray exposure. ABP levels in caput epididymidis remained normal or only slightly reduced up to 30 days following irradiation, at a time when the germinal cells were completely deteriorated. The ABP concentration in the testis was rapidly increasing, probably due to removal of ABP-free cells (germ cells) and 30 days after X-irradiation there is several times more ABP than in the normal controls (3,6, 7). These studies might indicate that X-irradiation has relatively little effect on the Sertoli cells and that the main damage of such treatment is due to a direct effect on the germinal cells.

EFFECTS OF DRUGS

Drugs like nitrofurazone and ethionine are strong inhibitors of spermatogenesis. When nitrofurazone was added to the food given to adult rats for 30 days, there was an almost complete destruction of germinal elements within the seminiferous tubules (6). Ethionine added to the drinking water in a concentration of 1% also had a dramatic effect on the production of germ cells (Hagenas and Ritzen, unpublished). Measurement of the rate of ABP production in nitrofurazone and ethionine treated rats shows that both these drugs have a slight inhibitory effect on the secretory function of the Sertoli cell, but it can hardly be the only reason for the dramatic failure in the proliferation of germinal cells. It is therefore probable that these drugs might have additional effects directly upon the germ cells as well.

SUMMARY

Using ABP as an index of Sertoli cell secretory function, several important features of the Sertoli cell have emerged:

1. The stimulation of ABP production by FSH clearly points to the Sertoli cell as a target cell for FSH (3,4,9-16,21,24).

2. The dramatic effects of androgens on ABP production both in immature and mature rats also suggest that the Sertoli cell is a target cell for androgen (3,12,14,16,25).

3. The striking reduction in ABP production in the cryptorchid testis raises the question whether impairment of Sertoli cell function is the primary reason for the loss of germ cells that occurs in this condition (20).

4. Drugs like nitrofurazone or ethionine, or X-irradiation only slightly affect the secretory function of the Sertoli cells (ABP production), indicating that these treatments most probably have direct effects on the germ cells as well.

Thus, measurement of ABP production rate is a very important tool in order to evaluate how hormones, drugs, and physical injuries might affect the secretory function of the Sertoli cell. This test system might be of great use in order to study the physiology and hormonal regulation of the Sertoli cells. It might also be valuable in pharmacological and toxicological studies.

REFERENCES

1. Ritzen, E.M., Nayfeh, S.N., French, F.S., and Dobbins, M.C., Endocrinology 89: 143, 1971.

2. Hansson, V., and Tveter, K.J. Acta Endocrinol. (Kbh) 66: 745, 1971.

3. Hansson, V., Ritzen, E.M., French, F.S., and Nayfeh, S.N., Androgen transport and receptor proteins in the testis and epididymis. Handbook of Physiology, Section 7, Endocrinology, Vol. 5, R.O. Greep and D.W. Hamilton (eds.), Amer. Physiol. Soc., 1975, p. 173.

4. Hansson, V., French, F.S., McLean, W.S., Smith, A.A., Tindall D.J., Weddington, S.C., Nayfeh, S.N. and Ritzen, E.M., J. Int. Res. Commun. 1: 26, 1973.

5. Guerrero, R., Ritzen, E.M., Purvis, K., Hansson, V., and French, F.S., this volume, p. 213.

6. Ritzen, E.M., Hagenas, L., French, F.S., and Hansson, V., II Int. Symp. J. Steroid Biochem., Paris, March 1974, J. Steroid Biochem. 5: Oct. 1974.

7. Hagenas, L., Ritzen, E.M., Ploen, L., Hansson, V., French, F.S., and Nayfeh, S.N., Mol. Cell. Endocrinol., in press.

8. Fritz, I.B., Kopec, B., Lam, K., and Vernon, R.G. In "Hormone Binding and Target Cell Activation in the Testis", M.L. Dufau and A.R. Means (eds.), Plenum Press, New York, 1974, p. 311 .

9. Vernon, R.G., Kopec, B., and Fritz, I.B., Mol. Cell. Endocrinol. 1: 167, 1974.

10. Sanborn, B.M., et. al., this volume, p. 293.

11. Hansson, V., Reusch, E., Trygstad, O., Torgersen, O., French, F.S., and Ritzen, E.M. Nature, New Biol. 246: 56, 1973.

12. Hansson, V., Trygstad, O., French, F.S., McLean, W.S., Smith, A.A., Tindall, D.J., Weddington, S.C., Petrusz, P., Nayfeh, S.N., and Ritzen, E.M. Nature 350: 387, 1974.

13. Hansson, V., Weddington, S.C., Petrusz, P., Ritzen, E M., Nayfeh, S.N., and French, F.S. Endocrinology, in press, 1975.

14. Ritzen, E.M., Hagenas, L., French, F.S., and Hansson, V., this volume, p. 353.

15. Fritz, I.B., Louis, G., Griswold, M., Rommerts, F., and Dorrington, J. this volume, p. 367.

16. Hansson, V., French, F.S., Weddington, S.C., Nayfeh, S.N., and Ritzen, E.M. In "Hormone Binding and Target Cell Activation in the Testis", M.L. Dufau and A.R. Means (eds.), Plenum Press, 1974, p. 287.

17. Steinberger, E., Physiol. Rev. 51: 1, 1971.

18. Ritzen, E.M., French, F.S., Weddington, S.C., Nayfeh, S.N., and Hansson, V., J. Biol. Chem. 46: 1523, 1974.

19. Steelman, S.L., and Pohley, F.M. Endocrinology 53: 604, 1953.

20. Hagenas, L., and Ritzen, E.M., submitted to Mol. Cell. Endocrinol.

21. Tindall, D.J., Schrader, W.T., and Means, A.R. In "Hormone Binding and Target Cell Activation in the Testis. M.L. Dufau and A.R. Means (eds.), Plenum Press, New York, 1974, p.167.

22. Dorrington, J.H., Roller, N.F., and Fritz, I.B. In "Hormone
     Binding and Target Cell Activation in the Testis, M.L. Dufau
     and A.R. Means (eds.), Plenum Press, New York, 1974, p. 237.

23. Means, A.R., and Huckins, C., In "Hormone Binding and Target
     Cell Activation in the Testis, M.L. Dufau and A.R. Means (eds.),
     Plenum Press, New York, 1974, p. 144.

24. Means, A.R., and Tindall, D.J., this volume, p. 383.

25. Weddington, S.C., Hansson, V., French, F.S., Nayfeh, S.N.,
     Ritzen, E.M., and Hagenas, L. Nature 254: 145, 1975.

HORMONAL REGULATION OF THE SEMINIFEROUS TUBULE FUNCTION

E. Steinberger

Department of Reproductive Biology and Endocrinology
University of Texas Medical School, 6400 West Cullen
Street, Houston, Texas   77025

Until the second half of the third decade of the twentieth century, questions concerning the controlling mechanisms in the development of the testes and in the maintenance of their function were frequently asked, but poorly understood. Numerous clinical and pathological observations led to a vague idea that these mechanisms may be located within the structure of the brain.

A series of simple but elegant experiments conducted by Smith (1) clearly established the pivotal role of the pituitary gland in the function of the testes. Numerous investigators rapidly confirmed and extended this concept. It could be considered as the first phase in the sequence of events leading to the elucidation of mechanisms concerned with the hormonal control of the seminiferous tubule and looked upon as the "gonadotropin → organ (testis)" phase. During this phase of investigations, the attention was focused on establishing a relationship between the pituitary gonadotropins and the growth and function of the testes.

The second phase of investigations dealt with formulation of a concept of dual control of testicular function. Greep and his coworkers (2) provided evidence that LH controls growth and function of the interstitial cells while FSH stimulated the growth of the tubules and the sperm production. This could be described as the "FSH → seminiferous tubule" phase.

At the time when evidence for the "FSH → seminiferous tubule" concept was being developed, it had been learned that testosterone, in the absence of gonadotropins, will also maintain the seminiferous tubule function (3). This could be considered as the third or "testosterone → seminiferous tubule" phase of the development of the concept of hormonal control of spermatogenesis.

The second phase concept was logical and simple. The discovery that testosterone will accomplish almost as much as the two gonado- tropins as far as spermatogenesis is concerned, and will definitely maintain sperm production and fertility created confusion and pro- vided the soil for controversy. It should be stressed that at this period of time the kinetics of spermatogenesis were appreciated only very general terms. The investigators utilized as the end points or primary parameters in interpreting their results fertility, testi- cular weights, or presence of qualitatively intact spermatogenic process. The idea that different hormones may be responsible for control of limited segments of the spermatogenic process was not appreciated.

For the next 25 years little progress was made. Except for sporadic studies suggesting that both FSH and LH (4,5) are essential for "spermatogenesis" or that LH alone (6,7) can accomplish this task, in other words studies confirming the confusion of the 1930's very little additional or new knowledge was acquired. In the mid 1960's, several investigators, some utilizing quantitative techniques for evaluation of spermatogenesis (7),concluded that FSH probably plays no role in the function of the seminiferous tubule and in the spermatogenic process (7,8,9). This fourth phase in the develop- ment of our knowledge could be designated as "anti-FSH" phase.

In the 1960's, we reexamined the role of FSH and androgens in the growth and function of the seminiferous tubule, utilizing a working hypothesis that these hormones may affect, whether by direct action on a specific type of germ cells or indirectly via the Sertoli cells, a specific segment of the spermatogenic process. Furthermore, we suggested that hormonal requirements for the first wave of spermatogenesis may differ from those required for its maintenance and/or reinitiation and that the hormonal requirements for quantitatively normal spermatogenesis may differ from those required for qualitative progression of the spermatogenic process (10-12). These considerations were essentially neglected by the early investigators (4,6,9) as well as by some in recent years (13,14). This fifth phase could be termed the "specificity and limited-target" phase. Numerous in vivo and in vitro studies pro- vided evidence that FSH is required for completion of the first wave of spermatogenesis, that androgens are essential for the com- pletion of the meiotic division, that some phases of spermatogenesis are probably hormone independent, and that the stem cells require no hormones for survival and multiplication (15).

The proposed idea for the role of FSH in spermatogenesis was based on the assumption that this hormone triggers an event in immature testes during the first wave of spermatogenesis which is essential for completion of spermiogenesis and its continuation in mature testes. Once this "event" is triggered, the process will

continue in absence of FSH as long as an uninterrupted supply of
testosterone is available. In other words, a concept of an
"obligatory but transitory role for FSH" was proposed.

This concept was confirmed in a series of elegant biochemical
studies demonstrating responsiveness of the testes to FSH with increase in RNA and protein synthesis occurring during the "sensitive"
or "receptive" stages of the first wave of spermatogenesis or during
reinitiation of spermatogenesis in posthypophysectomy regressed
testes (16,17). The role of FSH in the seminiferous tubule function
was further confirmed by the demonstration of specific localization
of FSH within the seminiferous tubules (18,19) and later the
demonstration of specific binding of FSH to seminiferous tubules (20-
22). These studies introduced the sixth phase or the "cellular
localization of molecular interactions" phase of investigations. The
work in a number of laboratories led to the discovery in the testes
of various components of the biochemical system classically involved
in the mechanism of polypeptide hormone action. Demonstration of
specific binding of FSH to seminiferous tubules extended the
earlier morphologic studies on localization of FSH within the seminiferous tubule and provided definite evidence for the cellular site
of FSH action in the testes. Biochemical evidence for FSH involvement in the molecular events triggering the chain of events
associated with the action of polypeptide hormones was provided by
demonstration of cyclic AMP in the tubules (23) and later demonstration of an increase in adenyl cyclase activity (24,25) and in the
levels of cAMP (24,26-28) in the seminiferous tubules in response
to FSH. The protein ABP in the testes (29-31) and the demonstration
of its dependence of FSH (31-33) related the androgens to the function of the seminiferous tubule and suggested a role for FSH in this
process. On the basis of this and above summarized information,
it has been suggested (31,32) that ABP is probably produced by the
Sertoli cells and a hypothesis to explain the hormonal control of
the seminiferous tubule function has been proposed (31,34) (Fig. 1).
This hypothesis suggests that FSH is bound specifically to the
Sertoli cells where it induces adenyl cyclase which stimulates production of cAMP. The cyclic AMP activates protein kinase which may
be involved in stimulating protein synthesis, one of the proteins
being ABP. Testosterone enters the Sertoli cells from the interstitial area and is bound by ABP. The ABP-T complex influences
spermatogenesis via an unknown mechanism.

Although we realized that this sequence of events may not be
accurate and the hypothesis naive, the proposed series of events
satisfied the available evidence and supported the earlier suggestions
that FSH is essential for initiation of first wave of spermatogenesis
(11) and that its role is "obligatory but transitory" in nature.

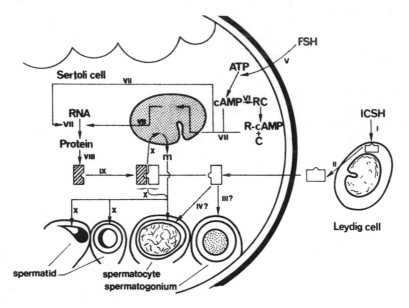

Figure 1. Hypothesis for the action of hormones on the seminiferous epithelium. For discussion of the diagram see text. From Steinberger et al., 1974 (31).

This was a plausible hypothesis but the major underlying assumption that the biochemical events described above indeed occur in the Sertoli cells was based entirely on indirect evidence and deductive thinking. To provide direct evidence for the involvement of the Sertoli cell, studies with a pure population of viable isolated Sertoli cells were indicated.

In the mid 1950's and early 1960's, we demonstrated that it is possible to produce experimentally testes with seminiferous tubules containing specific cell type populations, e.g. Sertoli cells only, Sertoli cells and spermatids, Sertoli cells, spermatogonia, and spermatocytes, etc. (35-38). This could be accomplished by various physical (x-ray, heat) or chemical (alkylating agents, vitamin deficiences, nitrofurans, etc.) agents. Utilizing a combination of these techniques, and specifically x-ray induced "Sertoli-cell only" testes, we localized the site of hyaluronidase production to the spermatids (35,36). During the first Testes Workshop (Washington, D.C., 1972), I suggested the employment of these techniques for localization of the above discussed molecular events to specific cell types in the testes and pointed out that x-irradiation, myleran or heat treatment could be utilized with advantage for obtaining "Sertoli cell only" seminiferous tubules. Upon further analysis of the possibility, however, we decided against this approach for the following reasons. While this approach was satisfactory in studies aimed for demonstrating that Sertoli cells do not contain a specific substance (e.g. hyaluronidase), it suffered from serious drawbacks in studies where a presence of a substance in the Sertoli cell was to be demonstrated and its possible dependence on hormones assessed. Firstly, x-ray, heat or treatment with alkylating agents-induced "Sertoli cell only" testis does not contain only Sertoli cells but also various cell types of the limiting membrane (myoid cells, fibroblast-like cells, endothelial-like cells, etc.) as well as cells found in the interstitial area, including the Leydig cells. Removal of the germinal elements induces hormonal changes in the pituitary-gonadal axis producing an abnormal hormonal milieu against which interpretation of studies involving hormonal treatments in vivo is difficult and frought with danger. Futhermore, the presence of Leydig cells in these preparations introduces a gonadotropin-dependent source of androgens which in turn may modify the responses of Sertoli cells to the experimental design created to investigate their behavior in response to hormonal treatment.

In view of these drawbacks, we abandoned the in vivo approach and concentrated on development of techniques which would permit in vitro isolation and later culture of relatively pure populations of Sertoli cells. Modifying a variety of mechanical and enzyme techniques developed in the past (39) and utilizing an observation made in the past that when dissociated testicular tissue is placed in culture the nongerminal cells attach to the glass surface of the culture vessel while germ cells fail to do so (40) we developed a technique for isolation and culture of relatively pure populations of Sertoli cells (41), germ cells and peritubular cells (42). In addition we utilized a technique developed in the past (43,44) to produce organ cultures of testes containing essentially only Sertoli cells and peritubular cells

Utilizing these techniques for preparation of populations of relatively pure testicular cell types, we examined the influence of hormones on a number of biochemical parameters. The details of the

biochemical techniques utilized in these studies are described
elsewhere (31,41,45,52).

    The Influence of Gonadotropins on cAMP in Testicular Cells

    Accumulation of cAMP was assessed in presence of 1 mM MIX
(1-methyl-3-isobutyl-xanthine) since it appeared to be a better
phosphodiesterase inhibitor than 5 mM theophylline (Fig. 2). A
word of caution concerning interpretation of these data is in order
since cAMP was measured only in the tissues or cells and not in the
incubation media.

    Both LH and FSH stimulated cAMP in homogenates of whole testi-
cular tissue from adult rats (Fig. 3). The striking difference in
the shape of the dose response curves and the additive effect of
the two hormones (when employed at maximum effective dose) (Fig. 4)
suggest that LH and FSH affect different cell types.

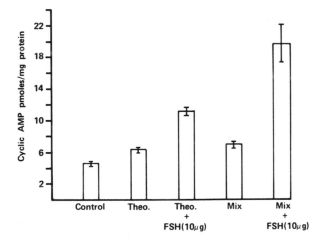

Figure 2.   Effect of 5 mM Theophylline or 1 mM MIX on the basal and
FSH stimulated cyclic AMP levels in whole testicular tissue.   Results are expressed as Mean ± S.E. (N=4).   From Heindel et. al.,
1975 (45).

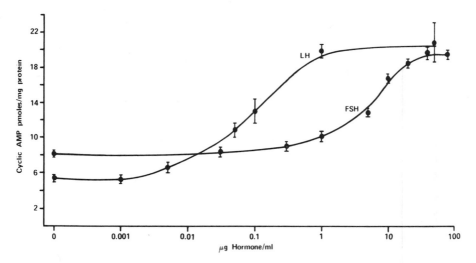

Figure 3.   Logarithmic dose response curves to LH and FSH on cyclic
AMP levels in whole testicular tissue.   Zero values were obtained
with 1 mM MIX alone.   Each point represents Mean ± S.E. (N=4).
From Heindel ct al., 1975 (45).

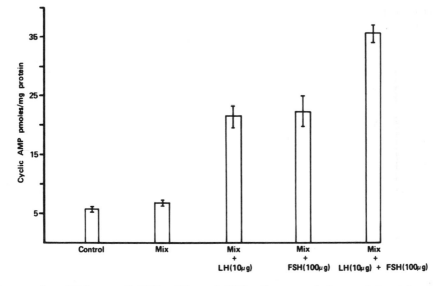

Figure 4.   Effect of MIX, LH and FSH alone and in combination on
cyclic AMP levels in whole testicular tissue.   Each value represents the Mean ± S.E. (N=4).   From Heindel et al., 1975 (45).

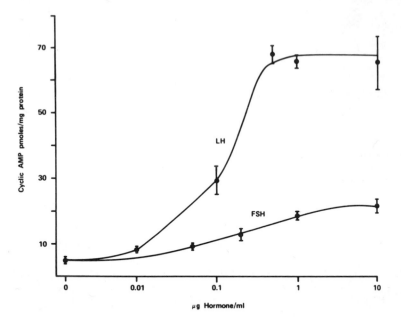

Figure 5.   Logarithmic dose response to LH and FSH on cyclic AMP
levels in isolated interstitial cells.   All samples were incubated
with 1 mM MIX.   The zero values were obtained with 1 mM MIX only.
Each point represents Mean ± S.E. (N=4).   From Heindel et al.,
1975 (45).

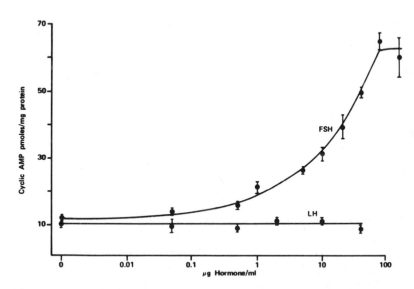

Figure 6.   Logarithmic dose response to LH and FSH on cyclic AMP
levels in isolated seminiferous tubules.   Each point represents
Mean ± S.E. (N=4).   The zero values were obtained with 1 mM MIX only.
From Heindel et al., 1975 (45).

It is of interest to note that in the Leydig cell preparations FSH also induced a slight but definite elevation of cAMP. This could be accounted for by minor contamination of this preparation with elements from the seminiferous tubules or by LH contamination of the FSH preparation (NIH-FSH-S1). However, the possibility that this response was a true reflection of an effect of FSH on the Leydig cells should not be totally discarded in light of reports suggesting effect of FSH on androgen synthesis (46,47).

In testes organ cultures containing only Sertoli cells and peritubular cells (Fig. 7) grown in vitro for 30 days, FSH produced striking elevation of cAMP while LH had no effect on androgen synthesis (Figure 8).

Freshly isolated Sertoli cells (containing over 90% of viable Sertoli cells and only occasional germ cells) responded with a 20-fold increase in cyclic AMP (Fig. 9).

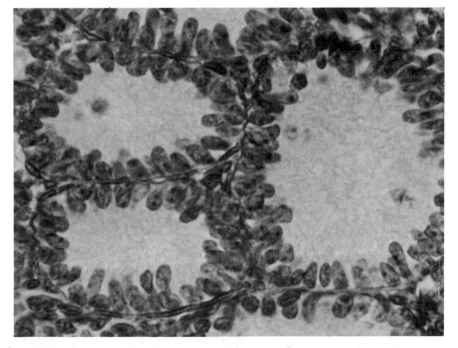

Figure 7. Three week old organ culture of rat testis. Note: tissue is composed only of Sertoli cells and peritubular cells.

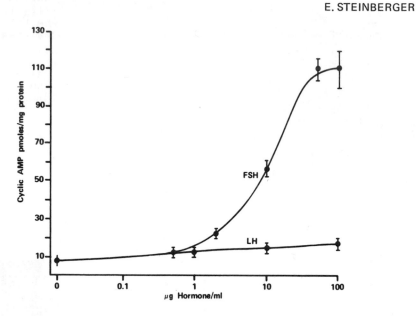

Figure 8.   Logarithmic dose response to LH and FSH on cyclic AMP
levels in testes organ culture grown for 30 days.   Approximately
10 mg of cultured tissue were incubated with 1 mM MIX and various
concentrations of hormones.   Values represent Mean $\pm$ S.E. (N=3).

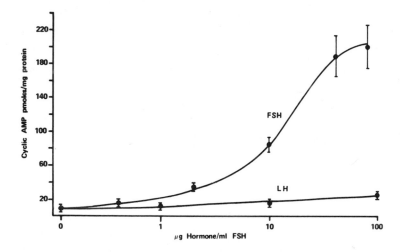

Figure 9.   Logarithmic dose response to LH and FSH on cyclic AMP in
freshly isolated Sertoli cells from a 21-day old rat.   Each point
represents Mean $\pm$ S.E. (N=3).   In a similar separate experiment a
26-fold increase in the cyclic AMP level was observed following
FSH stimulation.

In freshly isolated germ cells MIX alone increased the basal
cAMP levels. Both LH and FSH had an equally slight stimulating
effect (less than 2-fold). Most likely this slight stimulating effect
was due to contamination of this preparation with other cell types.
However, only further studies using more precise techniques will
determine whether this conclusion is warranted.

Preparations of freshly isolated peritubular cells as well as
cultures of peritubular cells failed to respond with significant
increases in cAMP to either LH or FSH at doses that produced maximal
stimulation in homogenates of whole testicular tissue. MIX, as expected, increased the basal levels of cAMP in both freshly isolated
cells and cell cultures.

In summary, experiments with various combinations of testicular
cell types as well as with relatively pure populations of each type ,
clearly indicate that the Sertoli cell is the only testicular cell
which responds to FSH, but not to LH, with a marked increase in cAMP
production   (Fig. 10).

Specific Binding of FSH to Sertoli Cells
and Stimulation of ABP Synthesis

As mentioned above specific binding of radiolabeled FSH to
whole testicular tissue and to seminiferous tubules has been previously demonstrated, and evidence was presented that the Sertoli
cell is most likely the site of the binding (48,49).

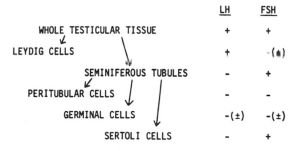

Figure 10. Production of cAMP by testicular cells in response to
gonadotropins (LH and FSH).

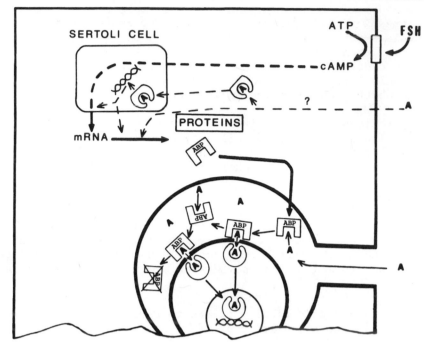

Figure 11. Updated hypothesis for the action of hormones on the seminiferous epithelium. For discussion of the diagram see text.

        Direct evidence for FSH binding to Sertoli cells was provided
by studies utilizing pure preparation of freshly isolated Sertoli
cells and Sertoli cell cultures. Study with the latter preparation
has also demonstrated that the Sertoli cells retain the capacity to
bind FSH after 11 days in culture (48). Utilizing these techniques
we have also demonstrated that FSH stimulates production of ABP in
Sertoli cells and that this capacity is retained for at least 11 days
in culture (41).

Testosterone Receptors

        Recently testosterone receptors have been demonstrated in testi-
cular tissue (50). This finding opened the door to elucidation of
the details of the mechanism of testosterone action in the testes.
Utilizing nuclear exchange technique (51) to measure the ability of
the nuclei to bind androgens we attempted to determine whether the
various cell types in the testes differ in their capacity for this

function (52). While some degree of exchange has been detected in several types of germ cells, the most effective exchange was observed in late spermatids and spermatozoa.

SUMMARY

Taking under consideration the new evidence available, a picture emerges concerning the molecular mechanism of hormone action on spermatogenesis (Fig. 11).

1. FSH is bound to a specific membrane receptor on the cytoplasmic membrane of the Sertoli cell where it activates the adenyl cyclase. Cyclic AMP, formed in response to this stimulus, promotes DNA-dependent RNA synthesis resulting in formation of proteins including a specific androgen binding protein (ABP).

2. ABP is transported into the intercellular spaces where it binds androgens which have diffused into the seminiferous tubules from the interstitial area. The ABP has a high affinity for androgens but a rapid dissociation rate constant.

3. The ABP-androgen complex comes in contact with the germ cell membrane where it facilitates the transfer of androgen to a cytoplasmic androgen receptor. The receptor-androgen complex is transported into the germ cell nucleus. The mechanisms of the action of androgens on the germ cells subsequent to this step are unknown.

4. The ABP after delivery of androgen to the germ cell can bind more androgens. The above described process may be repeated, the ABP-androgen complex may be secreted into the lumen of the seminiferous tubule or the ABP may be broken down by proteolytic enzymes within the germinal epithelium.

5. There is some evidence that an androgen receptor may be present in the Sertoli cells. Whether it plays a role in stimulating protein synthesis in the Sertoli cells is unknown.

ACKNOWLEDGEMENTS

I am grateful to my colleagues and collaborators for the time devoted to discussions which served as the basis for the concepts presented in this paper. This work was supported in part by USPHS grants HD 06319, HD 06316 and HD 08338.

REFERENCES

1. Smith, P.E., J. Amer. Med. Ass. 88:158, 1927.

2. Greep, R.O. and Fevold, H.L., Endocrinology 21: 611, 1937.

3. Walsh, E.L., Cuyler, W.K., and McCullagh, D.R., Amer. J. Physiol. 107: 508, 1934.

4. Woods, M. C. and Simpson, M. E., Endocrinology 69: 91, 1961.

5. Lostroh, A.J., Acta Endocr. (Kbh.) 43: 592, 1963.

6. Randolph, P.W., Lostroh, A.J., Grattarola, R., Squire, P.G., and Li, P.H., Endocrinology 65: 433, 1959.

7. Simpson, M.E., Li, C.H., and Evans, H.M., Endocrinology 35: 96, 1944.

8. Clermont, Y. and Harvey, S.C., Ciba Foundation Study Colloquia on Endocrinology 16: 173, 1967.

9. von Berswordt-Wallrabe, R. and Neumann, F., Proc. 5th World Congr. Fertility Sterility, 581, 1966.

10. Steinberger, E. and Duckett, G.E., Endocrinology 76: 1184, 1965.

11. Steinberger, E. and Duckett, G.E., J. Reprod. Fert. Suppl. 2: 75, 1967.

12. Steinberger, E. and Steinberger, A., In The Gonads, McKerns, K.W. (ed.), Appleton-Century-Crofts, New York, 1969, p. 715.

13. Go, V.L.W., Vernon R.G., and Fritz, I.B., Can. J. Biochem. 49: 768, 1971.

14. Vernon, R.G., Go, V.L.W., and Fritz, I.B., J. Reprod. Fert. 42: 77, 1975.

15. Steinberger, E., Physiol. Rev. 51: 1, 1971.

16. Means, A.R. and Hall, P.F., Endocrinology 82: 597, 1968.

17. Means, A.R., Endocrinology 89; 981, 1971.

18. Mancini, R.E., Castro, A., and Seiguer, A.C., J. Histochem. Cytochem. 15: 516, 1967.

19. Castro, A.E., Seiguer, A.C., and Mancini, R.E., Proc. Soc. Exp. Biol. Med. 133: 582, 1970.

20. Means, A.R. and Vaitukaitis, J., Endocrinology 90: 39, 1972.

21. Bhalla, V.K. and Reichert, L.E., In Hormone Binding and Target Cell Activation in the Testis, Dufau, M.L. and Means, A.R. (eds.), Plenum Press, New York, 1974, p. 201.

22. Steinberger, A., Thanki, K.H., and Siegal, B., In Hormone Binding and Target Cell Activation in the Testis; Dufau, M.L. and Means, A.R. (eds.), Plenum Press, New York, 1974, p. 177.

23. Sutherland, E.W. and Rall, T.W., J. Biol. Chem. 232: 1077, 1962.

24. Kuehl, F.A. Jr., Patanelli, D.J., Tarnoff, J., and Humes, J.L., Biol. of Reprod. 2: 154, 1970

25. Murad, F., Strauch, S., and Vaughan, M., M. Biochim. Biophy. Acta 177: 591, 1969.

26. Dorrington, J.H., Vernon, R.G., and Fritz, I.B., Biochem. Biophys. Res. Commun. 46: 1523, 1972.

27. Braun, T. and Sepsenwol, S., Endocrinology 94: 1028, 1974.

28. Cooke, B.A., Rommerts, F.G., Van der Kemp, J.W.C.M., and Van der Molen, H.J., Molec. and Cell. Endocrinol. 1: 99, 1974.

29. Ritzen, E.M., Dobbins, M.C., Tindall, D.J., French, F.S., and Nayfeh, S.N., Steroids 21: 593, 1973.

30. Hansson, V., Djoseland, O., Reusch, E., Attramadal, A., and Torgersen, O., Steroids 21: 457, 1973.

31. Steinberger, E., Steinberger, A., and Sanborn, B., In Physiology and Genetics of Reproduction Part A, Coutinho, E.M. and Fuchs, F. (eds.), Plenum Press, New York, 1974, p. 163.

32. Vernon, R.G., Kopec, B., and Fritz, I.B., Molec. Cell. Endrocr. 1: 167, 1974.

33. Hansson, V., Reusch, E., Trygstad, O., Torgersen, O., French, F.S., and Ritzen, E.M. Nature New Biol. 246:56, 1973.

34. Hansson, V., Trygstad, O., French, F.S., McLean, W.S., Smith, A.A., Tindall, D.J., Weddington, S.C., Petrusz, P., Nayfeh, S.N., and Ritzen, E.M., Nature 250: 387, 1974.

35. Steinberger, E. and Nelson, W.O., Endocrinology 56: 429, 1955.

36. Steinberger, E. and Nelson, W.O., Endocrinology 60: 105, 1957.

37. Steinberger, E., J. Reprod. Fertil. 3: 250, 1962.

38. Chowdhury, A.K. and Steinberger, E., Am. J. Anat. 115: 509, 1964.

39. Steinberger, E., Steinberger, A., and Ficher, M., Rec. Progr.
     Hormone Res. 26: 547, 1970.

40. Steinberger, A., Heindel, J.J., Lindsey, J.N., Elkington, J.S.H.,
     Sanborn, B.M., and Steinberger, E., 1975, this volume, p. 399.

41. Steinberger, A., Heindel, J.J., Lindsey, J.N., Elkington, J.S.H.,
     Sanborn, B.M., and Steinberger, E., 1975, this volume, p. 399.

42. Steinberger, A., In Methods in Enzymology, Vol. 39, Part D.,
     O'Malley, B.W. and Hardman, J.G. (eds.), Academic Press, New
     York, 1975 (in press).

43. Steinberger, A. and Steinberger, E., J. Reprod. Fertil. 9: 243,
     1965.

44. Steinberger, A. and Steinberger, E., J. Reprod. Fert. Suppl. 2:
     117, 1967.

45. Heindel, J.J., Rothenberg, R., Robison, G.A., and Steinberger,
     A., J. of Cyclic Nucleotide Research, 1975 (in press).

46. Johnson, B.H. and Ewing, L.L., Science 173: 635, 1971.

47. Steinberger, E. and Ficher, M., Steroids 22: 425, 1973.

48. Steinberger, A., Thanki, K.H., and Siegal, B., In Hormone Binding
     and Target Cell Activation in the Testis, Dufau, M.L. and Means,
     A.R. (eds.), Plenum Press, New York, 1974, p. 177.

49. Steinberger, A., Thanki, K.H., and Siegal, B., Abstract #21,
     Annual Meeting of the Society for the Study of Reproduction,
     Athens, Ga., 1974.

50. Hansson, V., McLean, W.S., Smith, A.A., Tindall, D.J., Weddington,
     S.C., Nayfeh, S.N., and French, F.S., Steroids 23: 823, 1974.

51. Anderson, J., Clark, J.H., and Peck, E.J. Jr., Biochem. J. 126:
     561, 1972.

52. Sanborn, B.M., Elkington, J.S.H., Steinberger, A., Steinberger,
     E., and Meistrich, M.L., 1975, this volume, p. 293.

IN VITRO SYNTHESIS OF TESTICULAR ANDROGEN BINDING PROTEIN (ABP):

STIMULATION BY FSH AND ANDROGEN

E. Martin Ritzen and Lars Hagenas

Pediatric Endocrinology Unit, Department of Pediatrics,
Karolinska Sjukhuset, Stockholm, Sweden

Vidar Hansson, Institute of Pathology, Rikshospitalet,
Oslo, Norway

Frank S. French

Department of Pediatrics and the Laboratories for
Reproductive Biology, University of North Carolina,
Chapel Hill, North Carolina, U.S.A.

INTRODUCTION

Androgen binding protein (ABP) was first demonstrated in the
rat epididymis (1,2). It was subsequently shown that it originates
in the testes, is secreted into the lumen of the seminiferous
tubule and transported to the caput epididymidis where it is
partially (in the rat) or completely (in the rabbit) degraded (3,4,5).
ABP is produced in the Sertoli cells (6-12) and specifically stimulated by FSH (6,7,9,10,13). Being hitherto the only well characterized specific product of the Sertoli cell, it offers itself as
an index of the functional activity of the Sertoli cell, as well
as a specific end point of FSH action in the testis.

In a recent report (14), the in vitro synthesis of rat ABP in
short time testicular organ cultures was described. The experiments to
be reported in the present paper will show that Sertoli cell function
as studied in vitro by the rate of ABP synthesis in whole testes
or testicular minces is responsive to hormonal stimulation in vitro,
as well as pretreatment of the animals in vivo. The details of the
methods used have been described elsewhere (14).

353

IN VITRO SYNTHESIS OF ABP IN THE ABSENCE OF HORMONES

When decapsulated but otherwise intact rat testes are cultured at 32°C in vitro, there is a continuous accumulation of ABP in the surrounding medium. In the adult testes, part of this is derived from preformed ABP in the lumen of the seminiferous tubules (14), part is due to active synthesis. The influence of preformed ABP on the rate of accumulation of ABP in the medium is minimized by preincubation or rinsing of minced tissue before the culture. The actual de novo synthesis of ABP by the testis in vitro was shown by the following findings (14): 1. ABP accumulation in the medium is greatly reduced at 0°C (Fig. 1). 2. No accumulation of ABP occurs in the absence of essential amino acids. 3. Specific inhibitors of protein synthesis prevent the accumulation of ABP in the medium (Fig. 2).

In the initial experiments, decapsulated but otherwise intact testes were used. However, the inter-animal variation in ABP content and production rate proved to be so large that one testis from each animal had to be used as control for the other. Thus, the number of variables to be studied was very limited, and in later experiments pooled testicular minces were used (14).

Since the tissue is studied directly after the removal and preparation of the testes, the state of ABP synthesis during the period immediately preceding the sacrifice of the rat is also reflected in the rate of ABP synthesis in vitro. The "baseline" (without additions to the medium) rate of ABP synthesis is highest during the first 4 hours period, and then remains at a constant but lower rate for at least the following 16 hrs (Fig. 1), which may reflect the disappearance of stimulatory factors.

During the first 4 hr of incubation, the rate of ABP production by the 21 day old testis was found to be 0.5 pmole/h/testis   (Fig. 1). This production rate is considerably greater than the in vivo rate of ABP transport into the epididymis at the same age, (0.04 pmole/hr) as measured by ligation of the efferent ducts (Svan and Ritzen, unpublished). These findings could be explained by a release from some control mechanism which might restrict the production of ABP in vivo, by leakage through the blood-testis barrier, or by a faster rate of ABP degradation as it accumulates in the ligated testis. It seems likely that ABP produced in vitro may escape degradation by diffusing into the medium from the site of production. The observations that some ABP is broken down or made

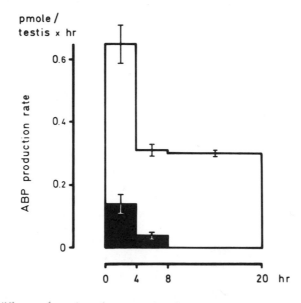

Figure 1. ABP production by testicular minces during 20 hr incubation. Testes from 21 day old rats were minced, pooled, and divided
into 100 mg aliquots that were incubated in Eagle's MEM (supplemented with L-glutamine and antibiotics) for 20 hr at 0^0 or 32^0C.
The medium was changed after 4 and 8 hr incubation. All media were
analyzed for ABP by steady state polyacrylamide gel electrophoresis
(16). Means ± S.E.M. N = 9 (0-4h), 6 (4-8h) and 3 (8-20h). Release
of preformed ABP at 0^0C is shown by the black columns. From
Ritzen et. al. 1975 (14).

inaccessible to hormone binding during the homogenization procedure
(14) and that the presence of certain sulfhydryl reagents seem to
enhance ABP binding activity in testis supernatant (Hansson, 1973)
also indicate that ABP degrading enzymes may be present in the
testis. Means and Tindall (15) reported that i.v. injection of FSH
to 16 day old "Sertoli-cell-only" rate resulted in a very rapid
increase in testicular ABP, followed by a similar rate decrease to
baseline levels within 4 hrs. Factors regulating the degradation of
ABP may prove to have important functions in the control of spermatogenesis.

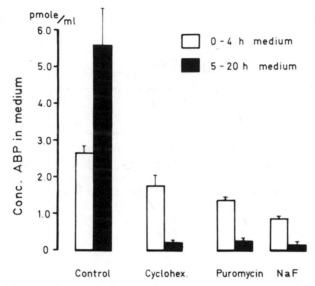

Figure 2. Effect of metabolic inhibitors on ABP synthesis. Twenty-one day old rat testes were minced, and 100 mg aliquots were incubated in 1.5 ml medium for 20 h, with change of medium after 4 h, without further additions, or in the presence of cycloheximide (0.05 mg/ml), puromycin (0.54 mg/ml)or NaF (75 mM). Mean ± S.E.M. of triplicate incubations. From Ritzen et. al., 1975 (14).

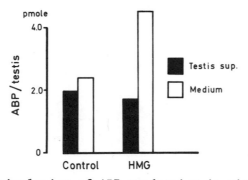

Figure 3.   HMG stimulation of ABP production in vitro.   One testis from each of four 21 day old rats was incubated in the presence of human HMG (7.5 IU/ml FSH, 2.5 IU/ml LH), the other testis serving as a control   All testes were rinsed by gentle shaking in the tissue culture medium for 2h at 0°C before the incubation at 33°C for 6h in HMG containing medium (2 ml/125 mg testis weight) was started.   At the end of the incubation, 105,000 x g supernatants were prepared as described elsewhere (16).   ABP in the incubation media and 105,000 x g supernatants was assayed by steady state polyacrylamine gel electrophoresis (SS-PAGE). (16)

GONADOTROPHIN STIMULATION OF ABP SYNTHESIS IN VITRO

When decapsulated testes from 21 day old rats were incubated for 6 hr at 33°C, ABP could be recovered in equal amounts from the medium and from the tissue that was homogenized after completed incubation (Fig. 3).   Addition of human postmenopausal gonadotrophin (HMG) caused an increase in ABP concentration in the medium, while ABP in the blotted tissue remained approximately unchanged, indicating a rapid release of newly formed ABP.   The increase in ABP production following HMG administration to the medium was dose dependent as measured by the accumulation of ABP in the medium (Fig. 4).

Addition of ovine FSH to the incubation medium of minced testes similarly caused a dose dependent increase in ABP accumulation in the medium (Table 1).   This response to added gonadotrophin was noticed at 37°C as well as 32°C, and was significant within the first 4 hours of incubation.   However, the response to stimulation with HMG or FSH is moderate (40-100% increase above baseline) compared

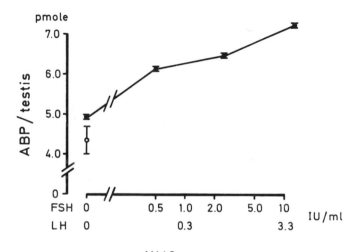

Figure 4. HMG stimulation of ABP production <u>in vitro</u>. Twenty-one
day old rats in groups of 4 were given one large dose (20 mg/rat)
of testosterone enanthate 3 days before the experiment. Decapsulated
but otherwise intact testes were preincubated for 1 h at 32°C,
followed by 6 h in the presence of increasing concentrations of HMG
(Homogonal[R] Leo) in tissue culture medium, 2ml/150 mg tissue, containing bovine serum albumin, 1 mg/ml. ABP was measured by SS–PAGE
in the final incubation media. Means and range of duplicate incubations. ABP production by testes from 4 parallel rats without
testosterone treatment (open circle) is included for reference.

TABLE I

Exp.	Age of Rats Days	Incubation Time, Hours	Concentration of NIH-FSH S-10			
			0	0.25	2.5	25 μg/ml
1	21	5-20	1.7 ± 0.17	2.4* ± 0.14	2.6* ± 0.12	2.8* ± 0.31
2	21(37°C)	0-4	2.8 ± 0.37	2.9 ± 0.56	3.7 ± 0.64	4.1* ± 0.17
		5-20	7.6 ± 1.2	9.8 ± 0.16	8.9 ± 1.06	10.2 ± 0.5
3	35	0-4	0.86 ± 0.11	C.94 ± 0.07	1.5 ± 0.14	1.1 ± 0.12
		5-20	2.3 ± 0.19	2.3 ± 0.39	2.7 ± 0.04	3.1 ± 0.31
	35(hypox at 28)	0-4	0.49 ± 0.18	0.60 ± 0.05	0.46 ± 0.10	0.59 ± 0.20
		5-20	1.3 ± 0.13	1.5 ± 0.13	1.5 ± 0.19	1.2 ± 0.15
4	70	0-4	0.47 ± 0.04	--	0.5 ± 0.09	--
		5-20	1.1 ± 0.05	--	1.5 ± 0.48	--
	70 (hypox at 50d)	0-4	0.42 ± 0.14	--	0.48 ± 0.04	--
		5-20	1.2 ± 0.20	--	1.5 ± 0.36	--

Effect of NIH-FSH S-10 on ABP production by testicular minces in vitro. Exp. 2 was performed at 37°C, the others at 32°C. Decapsulated testes from 4-8 rats were minced, pooled, and divided into 100 mg aliquots for incubation in the presence or absence of NIH-FSH S-10 in the medium. Means ± S.E.M. of ABP recovered from the medium (pmole/100 mg tissue) of triplicate incubations.

*Significantly (p<0.05) different from control without added FSH.

to that found in vivo (Hansson et al., 1973, 1974). Whether this
is due to a higher baseline production or the absence of other hormones acting synergistically with FSH remains to be shown.

No significant effect of FSH addition on the low baseline production of ABP was seen in testes obtained from intact or hypophysectomized 35-70 day old (Table 1) rats. This is in agreement with
the lack of stimulation of cyclic AMP production (17) or protein
synthesis (18) in testes of rats older than 35 days. The latter
responses to FSH, however, could be observed in mature testes
following hypophysectomy, which was not the case with ABP response
to FSH in vitro. This discrepancy may be due to the relatively short
period of time following hypophysectomy in our experiments. The
decrease in ABP production per 100 mg of tissue with increasing age
was observed previously (14), and may be explained by "dilution" of
Sertoli cells with cell types not involved in ABP production.

Addition of LH to testicular organ cultures is known to result
in a rapid release of testosterone to the medium (19,20). This could
explain preliminary observations that LH had a significant stimulatory effect on ABP synthesis by testicular minces in vitro. Also,
the combination of LH and FSH in the form of HMG gave less variation
than with FSH alone. Since testosterone is able to maintain ABP
production in hypophysectomized rats, and also potentiate the
effect of FSH on ABP synthesis (21-23), the combination of LH and
FSH in vitro may serve to increase the androgen concentration around
the tubules and augment the FSH response. This prompted us to examine
the direct effect of androgens on ABP synthesis in vitro.

EFFECTS OF TESTOSTERONE ON THE RATE OF ABP SYNTHESIS IN VITRO

In vivo administration of testosterone propionate to 18 day old
rats for 6 days caused a dose dependent decrease in the in vitro ABP
production rate up to a dose of 50 µg/day, while a larger dose resulted in a complete recovery to control levels. Estradiol given
to a parallel group of rats resulted in a dose-dependent decrease
in ABP production rates up to the largest dose given, 100 µg/day
(Fig. 5). The suppression of in vitro ABP synthesis may be explained by a suppression of the endogenous FSH levels in vivo. The
finding that administration of large doses of testosterone in vivo
caused the synthesis of ABP in vitro to continue at or above the
control levels (Fig. 5) is in agreement with similar studies in vivo
Androgenic hormones act synergistically with FSH in stimulating ABP
production, and treatment with testosterone alone maintains ABP
production in vivo after hypophysectomy (21-23).

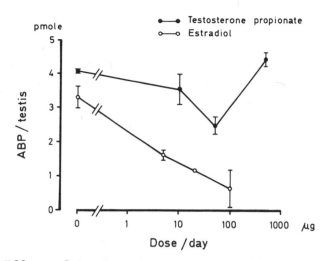

Figure 5.   Effect of in vivo testosterone or 17β-estradiol treatment on the in vitro ABP synthesis by prepubertal rat testis.   Immature male rats were given daily i.m. injections of testosterone
propionate (0,10,50 or 500 µg/rat x day) or 17β-estradiol (0,5,20
or 100 µg/rat x day) in oil from 18th to the 24th day of age.
Twentyfour hours after the last injections the testes were removed, minced, washed twice, and incubated in duplicates for 5 h
(estradiol experiment) or 6 h (testosterone experiment) at 32°C.
The media were analyzed for ABP, and the results expressed as ABP
produced by one testis (mean and range of duplicate incubations).

In vitro addition of testosterone to the incubation medium
caused assignificant increase in the ABP production rate by the 17
day old minced testes, 5-20 hr after the start of the incubation,
compared to controls (Fig. 6).   It is known that testosterone is
rapidly metabolized to 5α-reduced steroids by the immature rat testis
(24), and the stimulatory effect of added testosterone may well be
due to one or several of its metabolites.   However, these results
show that androgens have a direct action on the testis in stimulating ABP synthesis.

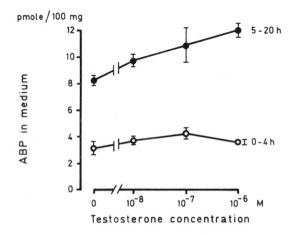

Figure 6. Effect of testosterone on ABP synthesis in vitro. Testes
from 17 day old rats were minced, pooled and divided into 60 mg
aliquots that were incubated in triplicates for 20 h at 32°C in the
presence of 0, 10^{-8}, 10^{-7}, or 10^{-6} M testosterone. Medium was
changed after 4 h. All media were analyzed for ABP by steady
state PAGE. Means ± S.E.M. of total ABP in the media for triplicate incubations.

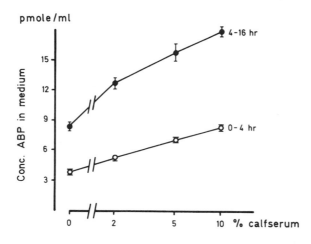

Figure 7. Effect of added calf serum on the rate of ABP synthesis
in vitro. Testicular minces from seven 21 day old rats were divided
into 100 mg aliquots and incubated with 0, 2, 5, or 10% serum for
20 h at 32°C. The calf serum had previously been heated to 70°C
for 30 min, which completely destroyed the testosterone binding
globulin (TeBG). The medium was changed after 4 h. All media were
analyzed for ABP, and results given as means ± S.E.M. of triplicate
incubations.

EFFECT OF CALF SERUM ON ABP PRODUCTION IN VITRO

    Addition of 2-10% heated calf serum to the incubation media had
a marked effect on the ABP production rate by 21 day old testicular
minces (Fig. 7), indicating that in addition to FSH and androgenic
hormones, other less specific factors may also act synergistically with
these hormones. Although the concentrations of gonadotrophins and androgens in this serum were not measured, the physiological levels are
low compared to the amounts of authentic FSH and testosterone used in
the previous experiments. Calf serum is known to contain several
other growth promoting components (25). A systematic study of
various serum factors is needed before the regulation of Sertoli
cell function will be fully understood.

CONCLUSIONS

1. Testicular androgen binding protein (ABP) is actively synthesized by immature whole testes or testicular minces in vitro
   at a higher rate than is measured in vivo.

2. The rate of in vitro ABP synthesis during the first 20 hr in
   culture reflects the rate of ABP production immediately before
   sacrifice of the animal.

3. ABP synthesis in vitro by immature testis tissue is stimulated
   by addition of human postmenopausal gonadotrophin (HMG),
   FSH or testosterone to the medium.

4. The stimulationoof ABP synthesis by added calf serum indicates
   that other factors than FSH and androgens may be important for
   the regulation of in vivo production of ABP.

ACKNOWLEDGEMENTS

The authors are indebted to the National Institute for Arthritis and Metabolic Diseases and to A.B. Leo, Sweden, for generous
gifts of LH-FSH and HMG (Homogonal), respectively.

Supported by the Swedish Medical Research Council (project 3168),
WHO (project H9-181-135), NIH (project HD04466) Nordic Insulin
Foundation and the Norwegian Research Council (NAVF) for Science
and the Humanities.

REFERENCES

1. Ritzen, E.M., Nayfeh, S.N., French, F.S. and Dobbins, M.C
   Endocrinology 89: 143, 1971.

2. Hansson, V. and Tveter, K.J., Acta Endocrinol. (Kbh) 66: 745, 1971

3. French, F.S. and Ritzen, E.M., Endocrinology 95: 88, 1973.

4. Ritzen, E.M., Dobbins, M.C., Tindall, D.J., French, F.S., and
   Nayfeh, S.N. Steroids 21: 593, 1973.

5. Ritzen, E.M. and French, F.S., J. Steroid Biochem. 5: 151, 1974.

6. Hansson, V., Reusch, E., Trygstad, O., Torgersen, O., French,
    F.S., and Ritzen, E.M. Nature, New Biol. 246: 56, 1973.

7. Hansson, V., Trygstad, O., French, F.S., McLean, W.S., Smith,
    A.A., Tindall, D.J., Weddington, S.C., Petrusz, P., Nayfeh, S.N.,
    and Ritzen, E.M. Nature 250: 387, 1974.

8. Ritzen, E.M., Hagenas, L., Hansson, V., French, F.S., and
    Nayfeh, S.N. Proc. of II Symp. of J. Steroid Biochem., March
    1974, in J. Steroid Biochem. 5:   , 1974.

9. Fritz, I.B., Kopec, B., Lam, K. and Vernon, R.G. In "Hormone
    Binding and Activation in the Testis" ed. M. Dufau and A. Means,
    Plenum Press, 1974.

10. Tindall, T.J., Schrader, W.T., and Means, A.R., In: "Hormone
    Binding and Target Cell Activation in the Testis", eds. Dufau,
    M.L., Means, A.R., Plenum Press, N.Y., 1974, p. 167.

11. Vernon, R.D., Kopec, B. and Fritz, I.B. Mol. Cell Endocrinology
    1: 167, 1974.

12. Hagenas, L., Ritzen, E.M., Hansson, V., French, F.S. and Nayfeh,
    S.N. Mol. Cell. Endocr., in press, (May 1975).

13. Sanborn, B.M., Eckington, T.S.H., and Steinberger, E. In: Hor-
    mone Binding and Activation in the Testis, eds. Dufau, M.L. and
    Means, A.R., Plenum Press, New York, 1974, p. 291.

14. Ritzen, E.M., Hagenas, L., Hansson, V., and French, F.S.
    Submitted to Mol. Cell. Endocrinology.

15. Means, A.R. and Tindall, D.J., this volume, p. 383.

16. Ritzen, E.M., French, F.S., Weddington, S.C., Nayfeh, S.N. and
    Hansson, V.   J. Biol. Chem. 249: 6597, 1974.

17. Dorrington, J. and Fritz, I.B. Endocrinology 94: 345, 1974.

18. Means, A. and Huckins, C., In: "Hormone Binding and Target Cell
    Activiation in the Testis", eds. Dafau, M.L. and Means, A.R.,
    p. 143, Plenum Press, 1974.

19. Dufau, M.L., Catt, K.T. and Tsuruhara, T.   Biochim. Biophys.
    Acta (Amst.) 252: 574, 1971.

20. Van Damme, M.P., Robertson, D.M., Romani, P. and Diczfalusy, E.
    Acta Endocrinol. (Kbh) 74: 642, 1974.

21. Hansson, V., French, F.S., Weddington, S.C., Nayfeh, S.N. and Ritzen, E.M. In: "Hormone Binding and Target Cell Activation in the Testis", eds. Dafau, M.L. and Means, A.R., p. 287, Plenum Press, 1974.

22. Weddington, S.C., Hansson, V., French, F.S., Nayfeh, S.N., Ritzen, E.M. and Hagenas, L., Nature 254: 145, 1975.

23. Elkington, J.S.H., Sanborn, B.M. and Steinberger, E., Mol. Cell. Endocr. 2: 157, 1975.

24. Nayfeh, S.N., Barefoot, S.W. Jr., and Baggett, B. Endocrinology, 78: 1041, 1966.

25. Wolstenholme, G.E.W., Knight, J. (eds.) "Growth Control in Cell Cultures", Ciba Foundation Symp., Williams and Wilkins Co., Baltimore, 1971.

BIOCHEMICAL RESPONSES OF CULTURED SERTOLI CELL-ENRICHED PREPARATIONS TO FOLLICLE STIMULATING HORMONE AND DIBUTYRYL CYCLIC AMP

Irving B. Fritz, B. Gregory Louis, Pierre S. Tung, Michael Griswold, Focko G. Rommerts and Jennifer H. Dorrington

Banting and Best Department of Medical Research University of Toronto, Toronto, Canada M5G 1L6

INTRODUCTION

Dorrington et. al. (1) have reported previously that FSH increases cyclic AMP formation by cultured Sertoli cell-enriched preparations. More recently the preparative and culture procedures also have been improved so that Sertoli cells can be better maintained and characterized. This report presents an investigation of Sertoli cell responses to FSH and other hormones under defined conditions. Details of methodology and information on the structural characteristics of the Sertoli-cell preparations have been provided elsewhere (2-4).

Preliminary observations indicated that FSH treatment of Sertoli cell-enriched cultures resulted in an increased appearance of androgen binding protein (ABP) activity in the medium(5). Since then, we have explored this phenomenon in more detail. This paper will summarize some of the data documenting the conclusion that ABP is produced by Sertoli cell-enriched preparations, and that FSH or cyclic AMP derivatives regulates ABP production in vitro. In addition, we shall summarize other recently obtained information indicating that treatment with FSH or cyclic AMP derivatives increases amino acid incorporation into proteins (3), thymidine incorporation into nuclear DNA by cultured Sertoli cells (6), and the rate of conversion of testosterone to 17β-estradiol (7).

ANDROGEN BINDING PROTEIN PRODUCTION BY SERTOLI
CELL-ENRICHED PREPARATIONS

We have previously suggested that the production of ABP by
Sertoli cells provides a specific response of potential physiological significance with which to follow FSH actions on the Sertoli
cell (5). The tentative conclusion that ABP was probably produced
by Sertoli cells in vivo was based on the following: (a) The depressed testicular ABP levels in adult hypophysectomized rats are
increased following FSH administration (5,8); (b) ABP levels are
elevated in regressed cryptorchid testes, when expressed as pmole
per mg testicular protein (5,8); (c) ABP capacity per mg protein
in testes from sex reversed adult female mice (Sxr mutants) are
within normal limits, even though these testes are completely devoid of germinal cells (5); and (d) little or no ABP could be detected in extracts from Leydig cells (8). Thus germinal cells
and Leydig cells appeared to be ruled out as a source for ABP. The
low testicular ABP levels in long-term hypophysectomized rats were
interpreted to indicate impaired Sertoli cell function (5,8).

Information published from other laboratories provides additional support to the hypothesis that ABP originates in Sertoli
cells. ABP levels are normal in testes partially depleted of
germinal cells by irradiation or treatment with nitrofurazon (9,10),
and has been in testes and epididymides of prenatally irradiated,
"Sertoli cell only" rats (11). This model is described in this
volume. There is ample evidence also from other laboratories that
in vivo FSH administration to hypophysectomized rats increases testicular ABP levels (9-12).

It was clearly desirable to test directly the hypothesis that
FSH stimulates Sertoli cells to produce ABP. Accordingly, we have
investigated ABP production by cultured Sertoli cell-enriched preparations. Stimulation by FSH of the appearance of ABP activity
in the medium of testicular cultures prepared from 20 day old rats
is shown in Fig 1. Methods used have been described in detail elsewhere (13). Neither synthetic ACTH (5 mg/ml) nor albumin (10 µg/ml)
influenced ABP production by cells cultured under identical conditions. Relatively impure FSH (NIH-FSH-S-10), at concentrations of
5.0 and 0.5 µg/ml, and a more purified FSH (G4-150c, kindly provided
by Dr. H. Papkoff) at a concentration of 0.2 µg/ml, were equally
effective in enhancing ABP production. In contrast, treatment of
cultures with HCG (NIH-HCG-CR 115) at concentrations up to 1 µg/ml
had no effect on ABP production (unpublished observations).

Within a given cell preparation, the initial ABP production per replicate vessel during the first 24 hours of culture is
relatively uniform. The coefficient of variation in a typical ex-

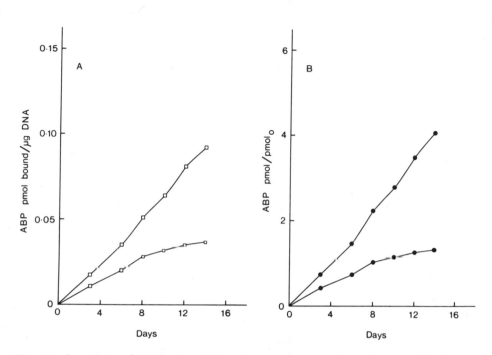

Figure 1. Stimulation by FSH of appearance of androgen binding activity in medium of cultured Sertoli cell-enriched preparations. Cells were cultured for 24 hrs in the defined medium alone, and then maintained for 14 days under identical conditions (lower curves); or in the presence of 5 μg/ml NIH-FSH-S10 (upper curves). At each point shown, the culture medium was removed from each flask for ABP assay, and fresh medium plus or minus FSH was added. The graphs are cumulative from the initial time of treatment. At the end of the experiments, cells were removed, and DNA content was determined. In panel A, data are expressed as pmole bound steroid in the medium per μg cell DNA. In panel B, the data are expressed as the ratio of the amount of steroid binding activity observed in medium from a given culture flask to the amount of steroid binding activity released into the medium in the same flask during the initial 24 hr culture period ($pmol_o$). Medium from each of four flasks was assayed separately, and the average androgen binding activity for the 4 determinations is represented by each point. In all cases, ABP activity was assayed by equilibrium dialysis against 1 nM (^{3}H)-dihydrotestosterone, as described in detail elsewhere (16).

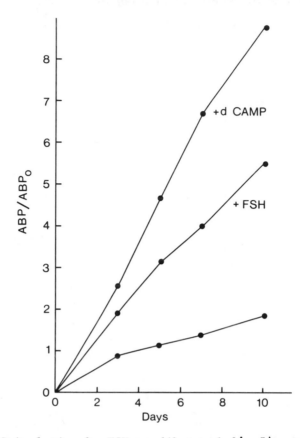

Figure 2.   Stimulation by FSH or dibutyryl 3', 5'-cyclic AMP of
appearance of androgen binding activity in medium of cultured
Sertoli cell preparations.   Data are expressed as in panel B of
Figure 1.   From Fritz et. al., 1975 (13).

periment with 24 culture flasks was 15.8%.   Cells subsequently
treated with dibutyryl cyclic AMP (0.1 mM) had higher rates of
production than did control cells or cells treated with FSH (Fig. 2).
Largest effects were evident in cells cultured in the presence of
dibutyryl cyclic AMP for several days (approximately a 3-fold increase after 4 days in culture).   Stimulation of ABP production
was also observed in cells treated with 0.1 mM N6-monobutyryl cyclic
AMP (Table 1).   A small increase (approximately 40%) was obtained
in cells treated with 1.0 mM cyclic AMP.   In contrast, there was
no effect on ABP production when cells were cultured under comparable conditions in the presence of 02-monobutyryl cyclic AMP
(0.1 mM) (Table 1).

TABLE I

Androgen Binding Protein (ABP) Activity
in the Medium of Sertoli Cell-Enriched
Preparations Cultured for 96 Hours

Treatment	ABP/ABP$_o$
Control	1.85 ± 0.034*(4)
N6-Monobutyryl cyclic AMP (10^{-4}M)	3.53 ± 0.159 (4)
02-Monobutyryl cyclic AMP (10^{-4}M)	1.78 ± 0.112 (4)
Sodium butyrate (10^{-4}M)	1.57 ± 0.251 (2)
5' Adenosine monophosphate (10^{-3}M)	1.90 ± 0.264 (2)

* Results are expressed as means ±SEM of the ratio of ABP activity
obtained in medium from cells cultured for 96 hours under conditions indicated, to the initial ABP activity (ABP$_o$), obtained during
the previous 24 hours, when cells were cultured in the defined
medium alone. ABP activities were determined by equilibrium
dialysis, by methods described elsewhere (13), using 1 nM 3H-dihy-
drotestosterone in the dialysis solution. In the experiment
indicated, ABP$_o$ levels were 1.38 ± 0.042 in 24 vessels. Numbers
within parentheses denote the number of replicate culture flasks
analyzed in the experiment.

K_d values and steroid specificity of ABP in the medium (13) were found to be similar to those previously reported for testicular ABP (5,8). The K_d for testosterone and dihydrotestosterone (DHT), calculated from Scatchard plots of results obtained with the charcoal-dextran method, were 2-3 nM for ABP present in concentrated medium in which Sertoli cell-enriched preparations had been cultured. When analyzed by steady-state polyacrylamide gel electrophoresis, according to the techniques of Ritzen et. al. (14), the (^{3}H)-DHT binding protein in the concentrated medium had a relative mobility identical to that obtained for ABP extracted from testis (13). ABP samples from the culture medium of control, FSH-treated and dibutyryl cyclic AMP-treated cells were observed to have identical electrophoretic mobilities in this system (13). ABP activity in the medium was destroyed following digestion with protease.

Intracellular ABP activity initially plated in culture flasks was less than 0.002 pmole/µgDNA, and this level did not appreciably change during culture under conditions described. In contrast, nearly 50 times this much ABP activity was released into the medium by cells cultured for 12 days in the presence of FSH (Fig 1A), and a greater amount by cells stimulated with dibutyryl cyclic AMP (Fig 2). These data indicate that ABP produced is rapidly secreted into the medium.

Addition of cycloheximide (1 µg/ml) to the medium reduced ABP production by approximately 60% in Sertoli cell-enriched preparations cultured for 48 hours. A similar degree of inhibition of incorporation of labeled amino acids into total proteins in the medium was also observed in these preparations (unpublished observations). Combined data are consistent with the conclusion that ABP released into the medium represents de novo protein synthesis.

INCORPORATION OF (^{3}H)-LEUCINE INTO PROTEIN BY SERTOLI CELL-ENRICHED PREPARATIONS

Means and Hall (15) demonstrated that FSH administration to immature rats increased the incorporation of labeled amino acids into proteins by whole testis preparations. The possible influence of FSH and dibutyryl cyclic AMP on the incorporation of (^{3}H)-leucine into proteins of cultured Sertoli cell-enriched preparations was therefore investigated (3). Preparations cultured in a protein free defined medium for 48 hours in the presence of FSH (5 µg/ml of NIH-FSH-S10) or dibutyryl cyclic AMP (0.1 mM) subsequently incorporated (^{3}H)- leucine into material precipitable by trichloroacetic acid (TCA) at a rate greater than that observed in cells cultured in the absence of FSH (Table 2). The increase in the specific activity of the TCA precipitate was highly reproducible, and was linear for the 2 hr period investigated (Fig 3). The rate

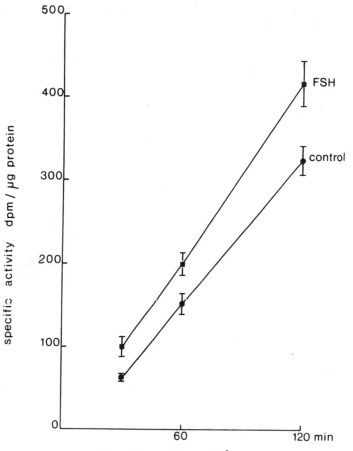

Figure 3.   Incorporation of (^{3}H)-leucine into TCA-precipitable material by Sertoli cell-enriched preparations previously cultured for 48 hr in MEM in the presence and absence of FSH (NIH-FSH S-10, 5 µg/ml). From Dorrington, et. al., 1975 (3).

of incorporation was linear for 48 hrs in culture when 0.4 mM (^{3}H)-leucine was present in the medium (unpublished observations). These data indicate sustained functional activity of preparations cultured in the presence or absence of FSH. In each experiment the total protein remaining in cells attached to the surface of the culture flasks was higher in those cultures to which either FSH or dibutyryl cyclic AMP had been added (Table 2).

The incorporation of (^{3}H)-leucine into TCA-insoluble material during the 2 hour incubation period was abolished by cycloheximide

TABLE II

The Incorporation of (^{3}H)-Leucine Into TCA-Insoluble Material By Sertoli Cells Previously Cultured For 48 Hr in the Presence of FSH (NIH-FSH-S10) or Dibutyryl Cyclic AMP

Additions to Culture Medium

Exp.	None protein (μg)	None S.A.[2] dpm/μg	FSH (5μg/ml) protein (μg)	FSH (5μg/ml) S.A.[2] dpm/μg	Dibutyryl Cyclic AMP (0.1mM) protein (μg)	Dibutyryl Cyclic AMP (0.1mM) S.A.[2] dpm/μg
1	821	296	863	466	972	465
2	462	282	602	373	610	320
3	702	324	1182	404	1022	467
4	684	370	898	475	812	428
5	550	342	718	428	702	489
Mean S.E.M.	644	323	853	429 ±19	824	434 ±30

1   After 48 hr in culture, the medium was replaced by Krebs-Ringer-bicarbonate buffer containing 1 mg/ml glucose and 0.1 the complement of amino acids in Eagle's MEM having 1.0 μCi (^{3}H)-leucine/ml. The final leucine concentration was 0.04 mM. The incubation was terminated after 2 hr by the addition of TCA. Aliquots of the TCA precipitate were assayed for protein and for radioactivity.

2   **$p < 0.02$, ***$p < 0.01$ (Aspin-Welch test of significance versus control).

(100 μg/ml) added 30 min before the addition of (^{3}H)-leucine (3).
The relatively small stimulation (30%) in (^{3}H)-leucine incorporation rates of Sertoli cell-enriched cultures treated with FSH or
dibutyryl cyclic AMP was highly reproducible. The mechanisms involved are being investigated. FSH effects are not evident until
cells have been cultured in the presence of FSH for 24 hours (3).
Similar results have been obtained with respect to ABP production
(13), indicating that complex intervening events must occur between
the time the cells first are stimulated by FSH or dibutyryl cyclic
AMP and the time specific proteins are synthesized.

The degree of stimulation by FSH of amino acid incorporation
into protein (approximately 30%) is considerably less than that
observed for stimulation of ABP production under identical conditions
(Figs 1,2) or of tubulin synthesis (unpublished observations). It
therefore appears that the Sertoli cell-enriched preparations preferentially synthesize particular proteins in response to FSH or
dibutyryl cyclic AMP stimulation.

CYCLIC AMP PRODUCTION BY ISOLATED SERTOLI CELL-ENRICHED PREPARATIONS

Addition of FSH to Sertoli cell-enriched preparations before
or after culturing them increased cyclic AMP levels (Table 3).
These data confirm and extend previous observations (1). Addition
of LH did not influence cyclic AMP levels in these preparations,
but LH did increase cyclic AMP in whole testis preparations from
20 day old rats (Table 3) (3). These data indicate that the Sertoli
cell-enriched preparations were essentially free of Leydig cells
(3).

OTHER BIOCHEMICAL PROPERTIES OF SERTOLI CELL-ENRICHED
PREPARATIONS UNDER INVESTIGATION

The increased conversion of testosterone to 17β-estradiol by
Sertoli cell-enriched preparations cultured in the presence of
FSH or dibutyryl cyclic AMP is published elsewhere in this book.
(7) In contrast, no influence of FSH on the conversion of (^{14}C)
testosterone to DHT and androstanediols is evident (2,16).

A greatly increased incorporation of (^{3}H)-thymidine into
nuclear DNA of Sertoli cell-enriched preparations has also been
recently observed in cultures treated with FSH or dibutyryl cyclic
AMP. These findings have been presented separately (6). The magnitude of FSH stimulation of DNA synthesis in treated cells is
considerably larger than that observed for other biochemical

TABLE III

Influences of FSH and LH on Cyclic AMP Formation by Whole Testis Preparations and Sertoli Cell-
Enriched Preparations From 20 Day Old Rats

Nature of Testicular Preparation	3'5' Cyclic AMP Levels (pmole/mg protein)			
	Control	FSH-NIH	FSH-Papkoff	LH-NIH
Whole Testis, Not Cultured	13*	110	56	54
Sertoli Cell, Not Cultured	17	94	110	11
Sertoli Cell, Cultured for 48 hr	17	233	220	12

* Cyclic AMP assays were performed in washed preparations, incubated for 20 mins at 32°C in 1 ml Krebs-Ringer bicarbonate buffer
containing 1 mg glucose/ml and 0.5 mM 3-isobutyl-1-methyl
xanthine. Concentrations employed were 10 µg/ml NIH-FSH-S10
0.5 µg/ml FSH (Papkoff G4-150C) and 10 µg/ml NIH-LH-S18. From
Dorrington et al., 1975 (3).

processes thus far examined, with the exception of the conversion
of testosterone to 17β-estradiol (7), and increased adenylate
cyclase activity (3).

GENERAL CONSIDERATIONS OF THE SERTOLI CELL-ENRICHED CULTURES

Differential cell counts of cultured Sertoli cell-enriched
preparations are shown in Table 4. A summary of the morphological
and ultrastructural characteristics of these preparations (4), on
which the counts in Table 4 are dependent, is given in Table 5.

TABLE IV

Differential Cell Counts in Sertoli
Cell-Enriched Preparations

Cell Type	Percentage Distribution* of Cells			
	Initial Aggregates	Cultured for 2-3 days	Cultured for 4-6 days	Trypsin-Removed Cultures
Sertoli Cells	70.3±2.6	85.0±2.9	88.0±0.7	93.0±1.3
Germinal Cells	23.1±4.2	8.7±1.4	10.5±1.1	3.7±1.4
Unidentified or Degenerating Cells	6.7±1.8	6.3±0.8	1.0±0.7	3.3±0.3

* Percentage distribution was obtained by identifying 470-1150 cells from each of 3 different preparations for each class listed, utilizing electron microscopy for structural identification.

Table 6 provides a comparison of the characteristics of the cultured Sertoli cell-enriched preparation which distinguishes them from cultured peritubular cell preparations. Finally, Table 7 summarizes the biochemical processes stimulated in Sertoli cell-enriched cultures by FSH which are referred to in this paper.

Two major unifying themes emerge from work summarized. The first involves the role of cyclic AMP in Sertoli cells. Increased cyclic AMP formation is elicited by FSH in Sertoli cell-enriched tubules obtained from hypophysectomized, cryptorchid or irradiated rats (17). The same response is observed in cultured Sertoli cell-enriched preparations (Table 3) (1,3). Treatment of cultured, Sertoli cell-enriched preparations with dibutyryl cyclic AMP results in the same responses as treatment with FSH. There is increased ABP formation (13), increased amino acid incorporation into proteins (3), increased conversion of testosterone to estradiol (7), increased incorporation of (^{3}H)-thymidine into nuclear DNA (6), and increased tubulin formation (unpublished observations). These findings strongly suggest that some or perhaps all of the FSH effects on Sertoli cells may be mediated via stimulation of adenylate cyclase activity.

TABLE V

Summary of Morphological and Ultrastructural
Characteristics of Cultured Sertoli
Cell-Enriched Preparations

I. General

    A. Homogeneous population of cells

        1. Light microscope level: Giemsa stain

        2. Transmission EM level: ≃ 90% similar appearance

    B. Ultrastructural characteristics

        1. Tight junctions

        2. Markedly indentated nucleus

        3. Satellite structures adjacent to nucleolus

        4. Well-developed Golgi apparatus

        5. Presence of other fine structures reported in
            Sertoli cells in situ

II. Structural Changes in Response to FSH

    A. Appearance of multiple cytoplasmic extensions

    B. Characteristic changes evident at scanning EM level

    C. Microtubule changes, with increased tubulin formation

The second theme involves the similarity between the biochemical behavior of Sertoli cell-enriched preparations in culture
and Sertoli cells in vivo. The structural properties of cultured
Sertoli cells are clearly not identical to those of Sertoli cells
in vivo, as is grossly evident from the tendency of the cultured
cells to flatten and lose the shape of elongated columnar epithelial
cells. Yet, the biochemical properties of the cultured cells
seem consistent with what is known about Sertoli cells in vivo.

TABLE VI

Summary of Characteristics of Cultured Sertoli Cell-Enriched Preparations which Distinguish Them from Cultured Peritubular Cell Preparations from Testes of 20 Day Old Rats

Property	Sertoli Cells	Peritubular Cells
General Shape	Squamous and polygonal in shape under most conditions	Shape variable, ranging from spindle, stellate to polyhedral
Growth Behavior in Culture	Forms monolayer only: mosaic-type cell borders.	Tendency to form multilayers, with frequent criss-crossing.
Mitotic Index	<0.03%	0.8-2.2
Structural Characteristics at Higher Magnification	1. Pleomorphic nucleus 2. Heterochromatin clumps in periphery of nucleus 3. Karyosomal structures seen around nucleolus. 4. Unique tight junctions 5. SER well developed, and RER not dilated. 6. Cytoplasmic filaments near plasma membrane rarely evident. 7. Very well developed Golgi apparatus. 8. Evidence of phagocytosis of foreign bodies	1. Nucleus oblong or slender. 2. Heterochromatin distributed more uniformly usually. 3. Nucleolus never tripartite. 4. Tight junctions never evident. 5. RER often dilated 6. Arrays of cytoplasmic filaments often appear near plasma membrane. 7. Interfilamentous dense bands frequent. 8. Autophagous bodies frequent
Responsiveness to FSH	Responds in defined medium, showing characteristic cytoplasmic extensions with arrays of parallel microtubules.	Non-responsive.

TABLE VII

Summary of Biochemical Processes Stimulated in
Sertoli Cell-Enriched Cultures by FSH

---

1. Increased cyclic AMP formation.

2. Increased incorporation of (^{3}H)-leucine into
    intracellular proteins.

3. Increased formation of extracellular ABP.

4. Increased (^{3}H)-thymidine incorporation into
    nuclear DNA.

5. Increased tubulin formation.

6. Increased conversion of testosterone to 17β-
    estradiol.

Administration of FSH in vivo has been shown to increase AMP production by testicular cells which have been inferred to be Sertoli
cells (5,9-12); to increase incorporation of amino acids into proteins (15) and to alter Sertoli cell morphology (18). These similarities encourage additional researches on the biochemical properties of the Sertoli cell-enriched cultures. The low rate of
mitosis in cultured cell preparations from testes of 20 day old
rats is consistent with the low mitotic activity of Sertoli cells
in vivo, and the diminished incorporation of (^{3}H)-thymidine into
Sertoli cell nuclear DNA with age (19,20). The higher levels of
incorporation of (^{3}H)-thymidine into nuclear DNA of cultured
Sertoli cells prepared from 10 day old rats than in those from
older animals (6) are also consistent with in vivo observations (20).

The interrelations of Sertoli cells with each other and with
germinal cells are multiple and complex (21). Germinal cell
development during spermatogenesis is doubtless dependent on hormones at more than one stage (22,23). It is conceivable that
hormonal regulation of Sertoli cell functions may provide one set
of important controls by which FSH and possibly androgens indirectly influence spermatogenesis.

ACKNOWLEDGMENTS

We are indebted to Ms. Krystyna Burdzy, Ms. Heather McKeracher and Ms. Eva Johansson for excellent technical assistance. We thank Mrs. Erene Stanley for typing the manuscript.

Supported by grants from the Canadian Medical Research Council and the Banting Research Foundation.

REFERENCES

1. Dorrington, J.H., Roller, N.F., and Fritz, I.B. In: Hormone Binding and Target Cell Activation in the Testis (eds) M. Dufau and A.R. Means, Plenum Press, 1974, p. 237.

2. Dorrington, J.H. and Fritz, I.B. Endocrinology 96: 1975. (in press).

3. Dorrington, J.H., Roller, N.F., and Fritz, I.B. Molec. Cell. Endocrinol., 1975 (in press).

4. Tung, P.S., Dorrington, J.H. and Fritz, I.B. Proc. Nat. Acad. Sci. (US) 1975, (in press).

5. Fritz, I.B., Kopec, B. Lam, K. and Vernon, R.G. In: Hormone Binding and Target Cell Activation in the Testis (eds) M. Dufau and A.R. Means, Plenum Press, 1974, p. 311.

6. Griswold, M., Mably, E. and Fritz, I.B. This Volume, p. 413, 1975.

7. Armstrong, D., Dorrington, J.H. and Fritz, I.B. This Volume p. 85, 1975.

8. Vernon, R.G., Kopec, B. and Fritz, I.B. Molec. and Cell. Endocrinol., 1: 167, 1974.

9. Hansson, V., Reusch, E., Trygstad, O., Torgersen, O., Ritzen, E.M. and French, F.S. Nature, New biology, 246: 56, 1973(b).

10. Hansson, V., Trygstad, O., French, F.S., McLean, W.S., Smith, A.A., Tindall, D.J., Weddington, S.C., Petrusz, P. Nayfeh, S.N. and Ritzen, E.M. Nature 250: 387, 1974.

11. Tindall, D.J., Schrader W.T. and Means, A.R. In: Hormone
     Binding and Target Cell Activation in the Testis, (eds) M.L.
     Dufau and A.R. Means, New York: Plenum Press, 167, 1974.

12. Sanborn, B.M., Elkington, J.S.H., Chowdhury, M., Tcholakian,
     R.K. and Steinberger, E. Endrocrinology, 96: 304, 1975.

13. Fritz, I.B., Rommerts, R.G., Louis, B.G., and Dorrington, J.H.
     (in press), J. Reprod. Fertil., 1975.

14. Ritzen, E.M., French, F.S., Weddington, S.C., Nayfeh, S.N., and
     Hansson, V. J. Biol. Chem., 249: 6597, 1974.

15. Means, A.R. and Hall, P.F., Biochemistry 8: 4293, 1969.

16. Dorrington, J.H. and Fritz, I.B. This Volume, p. 37, 1975.

17. Dorrington, J.H. and Fritz, I.B Endocrinology, 94:395, 1974.

18. Murphy, H.D. Proc. Soc. Exper. Biol. Med. 118: 1202, 1965.

19. Steinberger, E., Steinberger, A. and Ficher, M. Rec. Prog.
     Hormone Res. 26: 547, 1970.

20. Nagy, F.   J. Reprod. Fertil. 28: 389, 1972.

21. Fawcett, D.F. In: Handbook of Physiology. Male Reproduction,
     (eds) Greep, R.O. and Hamilton, D.W., Amer. Physiol. Soc.
     Washington, D.C., 1975 (in press).

22. Steinberger, E. Physiol. Revs., 51: 1, 1971.

23. Vernon, R.G., Go, V.L.W. and Fritz, I.B., J. Reprod. Fertil.,
     42: 77, 1975.

FSH—INDUCTION OF ANDROGEN BINDING PROTEIN IN TESTES OF SERTOLI CELL--ONLY RATS

A.R. Means and D.J. Tindall

Department of Cell Biology

Baylor College of Medicine, Houston, Texas   77025

Administration of a single dose of FSH to immature rats results in the initiation of a complex series of biochemical events within cells present in testicular seminiferous tubules (1).   In order to better define these events in chemically precise terms we have recently developed an animal model in which the tubules are devoid of all germ cells from birth. These Sertoli-cell only animals (SCO) respond to FSH in a manner which is indistinguishable from the effects noted in normal rats (2). Thus, after much indirect evidence the Sertoli cell emerges unequivically as a primary target cell for FSH.

Three of the initial events by which FSH initiates biochemical changes in the Sertoli cell include 1) binding to membrane-associated receptor proteins 2) stimulation of adenylate cyclase with a resultant increase in the intracellular concentration of cyclic AMP; and 3) activation of a specific soluble form of protein kinase (2). It is assumed that FSH-mediated phosphorylation of macromolecules underwrites a subsequent alteration in cell function. Indeed, FSH also stimulates a variety of transcriptional events which leads to an accelerated rate of protein biosynthesis (1,3,4). On the other hand, it has not been possible to directly link the membrane-associated events in a cause and effect manner with the later effects on nucleic acid and protein synthesis. One of the primary deterrents to such correlative studies has been the absence of a specific gene product to use as an endpoint to assess FSH action.

Studies from several laboratories have given us a likely candidate for an FSH--regulated protein (5-10). Androgen binding protein (ABP) is synthesized in the testis, secreted into the tubule lumen, and transported via the efferent ducts into the epididymis (7). Hypophysectomy results in the disappearance of ABP and levels

can be restored by chronic administration of FSH (6,8,9). We have
recently shown that the SCO-testis produces this protein and have
been able to duplicate the studies demonstrating responsiveness to
chronic FSH treatment previously documented for the normal rat
(10). Thus, ABP is a product of the Sertoli cell and appears to
be under the control of FSH. It was the purpose of the present
study to determine whether a single injection of FSH to SCO-rats
induced the synthesis of ABP and thereby establish a·specific endpoint marker for the acute effects of FSH on the Sertoli cell.

     The use of the SCO-model for ABP synthesis studies offers a
unique advantage. In these animals the blood-testis barrier does
not form until day 30 (11). This is a delay of 12 days compared to
tight junction formation in normal animals. Since blood-testis
barrier formation is required for complete canalization of the
tubules (13) and since a lumen is mandatory for transport of ABP
into the epididymis, ABP is restricted exclusively within the testis
prior to these events (11). Thus, by completing all experiments
prior to the 28th postnatal day, one is assured of measuring total
ABP. In the experiments to be reported all animals were SCO and
were used between days 14 and 18 postnatally.

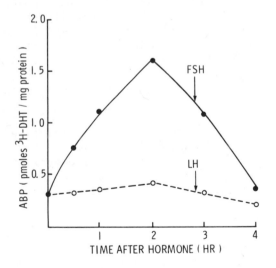

Figure 1. Stimulation of ABP production in testis of SCO-rats by
FSH. Rats, 14 days old, were given a single i.v. injection of 200 μg
of either NIH-FSH-S10 or NIH-LH-S18. Hormones were dissolved in
physiological saline and injected in 0.1 ml. At various times rats
were killed, testes removed and decapsulated and homogenized in
buffer (50 mM Tris-HCl, pH 7.4, 1 mM EDTA, 10% glycerol). ABP was
quantitated in the 105,000 xg supernatant fluid (cytosol) by the
steady state polyacrylamine gel electrophoresis techniques described
by Ritzen et al. (21).

Figure 1 reveals that a single intravenous injection of FSH to 14 day old rats causes a rapid increase in Sertoli cell ABP. Significant increases are seen within 30 minutes and the peak response occurs at 2 hr at which time a 5-fold stimulation over control values is achieved. A rapid decrease is then noted and by 4 hr ABP levels are once again at the control level. It can also be seen that a similar amount of LH was without a significant effect on ABP indicating the hormonal specificity of this response.

For any hormonal effect to be of physiological importance a dose response relationship must be established. The data in **Figure 1** were obtained by injecting 200 µg of NIH-FSH-S10, a preparation which is only about 2% FSH by weight. In order to explore the dose response a pure FSH preparation was needed. Such a preparation was kindly prepared and donated by Dr. Leo E. Reichert, Jr. of Emory University. Human FSH LER-1577 has an activity of 879 IU/mg and has been treated with chymotrypsin to remove most of the contaminating LH. As can be seen from Figure 2, a dose response does occur with as little as 200 ng LER-1577 resulting in a readily demonstrable stimulation of ABP. Maximal levels are achieved with 1 µg of hFSH and 13 times this amount of hormone failed to augment this concentration of ABP.

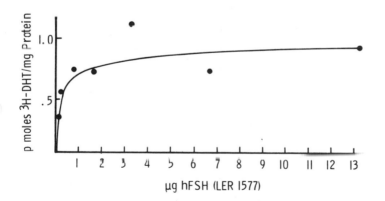

Figure 2. ABP production in response to various concentrations of FSH. Highly purified hFSH (LER-1577) was administered as a single intravenous injection to 16-day-old SCO rats. Testes were removed after 2 hr and ABP quantitated in cytosol (21).

As mentioned briefly above, it has been difficult to directly link the FSH-mediated effects on cyclic nucleotide metabolism with the subsequent effects on transcription and translation. Since the data reveal that the de novo synthesis of ABP is most likely stimulated by FSH we were interested to determine whether this effect could be mimicked by injection of cyclic AMP. Adminstration of exogenous cyclic AMP is not particularly effective. This is because the compound is rapidly metabolized by phosphodiesterase present in serum (as well as all cells) and it does not readily diffuse across the plasmalemma. Consequently the use of dibutyryl cyclic AMP has become popular. Several difficulties also exist with in vivo experiments involving this compound. First it is also hydrolyzed by phosphodiesterase with approximately the same kinetics as cyclic AMP. Secondly, although it apparently enters cells more readily, the compound will not activate protein kinase unless one of the butyric acid groups is first removed (13). Therefore, for our studies we have synthesized another analog 8-bromocyclic AMP. This compound enters the cell with considerable facility, activates protein kinase with the same kinetics as cyclic AMP, but is not hydrolyzed by phosphodiesterase (14).

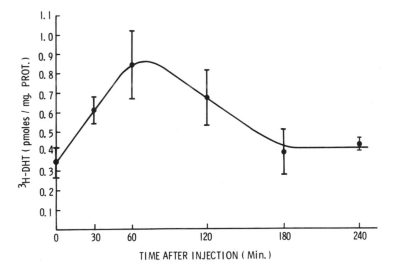

Figure 3.   Stimulation of ABP with 8 bromocyclic AMP. Protocols are the same as described in the legend to Figure 1 except that all rats were injected i.v. with 8 bromocyclic AMP (600 μg).   Each point represents the mean from five separate rats ± standard deviation.

Figure 3 illustrates the effect of a single intravenous injection of 8 bromocyclic AMP on ABP synthesis in testes of 16 day
old SCO rats. Stimulation is noted by 30 minutes and by one hour
ABP synthesis is increased 3-fold with respect to saline-injected
controls. Within 3 hr. the specific activity of ABP has again returned to control levels. Comparison of Fig. 1 and Fig. 3 reveals that maximal ABP levels are achieved earlier following 8-
bromocyclic AMP than following FSH. Thus cyclic nucleotides will
mimic the effect of FSH on testicular ABP synthesis. Moreover the
kinetics of the responses are compatible with an increase in intracellular concentration of cyclic AMP in response to FSH underwriting
the subsequent stimulation of ABP synthesis.

The transient nature of testicular responses to FSH has always
been somewhat puzzling. Since the apparent $t_{1/2}$ of ABP is only
approximately one hour, it was necessary to determine whether carefully timed multiple injections of FSH would either potentiate or
prolong the testicular concentration of ABP. An experiment of this
design is illustrated in Figure 4. The solid line shows the typical ABP response to a single injection of FSH with peak values at
2 hr and reestablishment of baseline values by 4 hr. However, if
a second injection of FSH is administered 90 min after the first,
ABP is slightly elevated after 30 minutes and is still at maximal
concentrations 2 hr later (i.e. 4 hr after the first injection).
This type of response is typical of inducible enzymes in many
systems and offers the first suggestive evidence that FSH may influence ABP by a mechanism involving induction of gene function.
Further such evidence can be obtained by the use of inhibitors of
protein and nucleic acid synthesis. Administration of cycloheximide
1 hr before injection of FSH completely inhibits the FSH-mediated
induction of ABP (Figure 5). These data reveal that the stimulation required continued elongation of peptide chains and argue for
a de novo synthesis of the binding protein. Actinomycin D administered similarly also abolished the FSH effect on ABP. The concentration of actinomycin D used in these experiments has been previously demonstrated to inhibit testicular mRNA synthesis (1). Thus,
ABP synthesis following FSH also required gene transcription. Our
results suggest that induction of ABP must occur subsequent to and
be dependent upon an effect of the hormone on gene transcription.

Previous studies on protein synthesis in the testis demonstrated
that FSH stimulates this parameter in immature or mature hypophysectomized rats (1,15,16). However, utilization of double labeling
techniques failed to reveal any qualitative differences (3). Since
ABP represents less than 0.1% of total testis protein, it is not
surprising that total protein synthesis assays failed to reveal
its presence. Another curious finding was that protein synthesis
was not demonstrably stimulated until 1 hr following FSH and once
maximal rates of synthesis were achieved they remained elevated for
at least 12 hr (1). Therefore, it was decided to assay ABP and

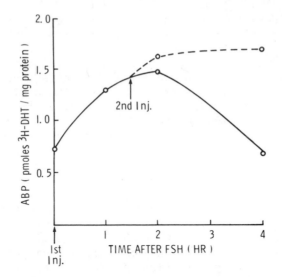

Figure 4.   Effect of multiple injections of FSH on testicular ABP
concentrations.   Protocols are exactly as described in the legend
to Figure 1 except that all rats received a second i.v. injection
of either FSH or saline 90 minutes after the first.

protein synthesis in the same tissue samples at various times after
administration of FSH.   These data are illustrated in Figure 6.
It is clear that the kinetics of ABP induction and disappearance
are different from the kinetics of overall protein synthesis in
Sertoli cells.   No increase in protein synthesis is observed until
1 hr after FSH.   Again, multiple injections of FSH do not effect
protein synthesis as was shown to be the case for ABP in Figure 4.
In addition, protein synthesis is still proceeding at a maximal
rate at 4 hr, a time when ABP levels have returned to control
values.   It is also interesting to note that FSH results in a 5-
fold increase in ABP but only a 0.6-fold stimulation in the rate
of total polysomal protein synthesis.   Once again, these data provide evidence that the effects of FSH on ABP is the result of a
selective induction process.

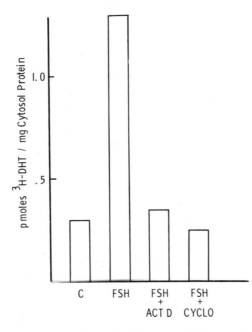

Figure 5. Effects of cycloheximide or actinomycin D on FSH-
mediated testicular production of ABP. Cycloheximide (500 µg) or
actinomycin D (100 µg) was administered intraperitoneally 1 hr
or 30 min respectively, before FSH. FSH was injected i.v. and
animals killed 2 hr later. ABP was quantitated in cytosol as
described by Ritzen et al. (21).

        Since the induction of ABP by FSH appears to be selective and
is inhibitable by Actinomycin D we decided to turn our attention to
possible alterations in Sertoli cell transcription in response to
this gonadotrophin. The first activity chosen was nuclear RNA polymerase activity since these enzymes are stimulated in normal immature testis by FSH (1). Figure 7 reveals that FSH administration
to 16 day old SCO-rats results in a rapid stimulation in the
activity of RNA Polymerase II. This response of heterogeneous
nuclear RNA synthesis increases linearly between 15 and 60 minutes

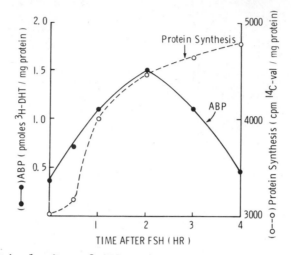

Figure 6.   Stimulation of ABP and protein synthesis by FSH.   FSH
was injected i.v. into 16-day-old SCO rats and animals were killed
at various times thereafter.   ABP was quantitated in cytosol as
described by Ritzen, et al. (21).   Rate of protein biosynthesis
was measured in tissue slices as previously documented (15,16).

following hormone, peaks at 1-2 hr and rapidly declines at times
thereafter.   On the other hand, no increase is noted in RNA Polymerase
I until 60 minutes after FSH.   Ribosomal RNA synthesis continues to
increase for 4 hr and apparently has still not reached a plateau.
These data fit with our previously reported results showing that
the maximal numbers of newly synthesized ribosomes appear in the
cytoplasm between 4 and 8 hr (1).   Taken together the results
point towards an initial effect of FSH on polymerase II activity.
Since this enzyme is responsible for transcription of unique
sequence DNA, we decided to measure mRNA activity at various times
after FSH injection.

     Total nucleic acid was extracted from testis of SCO-rats, and
Poly A-containing mRNA partially purified by the nitrocellulose
filter technique as previously described (17,18).   The wheat germ

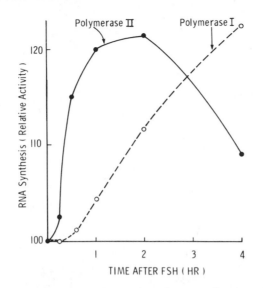

Figure 7. FSH stimulation of testicular nuclear RNA polymerase
activities. Sixteen-day-old SCO rats were injected i.v. with
FSH at various times before necropsy. Nuclei were isolated (3)
and assayed for RNA polymerase I and II as previously described (1).

translation system was chosen because of its low endogenous mRNA
levels and its ease of preparation and stability (19,20). Testicular mRNA promotes the synthesis of protein in a time-dependent
fashion as shown in Figure 8. Linear incorporation occurs for 90
minutes and a plateau is reached by 2 hr. This translation system
is also dependent upon the amount of mRNA added. Figure 9 reveals a linear increase in protein synthesis between 0.25 and 1.5
µg testicular mRNA. This system then is sufficiently sensitive
to detect quantitative changes in the activity of total poly A-
containing mRNA extracted from testis at various times after hormone administration.

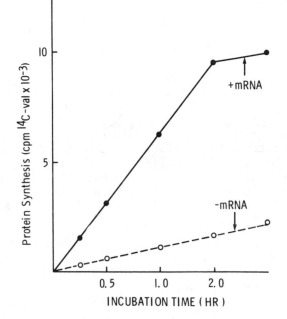

Figure 8.   Time course of protein synthesis in the testis mRNA-
directed wheat germ translation system.   Preparation of poly-A
containing mRNA was prepared as described by Means et al. (17).
The properties of the wheat germ system have also been reported
(20). Assays were performed in duplicate and each tube contained
either 1 μg of testis mRNA (+mRNA) or no exogenous mRNA (-mRNA).
Following incubation, the samples were centrifuged at 105,000 xg
for 1 hr.   TCA-precipitable radioactivity of this cytosol is a
quantitative measurement of complete newly synthesized proteins (20).

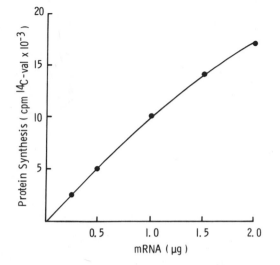

Figure 9.   The relation between the amount of testis mRNA added to
the wheat germ system and the amount of protein synthesized and
released.   Incubation in 50 µl reactions were for 2 hr at 25⁰. Details of the remaining protocols are described in the legend to
Figure 7.

        A single injection of FSH to 16-day-old SCO-rats results in
a demonstrable increase in testis mRNA activity assayed in the
heterologous protein synthesizing system (Figure 10).   Stimulation
is noted within 30 minutes, peaks between 1 and 2 hr and by 3 hr
has begun to decline.   Not only does FSH result in increased
activity of the mRNA fraction but it also promotes an increase in
the mass of mRNA recovered by nitrocellulose or oligo-dT cellulose
assays.   Table I illustrates that the recovery of total nucleic
acid from testis during the first 3 hours of FSH treatment does
not vary appreciably.   However, the percent of the total RNA
represented by poly A-containing mRNA increased from 1.4 to 2.5%.
Both the increases in activity and mass of mRNA could be prevented
by actinomycin D but not by cycloheximide.   Thus, FSH appears to
increase the synthesis of translatable mRNA in the Sertoli cell.

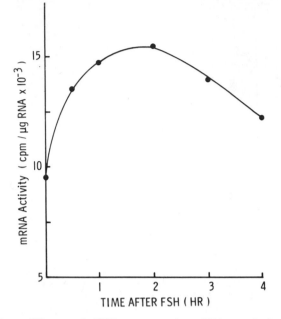

Figure 10.   The effect of FSH on testis mRNA activity.   Incubation
with 1 μg Poly A-containing mRNA was carried out for 2 hr at 25°.
Animals (16-day-old SCO-rats) were injected i.v. with FSH and
killed at various times thereafter.   Poly A-containing RNA was
isolated from total nucleic acid as described (20).

        A summary of the data is presented in Figure 11.   FSH induces
the synthesis of ABP in the Sertoli cell with very characteristic
kinetics.   Concomitant with (or proceeding) this induction, stimu-
lations of RNA polymerase II and translatable mRNA are noted.   Only
after these events have been increased does one detect an increase
in total cell protein synthesis.   A second injection of FSH pre-
vents the decline in ABP.   On the other hand little effect is
seen on the other events illustrated in Figure 10 upon multiple
injections of the hormone.   Thus, the effect of FSH appears to be
a selective induction of ABP.   At this juncture, however, other

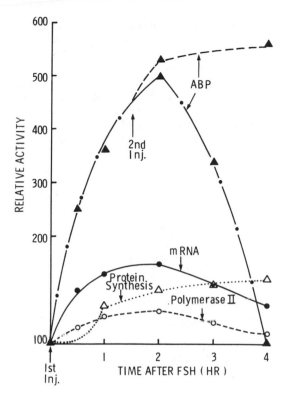

Figure 11. Summary of the effects of FSH on various biochemical events in the testis of SCO-rats. All data are prepared from previous figures in this paper but are expressed as relative activity with respect to the control value which is arbitrarily set at 100.

possibilities also must be considered. One possibility might be that ABP simply has a very short $t_{1/2}$. Indeed, if one assumes no new synthesis, a $t_{1/2}$ of 60 min can be calculated from the slope of Figure 1. Another consideration is that whereas ABP is normally

a secretory protein, under the conditions of our experiments, it is
retained in the testis due to the absence of tubule canalization.
Since the Sertoli cell is highly phagocytic, ABP (and other secretory proteins) may be selectively destroyed by specific proteases.
Nevertheless, a single injection of FSH results in a rapid nuclear-
dependent induction of a specific Sertoli cell protein, ABP. To
our knowledge, this marks the first demonstration of such an induction by a peptide hormone. The results presented here clearly
show that ABP can be utilized as a specific endpoint to assess the
effects of FSH on the Sertoli cell. These observations should now
allow elucidation of the precise temporal sequence of biochemical
events initiated by the interaction of FSH with its specific testicular target cell.

TABLE I

ISOLATION OF TESTICULAR mRNA FOLLOWING FSH ADMINISTRATION
TO 16 DAY OLD RATS

Time After FSH (hr)	Testis Weight (g)	Total RNA (mg)	Poly A-Containing mRNA	
			(μg)	(%)
0	4.04	3.14	44.3	1.41
0.5	3.93	3.19	61.2	1.92
1	4.07	3.47	86.4	2.49
3	4.44	3.43	62.4	1.82

FSH was injected i.v. to 16 day old SCO rats. At various
times following the injection, total nucleic acid was prepared as
previously described by Means et al.(17)   Poly A-containing mRNA
was then prepared following removal of DNA and 28S rRNA by sepharose
chromatography (16) by adsorption to and elution from oligo-dT
cellulose (20). RNA mass was quantitated spectrophotometrically
at $A_{260 nm}$ assuming 40 μg RNA per 1.0 A_{260} unit.

REFERENCES

1. Means, A.R. In: Handbook of Physiology Section 7: Endocrino-
    logy. (D. Hamilton and R. Greep, eds.) Academic Press, N.Y.,
    Vol V, p. 301, 1975.

2. Means, A.R. and Huckins, C. In: Hormone Binding and Target
    Cell Activation in the Testis (M. Dufau and A. Means, eds.)
    Plenum Press N.Y., p. 145, 1974.

3. Means, A.R. Endocrinology 89: 981, 1971.

4. Means, A.R. Life Sci. 15:371, 1974.

5. Ritzen, E.M., Nayfeh, S.N., French, F.S. and Dobbins, M.C. Endo-
    crinology 89: 143, 1971.

6. Vernon, R.G., Kopec, B and Fritz, I.B. Mol. Cell. Endocr. 1:
    167, 1974.

7. French, F.S. and Ritzen, E.M. Endocrinology 93:88, 1973.

8. Hansson, V., Reusch, E., Trygstad, O., Torgersen, O., Ritzen,
    E.M. and French, F.S. Nature New Biol. 246:56, 1973.

9. Sanborn, B.M., Elkington, J.S.H., Chowdhury, M., Tcholakian,
    R.K. and Steinberger, E. Endocrinology 96:304, 1974.

10. Tindall, D.J., Schrader W.T. and Means, A.R. In: Hormone
    Binding and Target Cell Activation in the Testis (M. Dufau
    and A. Means, eds.) Plenum Press, N.Y. p. 167, 1974.

11. Tindall, D.J., Vitale, R. and Means, A.R. Endocrinology 97:636,
    1975.

12. Vitale, R., Fawcett, D.W. and Dym, M. Anat. Rec. 176:333, 1975.

13. Neelon, F.A. and Birch, B.M. J. Biol. Chem. 248:8361, 1973.

14. Muneyama, K., Bauer, R.J., Shuman, D.A., Robins, R.K and
    Limon, L.N. Biochemistry 10:2390, 1971.

15. Means, A.R. and Hall, P.F. Endocrinology 81:1151, 1967.

16. Means, A.R. and Hall, P.F. Biochemistry 8:4293, 1969.

17. Means, A.R., Comstock, J.P., Rosenfeld, G.C. and O'Malley, B.W.
    Proc. Natl. Acad. Sci. U.S.A. 69:1146, 1972.

18. Woo, S.L.C., Rosen, J.M., Chan, L., Sperry, P., Means, A.R.,
     and O'Malley, B.W. Prep. Biochem. 4:555, 1974.

19. Roberts, B.E. and Patterson, B.M. Proc. Natl. Acad. Sci. USA
     70:2330, 1973.

20. Rosen, J.M., Woo, S.L.C., Holder, J.W., Means, A.R., and
     O'Malley, B.W. Biochemistry 14:69, 1975.

21. Ritzen, E.M., French, F.S., Weddington, S.C., Nayfeh, S.N.,
     and Hansson, V. J. Biol. Chem. 249:6597, 1974.

CULTURE AND FSH RESPONSES OF SERTOLI CELLS ISOLATED FROM SEXUALLY

MATURE RAT TESTIS

A. Steinberger, J.S.H. Elkington, B.M. Sanborn,
E. Steinberger

Program in Reproductive Biology and Endocrinology
University of Texas Medical School at Houston,
Houston, Texas   77025

J. J. Heindel

Program in Pharmacology
University of Texas Medical School at Houston
Houston, Texas   77025

J. N. Lindsey

Department of Human Biological Chemistry and Genetics
The University of Texas Medical Branch
Galveston, Texas   77550

We have previously provided evidence that ^{125}I-FSH specifically binds to various preparations of rat testis which contain Sertoli cells, e.g. isolated seminiferous tubules and organ cultures of testicular explants which have been depleted of most germinal elements and Leydig cells (1,2). On the other hand, isolated germinal cells, peritubular cells or interstitial cells show no binding of the labeled FSH. Subsequently, it was demonstrated that FSH also stimulates endogenous cAMP (3'5'-cyclic adenosine monophosphate) levels in the isolated seminiferous tubules and organ cultures, but has no effect on the isolated peritubular or interstitial cells and only a slight stimulatory effect on the germinal cells (3). These results provided suggestive evidence that of the various cell types

composing the testis, only the Sertoli cells possess the FSH binding
receptors and respond to FSH stimulation with increased levels of
cAMP. Since these two parameters are considered to be the initial
steps of gonadotropin action in the target cells (4), it appeared
that the Sertoli cells must represent the primary target site for
the biological action of FSH in the testis.

More direct evidence for this was obtained when Sertoli cells
which were isolated from 21 day rat testis were shown to respond
to FSH stimulation with dramatic increases (21-26 fold) in the
cAMP level (3). Similar results were reported by Dorrington et. al.
(5).

Isolation of Sertoli cells from immature rats and their maintenance in culture has been described by at least two groups of
investigators (5,6). Isolation of Sertoli cells from fully mature
animals, however, has not been reported. We like to describe
currently a method for the isolation and culture of essentially pure
populations of Sertoli cells from adult rat testes, and to illustrate
some of their responses to FSH.

MATERIALS AND METHODS

Adult rats of the Long Evans strain were used as the source
of testes for these studies.

The enzymes: trypsin (Difco 1:250) was purchased from Difco
Laboratories, Detroit, Michigan; collagenase (cl. histolyticum)
from Nutritional Biochemical Corp., Cleveland, Ohio; and DNAse
from Sigma Chemicals Corp., St. Louis, Missouri.

The culture dishes (Falcon plastics, 60 mm) and culture medium
(Eagle's Minimum Essential Medium) were obtained from Bioquest,
Cockeysville, Maryland. The culture medium was supplemented with
sodium pyruvate, the essential amino acids and 4 mM glutamine.
Penicillin 100 u/ml, streptomycin 100 µg/ml were added to the
medium to prevent microbial contamination. In some cases, the
medium also contained 10% fetal calf serum. The pH was adjusted
to 7.0-7.2 with sodium bicarbonate.

Procedures for ^{125}I-FSH preparation and hormone binding were
the same as used previously (1). The cAMP content in the cells was
measured by a radioimmunoassay procedure described in detail previously (3). The androgen binding protein (ABP) in the culture
media was assayed by the steady state polyacrylamide gel electrophoresis method described by Ritzen et al. (7).

Procedure for the Initial Isolation and Culture of Sertoli Cells

1.   Decapsulated testes are cut into 10-12 pieces, rinsed with Hank's balanced salt solution (HBSS), free of Ca^{++} ions, and incubated for 15 min at 37C in Ca^{++} free solution of 0.25% (w/v) trypsin, pH 7.4.   Approximately 15 ml of the trypsin solution is used per gram of testicular tissue.   The flask is agitated manually every 3-5 min.

2.   After the incubation, the contents are strained through a stainless steel sieve with a 100 μ opening size and rinsed with 100-200 ml of warm HBSS.

3.   The seminiferous tubules pieces retained by the grid are collected and incubated in a solution of collagenase (0.25%, w/v in HBSS containing Ca^{++}) at 37C for 1 hr (25 ml of collagenase solution per gram of original tissue).   The flask is frequently and vigorously agitated during the entire incubation period. Approximately 20 μg of DNAse is added to the flask 3-5 min before the end of incubation.

4.   The contents are then strained through a stainless steel grid with an opening of 74 μ and rinsed thoroughly with 100-200 ml of HBSS.   Cell aggregates, containing Sertoli cells and some germinal cells, which are retained by the grid are "backwashed" with culture medium or a suitable buffer.

5.   Cells obtained from a single testis are planted into 2-4 dishes with 5 ml/dish of culture medium with or without 10% fetal calf serum.

6.   The cultures are incubated at 31C in a humidified atmosphere of 5% CO_2 and 95% air.   The culture medium is replenished after the initial 24-48 hrs and at 3-4 day intervals afterwards.

RESULTS

Morphologic Characteristics

Appearance of the seminiferous tubules obtained after trypsin treatment and rinsing but before incubation with collagenase is shown in Fig. 1.   The tubules have been freed of interstitial tissue but still contain components of the tubule wall, as evident by a smooth outer layer of PAS positive material.   Flat nuclei of the peritubular cells in the boundary tissue are indicated by arrows.

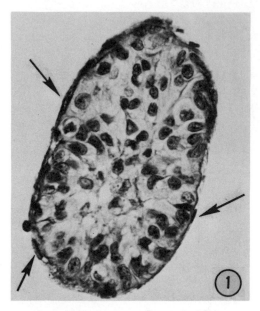

Figure 1. Microscopic appearance of seminiferous tubule after 15 min treatment with 0.25% trypsin and thorough rinsing with HBSS. The boundary tissue is still evident. Arrows point to nuclei of the peritubular cells. Bouin's fixative, PAS-H stain Magn.x600.

Appearance of the preparations following incubation with collagenase and rinsing with a large volume of HBSS is illustrated in Fig. 2. Chains of Sertoli cells with some germinal cells attached to them give a beaded appearance and are free of the boundary tissue layer (compare with Fig. 1). Thus, the treatment with collagenase followed by thorough washing, efficiently eliminates the peritubular cells from the remaining aggregates. Presence of the tight junctions (8) is believed to be responsible for the Sertoli cells remaining attached to each other.

When the cell aggregates are placed in culture dishes and incubated undisturbed for 24-48 hrs, the Sertoli cells attach to the surface and flatten out forming cell monolayer islands of different sizes. Most germinal cells remain floating in the medium and are eliminated during media changes. However, some germinal elements are also within the Sertoli cell cytoplasm (Fig. 3), most likely due to the phagocytic nature of these cells (9). When the Sertoli cell monolayers are examined by bright light microscopy, either in

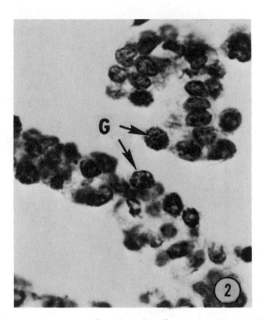

Figure 2. Cell aggregates obtained after consecutive treatment
with trypsin and collagenase followed by thorough rinsing with
HBSS. The Sertoli cells remain associated as "beaded" chains
with some germinal elements (G) attached to them. The peritubular
tissue has been completely eliminated. Bouin's fixative, PAS-H
stain, Magn.x720.

a living state or following in situ fixation and staining (Fig 3a),
they appear as syncytia with widely spread nuclei. The nuclei
contain a single prominent nucleolus which in many cases has the
characteristic tripartite structure. The cytoplasm contains numerous
vacuoles, lipid granules and ingested germinal cells or their
residues.

    Single Sertoli cells which are also present in the culture
appear pleomorphic with irregular outlines and numerous cytoplasmic
processes (Fig. 3b). Typical fibroblastic cells were found only
occasionally in some of the cultures and were believed to have
originated from the peritubular cells which may have contaminated
the initial preparation. These cells could be easily distinguished
from the Sertoli cells by having two or more nucleoli and a spindle-
shaped outline of the cytoplasm.

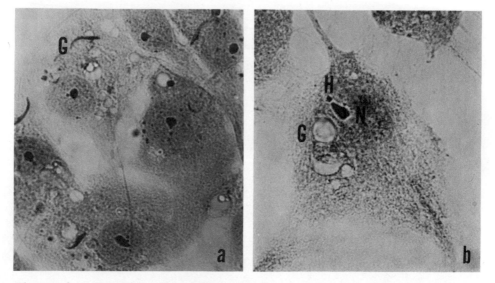

Figure 3. Sertoli cells after 11 days of cultivation fixed in situ
with formolsaline and stained with hematoxylin. The nuclei contain
single prominent nucleoli (N) with 1-2 lateral heteropyknotic bodies
(H). Ingested germinal elements (G), vacuoles and lipid droplets
are seen in the cytoplasm. Magn. a) x600, b)x900.

　　　　　Electron microscopic examination of the cultured Sertoli cells
(Fig. 4) revealed the following ultrastructural features: Abundance
of smooth and rough endoplasmic reticulum, well developed Golgi zone
and numerous lipid inclusions in the cytoplasm. The cytoplasm also
contained rod-shaped mitochondria with transverse tubular cristae.
Many adjacent cells had junctions similar to those observed between
mature Sertoli cells in vivo (8). The lobulated nucleus contained
a single nucleolus with one or two lateral heteropyknotic bodies.
Thus, the Sertoli cells cultured for 11 days (and possibly longer)
continued to exhibit many ultrastructural features which are characteristic for these cells in vivo.

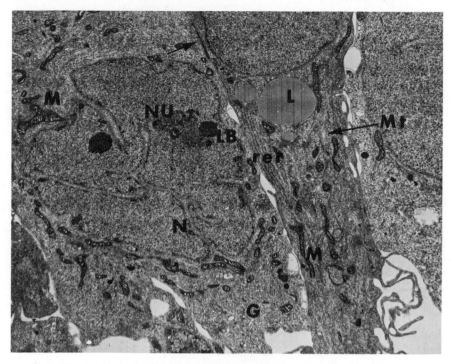

Figure 4. Electron micrograph of Sertoli cells in 11 day culture
fixed in situ. Nucleus (N), nucleolus (NU), lateral heteropyknotic
body (LB), mitochondria (M), microtubules (Mt), rough endoplasmic
reticulum (rer), Golgi (G), lipid droplet (L). Arrow points to a
specialized tight junction. Magn.x4,600.

        The Sertoli cells were maintained in culture for prolonged
periods of time (39 days was the longest period of observation)
without significant change in morphology or viability, as determined
by the exclusion of trypan blue dye (10). It is interesting that
during this period there was no evidence of cell division. In
addition, exposure of the cultures to ^{3}H-thymidine for periods of
up to 24 hr followed by radioautography, revealed no labeled Sertoli
cell nuclei. Occasionally observed labeled nuclei were always
associated with the fibroblastic cells, believed to be contaminating
peritubular cells.

TABLE I

Binding of ^{125}I-FSH to Freshly Isolated and Cultured Sertoli Cells

Sertoli cell preparation	Counts per minute/mg protein		
	Total binding	FSH[1]	LH[2]
Freshly isolated from 60d rats	2430 ± 150[3]	1391 ± 132	2512 ± 163
Isolated from 60d rats and cultured 11d	2871 ± 259	639 ± 81	2610 ± 320

The cells were incubated for 2 hrs at 37C with ^{125}I-FSH (LER 1366) in absence (total binding) or presence of 100-fold concentrations of unlabeled hormones. Protein was measured by the method of Lowry et al. (12)

[1] NIH-FSH-S1
[2] NIH-LH-S1
[3] Mean ± SE (N-3).

Sertoli Cell Responses to Gonadotropins

Freshly isolated or cultured Sertoli cells specifically bound the ^{125}I-FSH (Table I). The binding was specific in that it could be competitively inhibited by an excess of unlabeled FSH but not LH. Sertoli cells cultured for 11 days showed greater specific binding per mg protein than the freshly isolated cell preparations. This could have been due to elimination of many germinal cells present in the initial preparations or due to recovery of hormone binding activity after a partial receptor damage induced by the enzyme treatments. We observed recovery of ^{125}I-LH binding ability in cultures of interstitial cells isolated from rat testis with the aid of trypsin (11).

When the cultured Sertoli cells were incubated for 30 min at 34C with gonadotropins in presence of 1 mM MIX (1-methyl-3 isobutyl-xanthine) the cellular level of cAMP increased in a dose related fashion following stimulation with FSH. There was no response to LH under similar conditions (Fig. 5).

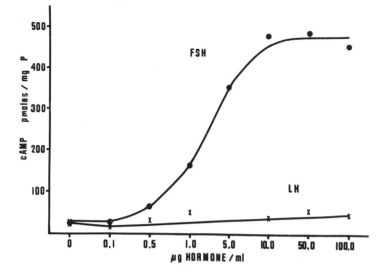

Figure 5. cAMP responses to various doses of LH (NIH-LH-S1) and FSH (NIH-FSH-S1) in 11 day Sertoli cell cultures. The incubation was carried out for 30 min at 34C in presence of 1mM MIX. The values represent means from two separate experiments using 2-3 cultures per each hormone dilution.

Maximum response was elicited in the cultured Sertoli cells by 10 µg FSH/ml compared to 100 µg of similar FSH preparation/ml required for maximum cAMP stimulation in all previously tested preparations (3).

The ability of the cultured Sertoli cells to secrete ABP and to respond to FSH stimulation with increased ABP secretion was investigated in the following experiment. Cultures of Sertoli cells were grown for 3 days in media containing 10% fetal bovine serum. On the third day, the culture dishes were rinsed twice with HBSS to eliminate the serum and non-attached cells and were given fresh serum-free media with or without 100 µg FSH/ml. The media in each group (3 cultures/group) were replenished at 3-4 day intervals and the spent media were assayed for ABP. The results are shown in Table II. Addition of FSH clearly stimulated ABP secretion throughout the treatment period whether the results were expressed as pmoles ABP per mg protein or per culture. In absence of FSH, the levels of ABP were much lower compared to the FSH-treated cultures in the 3-6 day media collections and became non-detectable after the 10th day.

TABLE II

Effect of FSH on ABP Secretion by Cultured Sertoli Cells

Age of culture (days)	pmoles ABP/mg protein		pmoles ABP/culture	
	FSH	Control	FSH	Control
3-6	3.96[1]	1.73	8.27	2.03
6-10	-	-	3.58	1.28
10-14	3.23	N.D.[2]	5.89	N.D.

The cultures were grown after the initial 3 days, in serum-free media with or without (control) 100µg/ml FSH (NIH-FSH-S1). The media in both groups of cultures (3 cultures/group) were replenished every 3-4 days and were assayed for ABP.

[1] Mean value of 3 cultures
[2] Non-detectable.

DISCUSSION

We have described here a method for the isolation and culture of Sertoli cells from sexually mature rat testis. The same method, however, can be used successfully for culture of Sertoli cells from 20-60 day old animals (13). We have also demonstrated that the Sertoli cells retain in culture many ultrastructural features which characterize them in vivo. The cultured Sertoli cells actively ingest degenerating germinal elements which are not eliminated from the cultures by media changes. Based on the exclusion of trypan blue dye (10), the Sertoli cells remained viable for at least 39 days but showed no evidence of replication. In addition, exposure to ^{3}H-thymidine for periods up to 24 hr, followed by radioautography, revealed no labeled Sertoli cell nuclei. The prolonged survival of the Sertoli cells, their highly phagocytic nature and lack of labeling have been previously observed in organ cultures of testicular explants (9,14,15). Whether DNA synthesis and cell division could be induced under certain conditions remains to be determined.

Indirect evidence has been provided suggesting that Sertoli cells may be a target site for the biological action of FSH in the testes, that they possess FSH binding receptors (16) and respond to FSH stimulation with increased levels of cAMP (17) and ABP (18, 19). Additional evidence supporting the Sertoli cells as the primary cell type responsive to FSH was provided by demonstrating that isolated interstitial (1,2,16) peritubular or germinal cells (1,2) do not bind labeled FSH, and show no increase of cAMP levels following FSH stimulation (3). Isolated Sertoli cells, on the other hand, were shown here to bind ^{125}I-FSH and to respond to FSH stimulation with dramatic increases in cAMP level. These results agree with other published reports on FSH induced cAMP production in isolated Sertoli cells from immature rats (3,5,13).

As demonstrated in this paper, and by Sanborn et. al. (20) the cultured Sertoli cells remain responsive to FSH for prolonged periods of time. This was evident from the binding of ^{125}I-FSH and stimulation of cAMP production in 11 day cultures and the stimulation of ABP secretion during 14 days of cultivation. Stimulation of ABP in immature Sertoli cells maintained in culture for 1-2 days has been described (21).

All of these results clearly establish the Sertoli cells as the primary and possibly only target site for FSH action in the testis. The prolonged viability and hormone responsiveness of the cultured Sertoli cells should encourage further in vitro studies on Sertoli cell metabolism and its regulatory mechanisms.

ACKNOWLEDGEMENTS

This work was supported by NICHHD Grant (HD08338) and Contract (N01-HD3-2783), National Science Foundation (GB-4133F) and the Faith Foundation. The authors acknowledge the competent technical assistance of Ms. R. V. Rodriguez and are grateful to NIAMDD for supplying the gonadotropins.

REFERENCES

1. Steinberger, A., Thanki, K.H., and Siegal, B.G. In: Hormone Binding and Target Cell Activation in the Testis, Eds. M. L. Dufau and A. R. Means, p. 177, Plenum Press, New York, N. Y., 1974.

2. Steinberger, A., Thanki, K. H., and Siegal, B. G., Abstract #21, Annual Meeting of the SSR, Ottawa, Canada, 1974.

3. Heindel, J. J., Rothenberg, R., Robison, G.A., and **Steinberger,** A., J. Cyclic Nucleotide Research 1: 1975.

4. Robison, G. A., Butcher, R. W., Sutherland, E. W., Cyclic AMP, Academic Press, N. Y., 1971.

5. Dorrington, J. H., Roller, N. F., and Fritz, I. B., In: Hormone Binding and Target Cell Activation in the Testis, Eds. M. L. Dufau and A. R. Means, p. 237, Plenum Press, New York, N. Y., 1974.

6. Welsh, M J. and Wiebe, J. P. Endocrinology 96: 618, 1975.

7. Ritzen, E. M. French, F. S., Weddington, S. C. Nayfeh, S. N. and Hansson, V., J. Biol. Chem. 249: 6597, 1974.

8. Dym, M., and Fawcett, D. W., Biol. Reprod. 3: 308, 1970.

9. Vilar, O., Steinberger, A., and Steinberger, E., Z. Zellforsh. 78: 221, 1967.

10. Girardi, A. J., McMichael, Jr., and Henle, W., Virology 2: 532, 1956.

11. Steinberger, A., Yang, K.P., and Ward, D. N., Abstract #447. Annual Meeting of the Endocrine Soc., 1973.

12. Lowry, O. H., Rosebrough, N. J., Farr, A. L., and Randall, R.J., J. Biol. Chem. 193: 265, 1951.

13. Steinberger A., Heindel, J. J., Lindsey, J.N., Elkington, J.S.H., Sanborn, B.M., and Steinberger, E., Endocrine Research Communications - in press.

14. Steinberger, A., and Steinberger, E., J. Reprod. Fertil. Suppl. 2: 117, 1967.

15. Steinberger, A., and Steinberger, E., Biol. Reprod. 4: 84, 1971.

16. Means, A. R., and Vaitukaitis, J., Endocrinology 90: 39, 1972.

17. Dorrington, J. H., and Fritz, I. B., Endocrinology 94: 345, 1974.

18. Hansson, V., Reusch, E., Trygstad, O., Torgersen, O., Ritzen, E., and French, F.S., Nature New Biology 246: 56, 1973.

19. Sanborn, B. M., Elkington, J.S.H., Chowdhury, M., Tcholakian, R.K., and Steinberger, E., Endocrinology 96: 326, 1975.

20. Sanborn, B. M., Elkington, J.S.H., Steinberger, A., and Steinberger, E., this volume, p. 293.

21. Fritz, I. B., Kopec, B., Lam, K., and Vernon, R. G., In: Hormone Binding and Target Cell Activation in the Testis, Eds. M. L. Dufau and A. R. Means, p. 311, Plenum Press, New York, N. Y., 1974.

STIMULATION BY FOLLICLE STIMULATING HORMONE AND DIBUTYRYL CYCLIC AMP OF INCORPORATION OF ^{3}H–THYMIDINE INTO NUCLEAR DNA OF CULTURED SERTOLI CELL-ENRICHED PREPARATIONS FROM IMMATURE RATS

Michael Griswold, Ellen Mably and Irving B. Fritz

Banting and Best Department of Medical Research

University of Toronto, Toronto, Ontario, M5G 1L6, Canada

During the neonatal period, Sertoli cells have been shown to proliferate rapidly within the seminiferous tubules. Between 12 and 14 days of age in rats, the mitotic activity of Sertoli cells becomes greatly diminished (1-3). Even though mitosis is very low by two weeks (<1%), the incorporation of ^{3}H-thymidine into DNA of Sertoli cells continues to be appreciable for an additional three to four weeks before reaching nearly undetectable levels (3). The physiological significance of the nuclear DNA synthesized in Sertoli cells during periods when the mitotic rate is low is unknown.

In this communication, we report studies on the incorporation of ^{3}H-thymidine into nuclear DNA of cultured Sertoli cell-enriched preparations, and present data indicating that treatment of cells with follicle stimulating hormone (FSH) or dibutyryl cyclic AMP (dcAMP) increases ^{3}H-thymidine incorporation into nuclear DNA.

METHODS

Procedures for Culturing Cells

Sertoli cell-enriched preparations from 20 day old rats were cultured as described by Dorrington et al. (4,5). The cells were initially maintained in modified Eagle's minimal essential medium (MEM) (4), supplemented with 1% rat serum. After culture for two

413

days, the medium was replaced with MEM alone and the preparation
was cultured for 1 day more. This time was then considered "time
zero". Fresh MEM alone was placed in flasks containing control
cells, and medium containing FSH (5 µg/ml of NIH-FSH-S10) or dcAMP
(0.1 mM) was added to others. After culture from this time (three
days after the initial preparation) for an additional 1 to 4 days,
control and treated cells were incubated in fresh MEM of the same
composition, but containing trace amounts of ^{3}H-thymidine (New
England Nuclear) (2 µg/ml, of specific activity 43.1 Ci/mmol). At
designated time intervals (usually 24 hrs) the medium containing
label was decanted, the cells were washed with fresh MEM and were
then removed from the culture flasks by sonication in a solution
of 1% SDS and 1 mM EDTA.

Determination of ^{3}H-Thymidine Incorporation into DNA.

The sonicated cells suspended in the SDS solution were treated
with trichloroacetic acid (TCA), filtered onto glass fiber discs
and washed by procedures similar to those described previously (6).
The discs containing the residue were placed in toluene scintillation
fluid containing Protosol, and radioactivity was determined. An
alternate procedure which provided identical data consisted of
binding the labeled DNA in sonicated cells to DEAE filter discs,
washing the filters with disodium phosphate and then counting the
filters as above (7).

In other experiments, radioautography was used to identify
cells which had incorporated ^{3}H-thymidine into nuclei. Conventional histological procedures were employed. Monolayers of the
cultured preparations were fixed in acidic ethanol (1 part acetic
acid to 3 parts ethanol, v/v for 30 mins), and stained after
radioautography with hematoxylin.

RESULTS

Sertoli cell-enriched preparations from 20 day old rats, cultured after "time zero" for 1 to 4 days in the presence and absence
of FSH, were incubated with ^{3}H-thymidine for the succeeding 24
hours, and the incorporation of ^{3}H-thymidine into DNA was determined.
Cells previously cultured in the presence of FSH for 24 hrs had a
greater incorporation than did untreated cells, and this stimulation
was larger in cells treated with FSH for longer periods prior to
incubation with ^{3}H-thymidine (Fig 1).

In extension of these studies, the incorporation of ^{3}H-thymidine
into cell DNA was investigated in Sertoli cell-enriched preparations
from 10, 20 and 30 day old rats. In experiments shown in Fig 2, all

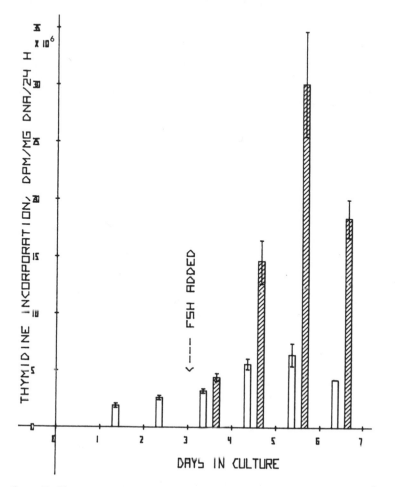

Figure 1.   Influence of FSH on in vitro incorporation of ³H-
thymidine into DNA in Sertoli cell-enriched preparations from 20
day old normal rats.   Cells were prepared and maintained in culture as described in the text.   FSH (NIH-FSH-S-10, 5 μg/ml) was
added to half the culture flasks at the time indicated ("time
zero" in the text).   Results shown (mean ± standard deviation)
represent the incorporation of ³H-thymidine into DNA per mg cell
DNA per 24 hr in 3 separate preparations. Hatched bars denote
results in cultures which were maintained in the presence of FSH,
while clear bars represent mean values in untreated preparations.
For each of the three experiments, mean values were obtained for
three separate culture vessels.   In all cases cells were incubated
with ³H-thymidine for 24 hrs, added to the culture medium at 1-4
days after "time zero".

cell preparations had been cultured for 72 hrs from "time zero" in the presence or absence of FSH or dcAMP. Control and treated cells were then incubated for 24 hrs in medium containing ^{3}H-thymidine. The incorporation of ^{3}H-thymidine into nuclear DNA from untreated control cells was greatest in preparations from 10 day old animals (Fig. 2). In contrast, in cells treated with FSH or dcAMP, the greatest relative stimulation of incorporation of ^{3}H-thymidine was observed in preparations from 20 and 30 day old rats (Fig. 2).

Radioautographs were prepared of cells cultured in the presence of ^{3}H-thymidine for 24 hours under conditions described above. In this type of preparation, an increased number of treated cells showed evidence of intensive ^{3}H-thymidine incorporation into nuclei. Data summarizing the percentage of labeled Sertoli cell nuclei, counted in radioautographs of various preparations cultured in the presence or absence of FSH or dcAMP, are presented in Table 1. In untreated control preparations, cells initially obtained from 10 day old rats had the highest proportion of labeled nuclei, while those prepared from older rats had a much lower percentage of labeled nuclei. In treated cells, cultured in the presence of FSH or dcAMP, the percentage of labeled nuclei was increased in preparations from 10,20 or 30 day old rats, with the greatest relative stimulation seen in cells from the older animals (Table 1). The data indicate that FSH or dcAMP increases the number of cultured cells capable of incorporating ^{3}H-thymidine into Sertoli cell nuclear DNA. Possible additional effects on spermatogonia have not been ruled out.

DISCUSSION

The incorporation of ^{3}H-thymidine into Sertoli cells cultured in the presence or absence of FSH was abolished by treatment with cytosine arabinoside or hydroxyurea (unpublished observations). These data are compatible with the assumption that incorporation studies reported provide measure of DNA synthesis from ^{3}H-thymidine.

Treated cells might have incorporated more ^{3}H-thymidine into DNA because different intracellular pool sizes of thymidine existed, or because ^{3}H-thymidine simply penetrated more rapidly into cells previously cultured in the presence of FSH or dcAMP. This appears unlikely because the number of nuclei labeled in treated cells (Table 1) is increased to an extent similar to the degree of stimulation of total incorporation of ^{3}H-thymidine into DNA (Fig 2). In addition, the degree of augmentation observed in cells treated with FSH or dcAMP was not reduced when varying amounts of unlabeled thymidine were added to lower the specific activity of the ^{3}H-thymidine (unpublished observations).

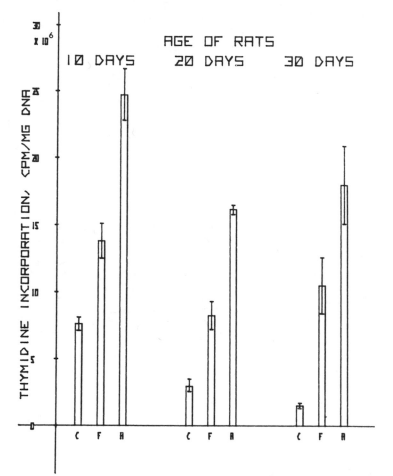

Figure 2. Influence of FSH and dcAMP on incorporation of ³H-thy-midine into DNA of Sertoli cell-enriched preparations from 10, 20, and 30 day old normal rats. Cells from 20 and 30 day old normal rats were maintained in culture as described in the text. The medium in which cells from 10 day old rats were cultured was supplemented with 1% homologous rat serum for the entire period until ³H-thymidine was added. In all vessels, cells were incubated with ³H-thymidine for 24 hrs, beginning three days after "time zero". FSH (NIH FSH S-10, 5 µg/ml) or dcAMP (0.1 mM) was added to some of the culture flasks at "time zero". Data are expressed as the mean of three experiments, each performed in triplicate. Values (mean ± S.D.) are given as DPM ³H-thymidine incorporated into DNA per mg cell DNA during the period from 72-96 hr after "time zero". "C" represents untreated control cells; "F" represents cells treated with FSH: and "A" represents cells treated with dibutyryl 3', 5' cyclic AMP.

TABLE 1

Effects of FSH and Dibutyryl 3', 5' Cyclic-AMP on Incorporation
of 3H-Thymidine into Nuclear DNA in Sertoli Cell-Enriched
Preparation from 10, 20 and 30 Day Old Rats

Percentage of Sertoli Cells
Containing Labeled Nuclei

Additions to Basic Medium at Time Zero	10	20	30 days old
None	3.7 ± 0.5*	0.9 ± 0.2	0.05 ± 0.02
FSH (5 µg/ml)	4.5 ± 0.7	3.7 ± 0.5	7.8 ± 1.0
dcAMP (0.1 mM)	14.7 ± 0.8	13.8 ± 0.8	not available

* Values are expressed as means ±S.D. of the percentage of Sertoli cells having labeled nuclei. Autoradiographs were prepared
of cell preparation cultured and treated as described in Fig. 2
and in the Text. Each percentage figure was obtained by counting
1000 cells in each of the three preparations for sets indicated, in
duplicate, by independent observers using a Zeiss microscope with
oil immersion objective (1000X). Cells were incubated with 3H-
thymidine during the period from 72 to 96 hr after "time zero".

In untreated control preparations from rats of varying ages,
the proportion of cells which incorporated 3H-thymidine into
nuclear DNA was greatest in cultured cells obtained initially from
10 day old animals and least in cells prepared initially from 30
day old rats (Table 1). These in vitro data parallel in vivo observations previously reported by others (2,3), which indicate
that Sertoli cell mitotic activity is severely reduced in rats
older than 10 days of age, and that the incorporation of 3H-thy-
midine into Sertoli cell nuclei tapers off after this period.
A quantitative discrepancy exists between the data reported by
Steinberger et al. (2) and those reported by Nagy (3). In the
latter studies, appreciable 3H-thymidine incorporation into nuclear
DNA of Sertoli cells persisted long after mitotic activity was
reduced (3). The basis for the quantitative discrepancy is unclear.
It would be of interest to know if plasma FSH levels differed in rats
from these two sets of studies, but this information is unfortunately
unavailable. The in vitro behavior of cultured Sertoli cell-enriched
preparations reported in Table 1 approximated that which would be
anticipated from the in vivo data of Nagy (3).

In cultured Sertoli cell-enriched preparations from 10,20 or
30 day old rats, prior treatment with FSH or dcAMP increased incorporation of 3H-thymidine into nuclear DNA, with greatest relative

stimulation in cells from older animals (Table 1 and Fig. 2).   The
degree of stimulation was increased in cells exposed to FSH for longer
time periods up to 96 hrs (Fig. 1).   Cells responding were identified
at a light microscope level as Sertoli cells.   Verification must
await radioautography at higher magnification, and experiments with
electron microscopy are now being conducted.   At the light microscope level, however, it is quite easy to rule out those labeled
cells which were germinal cells, and data reported in Table 1 exclude those few spermatogonia which continued to survive during
culture of the Sertoli-enriched preparation.   It is of interest that
effects of FSH were duplicated by dcAMP treatment of the cultured
cells (Fig. 2).   As discussed elsewhere in this book (8), all of the
biochemical effects on Sertoli cell-enriched cultures thus far
elicited by FSH treatment have been duplicated by the addition of
cyclic AMP or its derivatives.   In other cells such as fibroblasts,
cyclic AMP or dcAMP inhibits ³H-thymidine incorporation into DNA (9).
Experiments are in progress to determine if this is also the case
with cultured testicular peritubular cells.   In the Sertoli cell-
enriched preparation, FSH or dcAMP stimulation of ³H-thymidine incorporation into total DNA (Fig. 1, 2) and the discrete stimulation
of incorporation into particular Sertoli cell nuclei (Table 1) would
indicate that any peritubular cells which may be contaminating the
culture do not contribute to the ³H-thymidine incorporation experiments reported.

The nature of the newly synthesized nuclear DNA in the cultured
Sertoli cells is unknown.   It probably is associated at least in some
cases, with chromosomal DNA synthesized during the S phase in preparation for mitosis.   This is especially likely to be true in those
cells obtained from younger rats.   Mitotic activity remains relatively
high, both in vivo (2,3) and in vitro (unpublished observations) in
Sertoli cells of 10 day old rats when compared with mitotic activity
of cells from 20 and 30 day old rats.   Other types of ³H-thymidine
incorporation into DNA could be related to DNA repair mechanisms;
to partial DNA replication, as with satellite nucleolar heterochroma-
tin or gene amplification, and/or to an increase in ploidy of cultured Sertoli cells (10,11).   Which, if any, of these mechanisms is
involved when cells are stimulated by FSH remains to be investigated.

SUMMARY AND CONCLUSIONS

The incorporation of ³H-thymidine into DNA was investigated
in cultured Sertoli cell-enriched preparations from 10, 20 and 30
day old rats.   The amount incorporated per mg cell DNA during a 24
hr incubation period was far greater in Sertoli cells prepared
from younger rats than in those from 30 day old animals.   Prior
culture in the presence of FSH or dibutyryl cyclic AMP (dcAMP) increased the number of Sertoli cells whose nuclei were labeled.
This was evident in cultures of cells prepared from all ages cited,

but the most striking stimulation of DNA synthesis was observed in Sertoli cells initially prepared from testes of 30 day old rats. Data presented indicate that FSH or dcAMP stimulates nuclear DNA synthesis by Sertoli cells cultured under defined conditions.

ACKNOWLEDGMENTS

We express our indebtedness to Drs. J. H. Dorrington, B. G. Louis and P. S. Tung, with whom these data were frequently discussed. We thank Mrs. Erene Stanley for typing the manuscript.

Supported by grants from the Canadian MRC and the Banting Research Foundation.

REFERENCES

1. Clermont, Y. and Perey, B., Am. J. Anat., 100 : 241, 1957.

2. Steinberger, E., Steinberger, A. and Ficher, M., Rec. Prog. Hormone Res., 26 : 547, 1970.

3. Nagy, F., J. Reprod. Fert. 28 : 389, 1972.

4. Dorrington, J. H., Roller, N.F. and Fritz, I.B., Molec. Cell Endocrinol., 1975 (in press).

5. Dorrington, J.H., and Fritz, I.B., Endocrinology 96 : 1975 (in press).

6. Go, V.L.W., Vernon, R.G. and Fritz, I.B., Can. J. Biochem. 49 : 753, 1971.

7. Blatti, S.P., Ingles, C.J., Lindell, T.J., Morris, P.W., Weaver, R F., Weinberg, F. and Rutter, W.J., Cold Spring Harbor Symp. Quant. Biol. 35 : 649, 1970.

8. Fritz, I.B., Louis, B.G., Tung, P.S., Griswold, M., Rommerts, F.G. and Dorrington, J.H. This Volume, pg. 1975.

9. Wahrman, J.P., Winand, R. and Luzzati, D. Nature New Biol. 245 : 112, 1973.

10. Haver, C.W. Amer. Zool. 4 : 320, 1964.

11. Swift, H.H., Physiol. Zool., 23 : 169, 1950.

Purification of Testicular Proteins

ON THREE VARIETIES OF SPECIFIC BASIC PROTEINS ASSOCIATED WITH MAMMALIAN SPERMATOGENESIS

W. S. Kistler and H. G. Williams-Ashman

Ben May Laboratory for Cancer Research and Departments
of Biochemistry and of Pharmacological and Physiological
Sciences

University of Chicago, Chicago, Illinois 60637

The differentiation of haploid spermatozoa from diploid stem
cell spermatogonia in the mammalian germinal epithelium is an extremely complex process that remains very poorly understood. In
mammals spermatogenesis is clearly influenced not only by a variety
of hormones (especially FSH and androgens), but also by temperature
in most species. Elucidation of the mechanisms and regulation of
differentiation in eukaryotes is greatly aided where there exists
knowledge of macromolecular markers that are specifically produced
by one or more cell types that are intermediates and/or end products
of the overall differentiation process. As regards mammalian spermatogenesis, it would seem likely, for example, that there will be
specific macromolecules that play a role in meiosis, or alternatively
may be restricted in their occurrence to one or another phases of
spermiogenesis. Such testis-specific proteins might or might not
be found in fully differentiated spermatozoa.

In this respect, we have recently been concerned with the isolation and characterization of two specific small basic proteins
that seem to be uniquely associated with post-meiotic stages of
spermatogenesis in the rat (1 1). One of these proteins, which may
be designated as the spermatozoan basic chromosomal protein, is rich
in arginine, cysteine, and serine. It appears to have as its major
function the neutralization of the phosphate groups of the DNA that
is packaged into the head pieces of spermatozoa. The other protein,
which we have referred to as the testis-specific basic protein (1),
is rich in both arginine and lysine, and contains large amounts of
serine, but is devoid of cysteine and some other of the amino acids

423

commonly found in proteins. In contrast to the sperm chromosomal protein, the testis-specific basic protein is not detectable in epididymal spermatozoa.

A third protein that has been examined appears to be a lysine rich histone (Fl histone) component that is greatly enhanced during an early phase of spermatogenesis but may also be present in small amounts in other rat tissues besides the testis (4).

METHODS

The extraction from testis of proteins that are soluble in 3% trichloroacetic acid (TCA) has been described (1,3). Extraction of 0.5 N HCl-soluble proteins from testis following modification of sulfhydryl groups with ethylenimine (17) was as follows: Five grams of fresh decapsulated testis was homogenized in 3 volumes of cold 0.15 M NaCl, 0.01 M Tris-HCl at pH 7.5. The homogenate was centrifuged at 1,000 x g for 10 min at 4 C, the supernatant fraction discarded, and the pellet suspended in 6.4 ml of 0.1 M Tris-HCl at pH 8.5. Dithiothreitol was added to the suspension to give a final concentration of 0.01 M. After incubation in a covered tube for 30 min at room temperature, ethylenimine was added to give a concentration of 0.1 M. After 45 min further incubation at room temperature, the contents of the tube were poured into 10 volumes of cold acetone and kept at -20 C for 1 hr. The precipitate was collected by centrifugation, and the pellet was immediately homogenized in 10 ml of cold 0.5 N HCl. After standing on ice for 30 min, the acid homogenate was· centrifuged at 30,000 x g for 10 min. The supernatant fraction, containing the acid-soluble proteins, was mixed with 10 volumes of cold acetone and left at -20 C for 1 hr. The precipitated proteins were collected by centrifugation, washed once with ethanol/ether (50/50), dried under a gentle stream of N_2, and finally dissolved in 2 ml of 0.01 M acetic acid.

Electrophoretic separation was on polyacrylamide gels containing 0.94 M acetic acid, 6 M urea, and 20% acrylamide (4,15). Detection of protein bands by staining with amido black 10B has been described (1).

SPERMATOZOAN BASIC CHROMOSOMAL PROTEIN

During spermiogenesis in many forms of animal life the histones characteristic of somatic cells are replaced by a different class of basic proteins that have been referred to collectively as sperm histones (5). The protamines found in the spermatozoa of certain fish species (6,7) are perhaps the best known examples of such proteins.

Extraction of large quantities of the basic chromosomal protein associated with the headpieces of rat sperm cells has been accomplished by a number of techniques (1,8,9). Upon purification of the basic protein material released, its amino acid composition was found to consist of over 60% arginine and approximately 10% cysteine (1). Its composition is thus quite similar to that of a number of other mammalian sperm basic chromosomal proteins including those of the bull (10), stallion, ram, and boar (11).

In mature spermatozoa obtained from the cauda epididymis of the rat, or by ejaculation from the bull, it appears that nearly all of the cysteine residues of the sperm chromosomal proteins are involved in disulfide linkages, at least a portion of which are probably intermolecular (12,13). The functional basis for the presence of numerous disulfide bonds in the chromosomal proteins of eutherian mammals is not readily apparent, although it has been suggested that the reason may be a requirement for unusual rigidity in the sperm head during the penetration of the zona pellucida of the ovum during fertilization (14).

Our interest in the biosynthesis of the sperm chromosomal protein led us to devise procedures for its extraction and identification from rat testis. The detection of this protein among acid soluble proteins obtained from the testis is complicated, however, by the presence of the testis-specific basic protein. Thus, in the commonly used polyacrylamide gel electrophoretic systems of Panyim and Chalkley (15) or of Reisfeld et al. (16) as used in this laboratory (1,4), these two proteins are barely resolved from one another. One solution to this problem is to use a gel system that cleanly separates both proteins (system 2 of ref 1). An alternative approach is to modify the free sulfhydryl groups of the sperm chromosomal protein with ethylenimine to give product(s) of altered electrophoretic mobility due to the introduction of a substantial number of positively charged S-β-aminoethyl groups (17). The electrophoretic mobility of the testis-specific basic protein is not altered by such treatment as it contains no cysteine (1). When homogenates of adult testis are treated with ethylenimine under appropriate conditions, subsequent extraction of the preparation with 0.5 N HCl does in fact yield the sperm chromosomal protein in a form that separates from the testis-specific basic protein during electrophoresis in the system of Panyim and Chalkley (4,15) (Fig 1, Gel C).

The availability of techniques for the extraction of both of these proteins at the same time in electrophoretically resolvable forms should permit unambiguous studies on the incorporation of radiolabeled percursors into each of them simultaneously, and hence studies on the regulatory overtones of these processes.

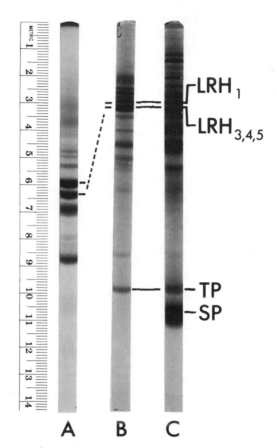

Figure 1. Electrophoretic separation of basic proteins from adult
rat testis. Gels A and B each contained the material from 100 mg
of decapsulated testis tissue that is soluble in 3% TCA (1,3). Gel
C contained the material soluble in 0.5 N HCl from 100 mg of decapsulated testis after modification of free sulfhydryl groups with
ethylenimine as described in "Methods." The cylindrical gels
measured 0.5 x 11 cm prior to staining and were run for 12 hr (A)
or 6.5 hr (B,C) at 150 V at room temperature with the negative elec-
trode at the bottom. The bands identified are: "HR,' Lysine rich
histones numbered as described in ref. 4; "TP", testis-specific basic
protein; "SP", sperm basic chromosomal protein.

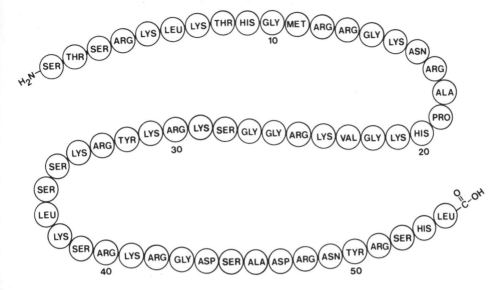

Figure 2. The complete amino acid sequence of the testis-specific basic protein from the rat (18).

TESTIS-SPECIFIC BASIC PROTEIN

Extraction of decapsulated testis tissue from sexually mature rats with cold 0.4 N H_2SO_4, followed by selection of those proteins that remain soluble in 3% TCA, yields acid extracts that contain the testis-specific basic protein, but none of the sperm basic chromosomal protein (Fig. 1, Gel B). Using such an extraction procedure the testis-specific basic protein has been identified in the sexually mature testes of a variety of eutherian mammals including rat, mouse, hamster, cat, bull (1), monkey, and man (3). The complete amino acid sequence has been established for the rat form of this protein (18) (Fig. 2). The protein from the human has been purified and the composition found to differ from that of the rat in the case of four amino acids (3). These differences are such that it is possible that the proteins from rat and man are differentiated by changes at only two residues out of 54 (Table 1). A similar protein was earlier isolated from mouse testis by Lam and Bruce (19). (We have confirmed their observations on mouse testis but could not substantiate their claim that this basic protein is also present in murine spermatozoa.)

TABLE 1

Amino Acid Composition of Human Testis-Specific
Basic Protein Compared to That of the Rat

Amino Acid	Specific Basic Protein From:	
	Human Testis (3)	Rat Testis (2)
Aspartic acid, Asparagine	5 (+1)	4
Threonine	1 (-1)	2
Serine	9 (+1)	8
Proline	1	1
Glycine	6	6
Alanine	1 (-1)	2
Valine	1	1
Methionine	1	1
Leucine	3	3
Tyrosine	2	2
Histidine	3	3
Lysine	10	10
Arginine	11	11
Try, Phe, Cys, Ile, Glu, Cln	0	0

The function(s) of the testis-specific basic protein is unknown, but a considerable body of indirect evidence suggests that
it is associated with the normal development of spermatids. During
development of the young male rat this protein is first detectable
in the testis about 34 days of age; at this time most seminiferous
tubules contain large populations of cells undergoing meiosis, and
the most advanced cell types in the germinal epithelium appear to
be spermatids undergoing nuclear elongation and condensation (1).
In all cases thus far examined the presence of this protein correlates with the occurrence of spermatids of this type in the tubules.
Thus, when the rat testis is rendered artificially cryptorchid, the
more advanced cell types of spermatogenesis disappear rather rapidly,
and after the testis has resided in the abdomen for 10 days, the
testis-specific basic protein is no longer detectable (1). In
this connection it should be noted that the function of interstitial
tissue is relatively little affected by the short term abdominal location of the testis (20). Similarly, none of this protein could be
detected in the abdominal testes of the Stanley-Gumbreck male
pseudohermaphrodite rats (2), which are characterized by hypertrophied
Leydig cells but no traces of spermatogenesis (21).

Although the presence of this protein correlates well with the
presence of maturing spermatids, there is as yet no direct evidence
that this protein is actually present or synthesized in spermatids.
Conceivably, the testis-specific basic protein could be a product
of the Sertoli cell that is in some way associated with the maturation of spermatids.

When rat testicular subcellular organelles are fractionated by differential centrifugation, the testis-specific basic protein is found associated with the nuclear fraction (unpublished). If chromatin is prepared from detergent-washed testicular cell nuclei by the procedure of Panyim et al. (22), the testis-specific basic protein is found as a prominent component of the histones extracted with acid from such chromatin. These observations suggest but do not prove that the testis-specific basic protein is bound to DNA. If this is the case, then perhaps it plays a role in the ordered replacement of histones by the cysteine-containing sperm chromo-somal protein finally found in the sperm nucleus. In this connec-tion it is interesting that Marushige and Marushige (13) have recently presented suggestive evidence that this protein is associated with the condensing fraction of spermatid chromatin.

ENHANCEMENT OF A SPECIFIC TESTICULAR LYSINE RICH HISTONE COMPONENT

During the course of studies of the testis-specific basic protein, we have frequently examined electrophoretically those pro-teins from the testis and other organs that are soluble in 3% TCA. Such extracts, when separated on gels containing 0.94 M acetic acid and 6 M urea, are found to contain a relatively slowly mi-grating but prominently stained band (Fig. 1) that is present only in trace amounts in other rat tissues (4). More detailed study of the material making up this band (indicated as LRH_1 in Fig. 1) has revealed that it is in fact composed of two different proteins. One of them is not as yet well characterized but appears to be specific to the testis. The other has been identified as a lysine rich histone component (LRH_1) (4).

The lysine rich histones of rat tissues comprise at least five separate species that are likely to consist of distinct proteins irrespective of post-translational modifications such as phosphory-lation (23). It appears that one of these components (LRH_1), which in many other rat organs is at most a very minor species, assumes in the testis the role of a major constituent. This phenomenon is associated with spermatogenesis since the quantity of LRH_1 diminishes rapidly in the cryptorchid testis and is also much reduced in the testis of the neonatal rat (4). The time at which LRH_1 attains its adult prominence in the developing rat testis has not been precisely determined, but probably occurrs by 20 days of age (4), a point at which spermatogenesis has not progressed past the prophase of the first meiotic division. Whether LRH_1 is associated in some way with the series of mitotic divisions preceeding meiosis, or perhaps with an early aspect of meiosis itself, remains uncertain.

CONCLUSIONS

We have identified two specific proteins in the rat testis
that appear to be confined to haploid cells of the germinal
epithelium, and in the case of LRH_1, a histone component that is
extraordinarily enriched in the testis compared to many other organs.
It is not yet known whether the synthesis of one or another of
these proteins is subject to endocrine regulation in a more direct
way than via the well known overall dependence of spermatogenesis
upon hormonal influences; however, this will be an interesting topic
for future study.

It is likely that both the testis-specific basic protein and
the sperm basic chromosomal protein are synthesized in maturing
spermatids on long-lived messenger RNA templates, because once
meiosis is completed, RNA synthesis in the developing spermatids
is rather quickly reduced to a very low level if not entirely
prohibited (24). Because the informational segments of the
messenger RNAs for these proteins are presumably relatively small
(roughly 150 to 170 nucleotides in length), it might be fairly
easy to separate them from most other testicular mRNA molecules.
Whether or not such studies of specific testicular messenger RNA
function should prove possible, the availability of the three
specific proteins described above may well prove useful in further
probes of the causative factors at the molecular level that under-
lie the precisely programmed transformations that accompany the
differentiation of the male gamete in eutherian mammals.

ACKNOWLEDGMENTS

This work was supported by United States Public Health Service
Grants HD-04592 and HD-07110.

REFERENCES

1. Kistler, W.S., Geroch, M.E., and Williams-Ashman, H.G., J.
    Biol. Chem., 248: 4532-4543, 1973.

2. Kistler, W.S., Noyes, C., and Heinrikson, R.L., Biochem. Biophys.
    Res. Commun., 57: 341-347, 1974.

3. Kistler, W.S., Geroch, M.E., and Williams-Ashman, H.G., Invest.
    Urol., 12: 346-350, 1975.

4. Kistler, W.S., and Geroch, M.E., Biochem. Biophys. Res. Commun.,
    63: 378-384, 1975.

5. Bloch, D.P., Genet. Suppl., 61 : 93–111, 1969.

6. Felix, K., Advan., Protein Chem., 15 : 1–56, 1960.

7. Ando, T., Yamasaki, M., and Suzuki, K., Protamines : Isolation, Characterization, Structure, and Function, Springer-Verlag, New York, 1973.

8. Coelingh, J.P., Rozijn, T.H., and Monfoort, C.H., Biochim. Biophys, Acta, 188 : 353–356, 1969.

9. Calvin, H.I., and Bedford, J.M., J. Reprod. Fert. Suppl., 13 : 65–76, 1971.

10. Coelingh, J.P., Monfoort, C.H., Rozijn, T.H., Gevers Leuven, J.A., Schiphof, R., Steyn-Parve, E.P., Braunitzer, G., Schrank, B., and Ruhfus, A., Biochim. Biophys. Acta, 285 : 1-14, 1972.

11. Monfoort, C.H., Schiphof, R., Rozijn, T.H., and Steyn-Parve, E.P., Biochim. Biophys. Acta, 322 : 173–177, 1973.

12. Marushige, Y., and Marushige, K., Biochim. Biophys. Acta, 340 : 498–508, 1974.

13. Marushige, Y., and Marushige, K., J. Biol. Chem. 250 : 39–45, 1975.

14. Bedford, J.M., and Calvin, H.I., J. Exp. Zool., 188 : 137–156, 1974.

15. Panyim, S., and Chalkley, R., Arch. Biochem. Biophys., 130 : 337–346, 1969.

16. Reisfeld, R.A., Lewis, U.J., and Williams, D.E., Nature, 195 : 281–283, 1962.

17. Raftery, M.A., and Cole, R.D., J. Biol. Chem., 241 : 3457–3461, 1966.

18. Kistler, W.S., Noyes, C., Hsu, R., and Heinrikson, R.L., J. Biol. Chem., 250 : 1847–1853, 1975.

19. Lam, D.M.K., and Bruce, W.R., J. Cell. Physiol., 78 : 13 24, 1971.

20. Nelson, W.O., C.S.H. Symp. Quant. Biol., 5 : 123–135, 1937.

21. Stanley, A.J., Gumbreck, L.G., Allison, J.E., and Easley, R.B. Rec. Prog. Horm. Res., 29: 43–64, 1973.

22. Panyim, S., Bilek, D., and Chalkley, R., J. Biol. Chem., 246 : 4206–4215, 1971.

23. Kinkade, J.M., Jr., J. Biol. Chem., $\underline{244}$: 3375-3386, 1969.

24. Monesi, V., J. Reprod. Fert. Suppl., $\underline{13}$: 1-14, 1971.

PURIFICATION AND CHARACTERIZATION OF RABBIT TESTICULAR ANDROGEN

BINDING PROTEIN (ABP)

S.C. Weddington, P. Brandtzaeg, K. Sletten, T.
Christensen and V. Hansson
Institute of Pathology, Rikshospitalet, Oslo, Norway;

F.S. French, P. Petrusz and S.N. Nayfeh
Departments of Pediatrics, Biochemistry and The Labor-
atories for Reproductive Biology, University of North
Carolina, School of Medicine, Chapel Hill, N.C. U.S.A.

E.M. Ritzen
Pediatric Endocrinology Unit, Clinical Research
Laboratory, Karolinska Sjukhuset, Stockholm, Sweden

INTRODUCTION

We have reported the presence of an androgen binding protein
(ABP) in the cytosols of testis and epididymis of several mammalian
species (1). ABP in cytosol preparations has been shown to have a
sedimentation coefficient of 4.6 S, an isoelectric point of 4.5-5.2,
a Stokes radius of 43 (rabbit) and 47 Å (rat), and a frictional ratio
of 1.6, indicating a molecular weight of about 70,000 and 90,000
respectively.

ABP is produced by the Sertoli cells (2,3,5,7-9) and specifically
stimulated by FSH (2-4, 6-10). It is secreted in the epididymis by
way of the efferent ducts (11,12). In the epididymis, ABP concentration decreases rapidly from caput to cauda, reaching a very low
level in rat or undetectable level in rabbit (1,12,13). The exact
fate of ABP in the testicular and epididymal lumina is not known,
although it may either be taken up by pinocytosis by the lining
epithelial cells or inactivated in the lumen. A monospecific antibody against ABP would allow immunohistochemical examination of the
origin and fate of ABP in the testis and epididymis independent
of its binding activity.

433

The observation that ABP is an FSH-dependent product of Sertoli cells has made it a valuable tool both as a specific endpoint for FSH action (23) and as an index of the secretory function of the Sertoli cell (15). A specific and sensitive ABP radioimmunoassay will undoubtedly be very useful for detecting early changes in ABP concentration in response to FSH or other hormonal treatments.

Rabbit serum also possesses a serum androgen binding protein (TeBG) with properties very similar to ABP (13,16-19). Since both TeBG and ABP are also present in man, it is possible that the rabbit might be used as a model for studying the possible functions of and interrelationships between these two proteins in man. In rabbits ABP and TeBG are indistinguishable by size, stability and steroid binding properties (20). Thus, since careful investigations of physical characteristics revealed no decisive differences, antisera raised against ABP might be used to establish whether or not ABP and TeBG show immunological cross-reactivity.

PURIFICATION OF ABP

Epididymal 105,000 x g supernatant was labeled with ^{3}H-DHT in order to follow ABP binding activity. Measurement of binding of ^{3}H-DHT to ABP by SS-PAGE (21) was used for monitoring the percent yield of ABP after each purification step.

Ammonium Sulphate Precipitation

ABP was first precipitated from ^{3}H-DHT labeled supernatant with 50% ammonium sulphate and the sediment was subsequently washed 3 times with 50% $(NH_4)_2SO_4$ solution. This treatment reduced the volume by a factor of 5 and separated ABP from a large portion of the major bulk proteins. About 60-100% ABP activity was recovered with a two-fold increase in specific activity. Best recoveries were obtained by the slow addition of finely powerded $(NH_4)_2SO_4$ (over an 8 hour period). Addition of 10-20% glycerol to the resuspension buffer appeared to stablize ABP binding activity.

DEAE-cellulose Chromatography

After $(NH_4)_2SO_4$ precipitation, the sample was redissolved in 10 mM Tris-HCl buffer, pH 7.4, containing 10% glycerol and desalted by gel filtration on a Sephadex G-25 column. The desalted fraction was next applied to a DEAE-cellulose column, and the proteins were eluted from the column using a linear gradient from 0-0.4 M KCl. We have previously shown that ABP is eluted from DEAE cellulose at about 0.17 M KCl (20). As seen in Figure 1, ABP, as measured by ^{3}H-DHT binding activity, was eluted as a symmetrical peak between 11 and

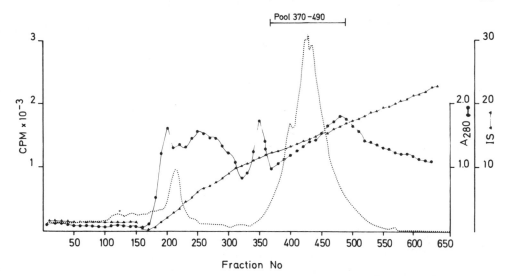

Figure 1.   Chromatography on Whatman DEAE-Cellulose (DE-52) of 1000
ml dissolved and desalted $(NH_4)_2SO_4$ precipitate.   The $(NH_4)_2SO_4$ precipitate was dissolved in 10 mM Tris-HCl buffer containing 1 mM EDTA
and 10% glycerol and desalted on a Sephadex G-25 column.   The area
of the eluate from the DEAE cellulose column was pooled for further
purification as indicated in the figure.   Column dimensions: 5.0
x 80 cm; flow rate: 300 ml/hour; temperature: 2-4°C.   Fractions were
14.6 ml each and aliquots of 200 µl were taken for counting.   Con-
ductivity mMHO/cm: ▲ ——— ▲; Absorbance at 280 mm (A_{280}): ●——●;
Radioactivity: • • • • • • • • • • • •

18 mMHO/cm.   Due to its high capacity, DEAE cellulose chromatography
was a desirable step.   However, this step gave only about 50% recovery with 2-6 fold increase in specific activity.   The low recovery probably resulted from denaturation of ABP on the column.

Gel Filtration on Sephadex G-200

The pooled fractions from the DEAE-cellulose were concentrated
by ultrafiltration in a Amicon stirred cell using a PM-10 filter.
Following this step, the sample was reprecipitated with 50% $(NH_4)_2SO_4$
and redissolved in 75 ml of 10 mM Tris-HCl buffer containing 1 mM
EDTA and 10% glycerol, and applied in portions of 25 ml to a
column of Sephadex G-200.   The radioactivity was eluted as a single

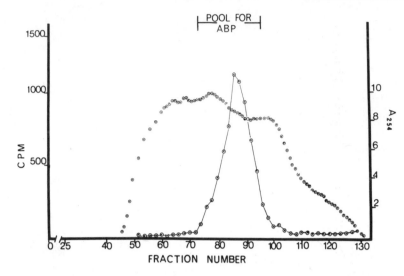

Figure 2. Gel filtration on Sephadex G-200 of the pooled ABP
containing fractions from the DEAE-cellulose column. Before G-200
chromatography, the eluate was concentrated to 75 ml with an Amicon
ultra-filter using a PM-10 membrane. Samples were chromatographed
on G-200 in 3 runs of 25 ml each. The fractions pooled for further
purification are indicated in the figure. Column dimensions: 3.3 x
93 cm; flow rate: 18 ml/hour (upwards); temperature: 2°C; elution
buffer 10 mM Tris-HCl, pH 7.4. Fractions were 6 ml each and aliquots
of 25 μl were taken for counting. Absorbance at 280 nm (A_{280}):
⊖⊖⊖⊖⊖; Radioactivity: ⊖—⊖.

peak having a distribution coefficient (Kav) of 0.30 (Fig. 2). This
step resulted in a 3-4 fold increase in specific activity and almost
100% recovery of ABP binding activity.

Hydroxyl-apatite Chromatography

The fractions corresponding to the ABP peak from the 3
columns of Sephadex G-200 were pooled, concentrated by ultrafiltration
and chromatographed on a hydroxyl-apatite (Bio-Rad-HT) column previously equilibrated with 10 mM Tris buffer, pH 7.4. The column was
washed with starting buffer and eluted stepwise with increasing concentrations of phosphate buffer. As can be seen in Fig. 3, the ABP

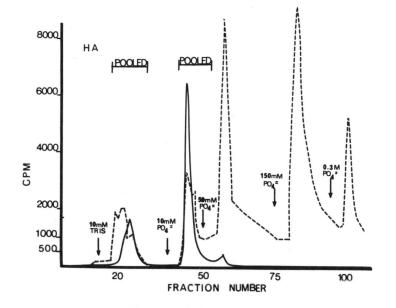

Figure 3. Chromatography on hydroxyl-apatite (Bio-Rad-HT) of the pooled G-200 eluate from 3 columns after concentration to a volume of 50 ml. The fractions containing ABP were pooled for further purification as indicated in the figure. The arrows indicate the buffer changes. Column dimensions: 2.5 x 38 cm; flow rate: 40 ml/hour; temperature: 2°C. Fractions of 10 ml were collected and aliquots of 25 µl taken for counting. Absorbance at 280 nm (A_{280}) -----; Radioactivity: _____.

activity was eluted as two sharp peaks, the first with the Tris-HCl buffer and the second with the 10 mM phosphate buffer. Most of the other proteins were retained by the hydroxyl-apatite column. This procedure resulted in a further 3-fold increase in specific activity and an approximately 60-90% recovery of ABP binding activity. To prevent packing and impaired flow the hydroxyl-apatite column had to be run at a low flow rate.

Following concentration of the pooled fractions (Fig. 3) by ultrafiltration the sample was again chromatographed on a Sephadex G-200 column using the procedure outlined above (Fig. 4). With this second gel filtration, ABP was eluted prior to the major protein band, and a further 2-3 fold increase in the specific activity with good recovery was obtained.

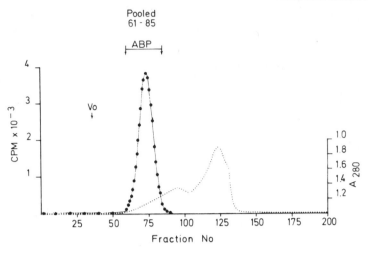

Figure 4.   Gel filtration on Sephadex G-200 (3.3 x 90 cm) of the
pooled fraction of hydroxyl-apatite eluate after concentration to a
volume of 17.5 ml.   The conditions are the same as in Figure 2.   The
fractions which were pooled for further purification are indicated
in the figure.   Absorbance at 280 nm (A_{280}):   -----; Radioactivity:
●————●.

Preparative Polyacrylamide Gel Electrophoresis

As a final purification step the eluate from the Sephadex G-200
column was concentrated and further purified by preparative
acrylamide gel electrophoresis.   The electrophoresis was carried
out in Tris-glycine buffer (pH 8.6), and a 13 mm inside diameter
glass column fitted with a special adaptor for continuous flow
of elution buffer across the bottom of the gel.   The protein was
eluted between 30 and 50 hours (Fig. 5).   This procedure gave only
a 10-30% recovery of ABP binding activity.   However, the major
fraction showed an additional increase of 4-10 fold in the specific
binding activity of ABP.   These fractions were pooled as indcated and
concentrated in a stirred Amicon cell to a protein concentration
of 0.5 mg/ml.

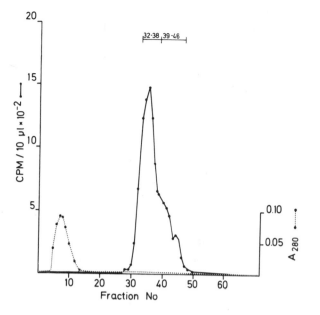

Figure 5. Preparative polyacrylamide gel electrophoresis of partially purified ABP obtained by $(NH_4)_2SO_4$ precipitation, chromatography on DEAE-Cellulose, Sephadex G-200 and hydroxyl-apatite. The gels contained 7% acrylamide (v/w) and 2% cross linking (bis-acrylamide). The separating gel measured 1.3 x 5 cm with 10 cm long stacking gel on the top. Electrophoresis was run in Tris-glycine buffer, pH 8.6 (measured at 25°C) and with the gel completely immersed in the lower buffer, which was kept at 0°C. Flow rate of elution buffer: 1 ml/hour; Current: 3 mA; One ml fractions were collected. Absorbance at 280 nm (A_{280}): ●——●; Radioactivity: ○————○.

CHARACTERIZATION OF PURIFIED ABP

Analytic gel electrophoresis

The purified ABP (∿ 1000 pmoles/mg protein) was homogeneous when analyzed by polyacrylamide gel electrophoresis in 6.5% polyacrylamide gels, pH 8.6. It showed a mobility of 0.4 relative to Bromphenol Blue (BPB) and the protein band stained with Coomassie Blue was concurrent with the peak of ABP binding activity (Fig. 6). However, since preparative polyacrylamide gel electrophoresis had

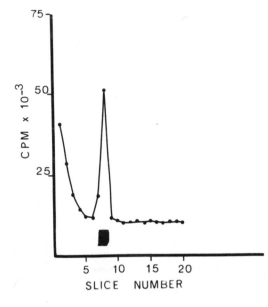

Figure 6.   Analytical polyacrylamide gel electrophoresis of 50 µg purified ABP in 6.5% polyacrylamide gels.   Note the activity band corresponds to that of the stained protein band.   Sample volume: 100 µl; Voltage: 100–150 V; Current: 1.5 mAmp/tube; Gel dimensions: 0.5 x 7 cm (i.d.).   Temperature: 0°C.

been used in the purification procedure, the purity of the ABP preparation was further examined by electrophoresis in 10% polyacrylamide gels containing 0.1% SDS.   This procedure yielded a major protein band migrating with a mobility of 0.25 relative to Bromphenol Blue (BPB).   Three minor bands moving with a relative mobility of 0.16, 0.35, and 0.40, respectively were also found (Fig. 7).   Figure 7 shows the plot of the mobility of ABP compared to known protein standards.   As seen, the mobility of ABP was almost identical to that of bovine serum albumin, indicating a molecular weight of about 68,000.

Analytical ultracentrifugation

Another ABP preparation with a higher specific binding activity ($\sim$ 2500 pmoles/mg protein) was analyzed by analytical ultracentrifugation.   ABP was found to have a sedimentation coefficient ($S_{20,w}$) of 4.5 S as calculated from the plot of the log of the distance

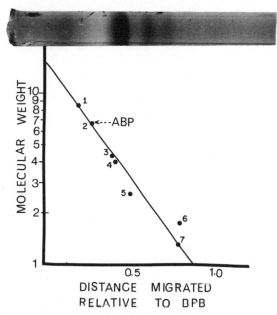

Figure 7.   Analytical polyacrylamide gel electrophoresis in 10%
gels (0.5 x 9 cm) containing 0.1% of sodium dodecyl sulphate (SDS)
(23).   Current: 5 mA/tube; Voltage: 200-300.   Samples of 100 µl
(50 µg, ABP and standards) were layered on the top of 3% stacking
gels and electrophoresis run for 6 hours at room temperature.   Gel
is stained with Coomassie Blue (insert).   Mobility of ABP compared
with the standard proteins: (1) ovalbumin dimer, (2) Bovine serum
albumin, (3) Ovalbumin, (4) Aldolase, (5) Chymotrypsinogen, (6)
Myoglobin, (7) Cytochrom C.

migrated versus time in minutes (Fig. 8A).   Equilibrium ultracentrifugation data plotted as log of optical density versus the square
of the radius, gave a straight line indicating a homogeneous protein
with a molecular weight of 65,500 (Fig. 8B).   A partial specific
volume of 0.70 cm^3/g was used in the calculations.

Chemical composition

, The ABP preparation examined by analytical ultracentrifugations
was further studied for its content of carbohydrates and amino
acids.   Results from chemical analysis are shown in Table 1.   Acid
hydrolysed ABP showed a relatively high content of aspartic and
glutamic acids, proline, glycine and half cyteines, whereas the
content of methionine and tyrosine is low.   The protein portion of
the purified ABP preparation accounts for approximately 70% of the
total weight and the carbohydrate moiety for the remaining 20-30%.

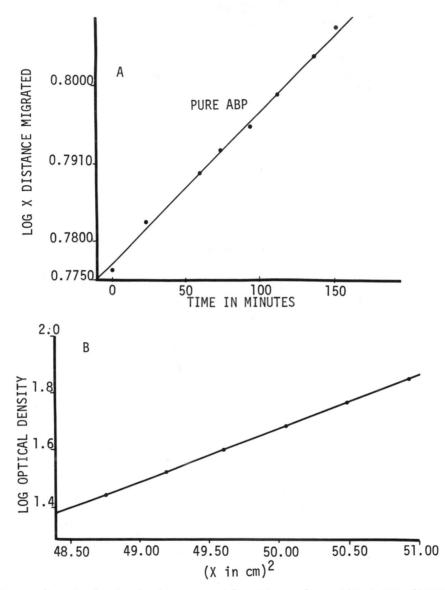

Figure 8.   Analytical ultracentrifugation of purified ABP (2500 pmoles/mg protein) in a Beckman (Model E) centrifuge with a double beam photoelectric scanner dissolved in 10. mM Tris–HCl buffer, pH 7.4.   Protein concentration of sample was 0.5 mg/ml.
A.   Sedimentation velocity run at 40,000 rpm/min and 20°.
B.   Sedimentation equilibrium centrifugation at 10,000 rpm for 48 h. at 20°C.

Table 1

CHEMICAL COMPOSITION OF RABBIT
TESTICULAR ANDROGEN BINDING PROTEIN (ABP)

Carbohydrate analysis of purified ABP (2500 pmol/mg protein) was
carried out according to the method of Chambers and Clamp (24) using
gas liquid chromatography in conjunction with the silyl derivatives
of methyl glycosides released from the protein by methanolysis. The
precipitate after methanolysis was subjected to acid hydrolysis and
amino acid analysis was performed as described elsewhere (25).

AMINO ACIDS		CARBOHYDRATES	
RESIDUE	No. of resi-dues/100[*]	RESIDUE	percent of total (w/w)
Asp	8.7	Mannose	3.2
Thr	5.1	Galactose	1.9
Ser	7.7	N-acetyl-galactosamine	17.1
Glu	12.2		
Pro	6.4	N-acetyl glucosamine	2.8
Gly	15.4		
Ala	9.5	Sialic acid	<1
1/2 Cyst[**]	3.1		
Val	6.3		
Met	(+)	Total carbo-hydrates	25
Ile	2.9		
Leu	9.3		
Tyr	(+)		
Phe	4.0		
His	2.4		
Lys	3.8		
Arg	3.6		
Trp[***]	N.D.		

[*] Mean of 2 separate determinations (130 μg ABP each)

[**] Determined as cysteic acid

[***] Not determined

(+) Little but present

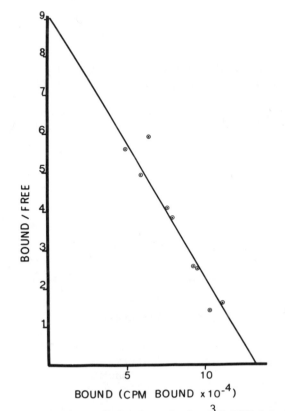

Figure 9.   Scatchard plot analysis of the ^{3}H-DHT binding to ABP.
Data were obtained from SS-PAGE at 0°C keeping the concentration of
ABP constant and varying the ^{3}H-DHT concentration (0.5 to 8 nM in
the polyacrylamide gel.   The straight line was obtained by regression analysis of the points.   Ordinate: Bound/Free.   Abcissa;
[3]H-DHT bound to ABP.

                        Iso-electric Focusing

        As an additional criterion of purity, ABP ($\sim$ 1000 pmoles/mg pro-
tein) was focused in a 3-10 pH gradient of 6.5% polyacrylamide gel.
The activity focused as a broad peak around pH 4.8.   When the gel
was sliced longitudinally and half the gel stained and the other
half sliced for counting, the Coomassie Blue stained band corresponded to the band of ABP binding activity.

        Purified ABP ($\sim$ 1000 pmoles/mg protein) was also focused in
a sucrose column and was shown to focus as a broad band at pH 4.5-
5.0.   This is in agreement with our previous results on less pure
preparations (20).

Binding affinity

The equilibrium constant of dissociation (K_d) at 0°C of purified ABP ($\sim$ 1000 pmoles/mg protein) has been determined by the use
of SS-PAGE at 0-2°C. An average K_d 4.1 x 10^{-9} $\pm$ 0.4 (S.D.) was
found (Fig. 9). This is a higher value than that obtained for ABP
in rabbit efferent duct fluid, 1.9 x 10^{-9} M (derived from Fig. 6,
ref 21) using SS-PAGE and by Sephadex gel equilibration (0.72 x
10^{-9} M). In the present studies on rabbit ABP a K_d of 4 x 10^{-9}
M have been used for calculating data from SS-PAGE.

Stability

The purified ABP was stable after exposure to 1, 2 or 4 mM
p-chloromercuriphenyl sulphonate (PCMPS) and 10 mM 2-mercapto-
ethanol for 30 minutes at 0°C. However, the binding is reduced to
less than 20% by 100 mM 2-mercaptoethanol. Neither storage at 4°C
for up to 60 days nor freezing and thawing and dialysis against
10 mM Tris-HCl buffer, pH 7.4 at 2-4°C seemed to have any effect
on the binding of ^{3}H-DHT to purified ABP.

Immunological Studies

Antisera to ABP were prepared using the second G-200 eluate
(showing 5 bands by analytical polyacrylamide gel electrophoresis)
as an antigen. Each of 4 guinea pigs was injected intracutaneously
in multiple sites with 0.5 ml (12.2 mg/ml) of antigen emulsified in
0.5 ml of Freunds Complete Adjuvant. The animals were bled after
6 weeks and those showing an ABP titer were given one booster injection to increase the titer. Antisera were checked for precipitin
lines by double diffusion test in agar, and by inhibition of ABP
binding activity as measured by SS-PAGE (21). A standard solution
of partly purified ABP was used as an antigen.

Double diffusion tests in agar showed that three of the four
animals had produced antibodies against the G-200 eluate. All antisera had at least 2 precipitin lines in common, with 405 lines being
present in all antisera. When purified ABP ($\sim$ 1000 pmoles/mg
protein) was examined by double diffusion tests, 3-4 lines were seen,
indicating contaminants present in some of the purified ABP preparations. This was in agreement with the results from analytical
SDS polyacrylamide gel electrophoresis, showing three minor bands
in addition to the major ABP band (Fig. 7).

The degree of inhibition of binding of ^{3}H-DHT to ABP by ABP
antisera (1st bleeding) was determined by SS-PAGE following incubation of ABP with ^{3}H-DHT in the presence of the antisera. Normal
guinea pig serum at each dilution served as control. At a
dilution of 1:10, antisera 2 and 4 caused 100% inhibition of ABP

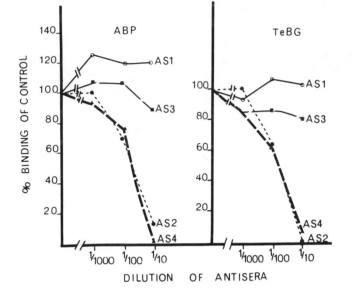

Figure 10.   Inhibition of ^{3}H–DHT binding to ABP (left) and TeBG
(right) by different dilutions of anti-ABP antisera.   Four guinea
pigs were injected with partially purified rabbit ABP in complete
Freunds adjuvant, and bled after 6 weeks.   Various dilutions of
antiserum (1/10, 1/100, 1/1000) were added to an equal volume of
partially purified ABP or immature rabbit serum (dil. 1:50, v/v).
Normal guinea pig serum in the same dilution served as controls.
After incubation for 48 h at 2–4°C the samples were centrifuged at
10,000 x g for 15 min and binding of ^{3}H–DHT to ABP and TeBG was
analyzed by SS-PAGE (21).   From Weddington et al., 1975 (26).

binding activity.   Some inhibition was also observed at dilutions
of 1:100 but none at 1:1000 (Fig. 10).   Antisera from animal 1 and
3 showed little or no inhibition of binding activity, although they
had activities against other antigens in the G-200 eluate as
demonstrated by double diffusion tests in agar.   These latter antisera might be valuable as immunosorbents in order to remove the
major contaminants from the second G-200 eluate.   After one booster
dose, the titer against ABP increased about 10-fold giving 100%
inhibition of ^{3}H-DHT binding to ABP at a dilution of 1:100.

Figure 10 shows that the ABP antisera 2 and 4 also inhibited
binding of ^{3}H-DHT to TeBG and that the inhibition at different
dilutions of the antisera was identical to the inhibition of binding

to ABP. The finding that all 4 antisera showed precipitin lines
in double diffusion tests and only 2 had a detectable titer against
ABP and TeBG, suggests that the inhibition is caused by a specific
antibody against ABP and is not an artifact due to co-precipitation
with contaminating antigens.

DISCUSSION

In the present study we have purified ABP from rabbit epididymis, in some experiments approaching a specific activity of some
2500 pmoles/mg protein. This represents approximately 20% of the
theoretical maximum (14,000 pmoles/mg protein), assuming 1 binding
site per molecule of ABP. The best ABP preparation obtained was
apparently homogenous by equilibrium ultracentrifugation and was
used for amino acid and carbohydrate analyses. In subsequent
purifications, we obtained ABP preparations with specific activities
of 800-1200 pmoles/mg protein. These preparations were shown by
SDS electrophoresis to contain one major band with a molecular
weight (MW) of 68,000 (ABP) and 3 minor bands with MW of 100,000,
50,000, and 40,000, respectively (Fig. 7). These preparations also
contained 3-4 precipitin lines in double diffusion tests in agar
with antisera raised against an impure ABP preparation.

It is apparent from these studies that it might be difficult
to obtain 100% pure preparations of ABP, as evaluated by binding
activity, using conventional techniques. Some of the ABP may lose
its binding activity during the various steps in the purification.
It might be possible to increase the yield of active ABP by including
affinity chromatography and immunological methods in the purification scheme.

The present study showed that ABP is a glycoprotein containing
20-30% carbohydrates, and 70-80% aminio acids. Preliminary amino
acid composition data (Table 1) indicated a high content of aspartic
and gluamic acid, proline, cysteine (identified as cysteic acid)
and glycine, whereas the content of methionine and tyrosine was low.
The amino acid analysis was performed on the precipitate after
release of the carbohydrates by acid methanolysis. Acid methonolysis
is a mild treatment, which is not supposed to hydrolyse the peptide
chains. It will, however, be of interest to compare the amino acid
composition of ABP preparations before and after acid methanolysis.
So far, we have not been able to provide enough highly purified ABP
to do such studies. The carbohydrate moiety contained mainly N-
acetylglactosamine and smaller amounts of mannose, galactose and
N-acetylglucosamine. Very low content of sialic acid (< 1%) was
also found.

Table 2

COMPARISON BETWEEN RABBIT TESTICULAR ANDROGEN BINDING PROTEIN (ABP)
AND TESTOSTERONE BINDING GLOBULIN (TeBG) IN RABBIT SERUM

	ABP	TeBG
Physical characteristics	----------Identical----------	
Immunological characteristics	----------Identical----------	
Origin	Sertoli cells	Liver (?)
Regulation of synthesis:		
FSH	↑	–
Androgens	↑	↓
Estrogens	↓	↑

One important observation from these studies was the immunological
cross-reaction between ABP and TeBG. The explanation for this
apparent immunological similarity could be that TeBG is one of the
proteins present in the ABP preparation used for immunization, and
that antibodies against both ABP and TeBG have been developed.
This is unlikely, however, since the maximal concentration of TeBG
in rabbit epididymal cytosol is only 1-2% that of ABP. Furthermore, the fact that the antisera having activity against ABP (2 and
4) also are the ones inhibiting ^{3}H–DHT binding to TeBG indicates
that binding to ABP and TeBG is being inhibited by the same
antibody population.

ABP is produced in the Sertoli cells and secreted into the
testicular fluid, while TeBG is present in the systemic circulation,
but of unknown origin. It is not likely that ABP originates in
serum and is concentrated by the Sertoli cells in the seminiferous
tubular fluid, since ABP is found in high concentrations in the rat,
which lacks serum TeBG (1). Neither is it likely that TeBG originates
in the testis, since high concentrations of TeBG are found in orchiec-
tomized males as well as in normal females (17). Furthermore, ABP
production is stimulated by FSH and androgens, while TeBG concentrations in serum are depressed by androgens and increased by
estrogens (Table 2). Thus, ABP and TeBG might well be the same
protein, but produced at two different sites in the body and
regulated by completely different hormonal mechanisms. Some

indication that there might be small differences in the carbohydrate
parts of the ABP and TeBG molecules arise from studies using
Concanavalin A (Con A) affinity chromatography. Rabbit TeBG is
constantly retained by the Con A columns, whereas ABP is more or
less excluded from such columns (Weddington, Hansson and French, unpublished).

SUMMARY

Testicular androgen binding protein (ABP) was purified from
the epididymis of 1500 adult rabbits by the sequential use of
ammonium sulphate precipitation, ion exchange chromatography on
DEAE cellulose, gel filtration on Sephadex G-200, hydroxyl-apatite
chromatography and preparative polyacrylamide gel electrophoresis.
This procedure yielded a 1000-fold increase in specific activity
compared to that of the 105,000 x g supernatant, and the recovery
of active ABP was about 3-5%. ABP is acid glycoprotein with a
molecular weight of 65-68,000 daltons.

Antisera to rabbit ABP raised in guinea pigs inhibit ^{3}H-
DHT binding to ABP as measured by SS-PAGE. When diluted rabbit
serum containing TeBG is treated with the same dilutions of these
antisera, identical binding inhibition curves are found. Thus,
ABP and TeBG in rabbits appear to possess identical immunological
determinants.

ACKNOWLEDGEMENTS

Financial support was given by National Institutes of Health,
USA (research grant HD04466 and training grant AM05330), The
Rockefeller Foundation, World Health Organization (grant H9/181/83),
Swedish Medical Research Council grant 3168), the Norwegian Research
Council for Sciences and Humanities, Nordic Insulin Foundation and
Norwegian Agency for International Development (NORAD). S.C.
Weddington is a predoctoral fellow from the University of North
Carolina, and V. Hansson, to whom correspondence should be
addressed, is a Career Research Awardee of Oslo University.

REFERENCES

1. Hansson, V., Ritzen, E.M., French, F.S., and Nayfeh, S.N.
    in: Handbook of Physiology, Section 7, vol. 5, eds. D.W.
    Hamilton and R.O. Greep, Amer. Physiol. Soc. 1975, p. 173.

2. Hansson, V., French, F.S., McLean, W.S., Smith, A.A., Tindall,
    D.J., Weddington, S.C., Nayfeh, S.N., and Ritzen, E.M.
    J. Int. Res. Commun. 1:26, 1973.

3. Hansson, V., Reusch, E., Trygstad, O., Torgersen, O., French,
    F.S., and Ritzen, E.M. Nature, New Biol. 246:56, 1973.

4. Hansson, V., Trygstad, O., French, F.S., McLean, W.S., Smith,
    A.A., Tindall, D.J., Weddington, S.C., Petrusz, P., Nayfeh, S.N.,
    and Ritzen, E.M. Nature 250:387, 1974.

5. Hagenas, L., Ritzen, E.M., Ploen, L., Hansson, V., French, F.S.,
    and Nayfeh, S.N. Mol. Cell Endocrinol. May, 1975.

6. French, F.S., McLean, S.W., Smith, A.A., Tindall, D.J.,
    Weddington, S.C., Petrusz, P., Sar, M., Stumpf, W.E., Nayfeh,
    S.N., Hansson, V., Trygstad, O., and Ritzen, U.M. in:
    Hormone Binding and Target Cell Activation in the Testis, eds.:
    M.L. Dufau and A.R. Means, Plenum Press, 1974, p. 265.

7. Tindall, D.J., Schrader, W.T., and Means, A.R. in: Hormone
    Binding and Target Cell Activation in the Testis, eds.: M.L.
    Dufau and A.R. Means, Plenum Press, New York, 1974, p. 167.

8. Vernon, R.G., Kopec, B., Fritz, I.B. Mol. Cell Endocrin.
    1:167, 1974.

9. Fritz, I.B., Kopec, B., Lam, K., and Vernon, G. in: Hormone
    Binding and Target Cell Activation in the Testis, eds.: M.L.
    Dufau and A.R. Means, Plenum Press, New York, 1974, p. 311.

10. Sanborn, B., Elinton, J.S.H., Steinberger, E., Steinberger, A.,
    and Meistrich, This Volume, p. 293.

11. French, F.S. and Ritzen, E.M. J. Reprod. Fert. 32: 479, 1973.

12. French, F.S. and Ritzen, E.M. Endocrinology 95:88, 1973.

13. Ritzen, E.M. and French, F.S. J. Steroid Biochem. 5:151, 1974.

14. Weddington, S.C., Hansson, V., French, F.S., Nayfeh, S.N.,
    Ritzen, E.M. and Hagenas, L. Nature 254:145, 1975.

15. Hansson, V., Weddington, S.C., Attramadal, A., Naess, O.,
    French, F.S., Nayfeh, S.N., and Ritzen, E.M. This volume,
    p. 323.

16. Hansson, V., Ritzen, E.M., French, F.S., Weddington, S.C.,
    Nayfeh, S.N., Reusch, E., and Attramadal, A. Steroids 22:
    185, 1973.

17. Hansson, V., Ritzen, E.M., Weddington, S.C., McLean, W.S.,
     Tindall, D.J., Nayfeh, S.N., and French, F.S. Endocrinology
     95:690, 1974.

18. Rosner, W.R., Darmstadt, A. Endocrinology 92:1700, 1973.

19. Mahoudeau, T.A. and Corvol, P. Endocrinology 92:1113, 1973.

20. Hansson, V., Ritzen, E.M., French, F.S., Weddington, S.C., and
     Nayfeh, S.N. Mol. Cell Endocrinol., May, 1975.

21. Ritzen, E.M., French, F.S., Weddington, S.C., Nayfeh, S.N.,
     and Hansson, V. J. Biol. Chem. 249: 6597, 1974.

22. Means, A.R. and Tindall, D.J., this volume, p. 383.

23. Webber, K. and Osborn, M. J. Biol. Chem. 244: 16, 1969.

24. Chambers, R.E. and Clamp, J.R. Biochem. J. 125:1009, 1971.

25. Sletten, K. and Husby, G. Eur. J. Biochem. 41:117, 1974.

26. Weddington, S.C., Brandtzaeg, P., Hansson, V., French, F.S.,
     Petrusz, P., Nayfeh, S.N., and Ritzen, E.M. Nature, 1975,
     in press.

Morphological Studies
on the Seminiferous Tubule

TRANSCRIPTION DURING MAMMALIAN SPERMATOGENESIS WITH SPECIAL REFERENCE TO SERTOLI CELLS

Laura L. Tres and A. L. Kierszenbaum

Laboratories for Reproductive Biology and Department of
Anatomy

School of Medicine, University of North Carolina,
Chapel Hill, North Carolina   27514, U.S.A.

INTRODUCTION

A differential transcription rate of distinct classes of RNA
is associated with an orderly series of cell differentiation processes occurring during spermatogenesis (25,26,27). Although the
mechanism underlying the transcription process during male gametogenesis is still unknown, experimental evidence indicates that
circulating hormones stimulate testicular transcription. Thus, FSH
stimulates testicular RNA and protein biosynthesis in immature and
mature hypophysectomized rats (34,49). RNA transcription in seminiferous tubules is induced by FSH (34,36,49) whereas similar synthetic activities in interstitial cells are hCG-dependent (49). FSH
effect is mediated by the adenyl cyclase-cyclic AMP system (7,12,
18) present in Sertoli cells (6,7) and presumably in spermatogonia
(6). Interstitial cells have a separate adenyl cyclase sensitive
to LH (6,7).

Testosterone is synthesized by interstitial cells (9) and can
maintain spermatogenesis in hypophysectomized animals (62). Rat
testis contains a cytosol androgen-binding protein (ABP) that binds
both testosterone and dihydrotestosterone (DHT) (17). This androgen
binding protein is secreted by Sertoli cells (17,60) after stimulation by FSH (17,35,60). It is concentrated within the lumen of
seminiferous tubules and subsequently transported toward the epididymis (14,50).

Specific intracellular receptor proteins for testosterone and
DHT have also been demonstrated in rat seminiferous tubules (17,41).

Despite this available information, the extent to which androgen-protein complexes influence specific cell types involved in spermatogenic events remains to be established. Some information regarding the localization of hormones in the testis has been provided by histological and cytological techniques. For instance, immunohistochemical (8) and autoradiographic experiments (3) in several species have indicated that the highest concentration of androgen is detected in interstitial cells although an appreciable amount of the hormone is also detected within the seminiferous tubules. Ferritin- and fluorescein-labeled FSH was localized selectively in the seminiferous tubular wall and cytoplasm of Sertoli cells (32). Similarly, in vitro binding analyses indicated that [^{125}I]-FSH has affinity for receptors associated with cells of the seminiferous epithelium, specifically those close to the tubular wall (11). [^{125}I]hLH was localized by autoradiography in rat interstitial cells (10).

Molecular organization and transcription have been studied during spermatogenesis (24,25,26,27) as a basis for later studies on hormonal factors controlling gene expression. In doing so, we used autoradiographic procedures and techniques for visualization of genome segments with the electron microscope. Some of the segments displayed transcription relationships. These procedures consume much time, but provide appreciable information on the structural organization and function of well characterized testicular cell types, otherwise difficult to identify by other procedures such as cell fractionation techniques.

In this paper, we summarize our data on meiotic and post-meiotic RNA synthesis. We also report recent findings on pre-meiotic transcription and discuss structural and transcription features displayed by Sertoli cells as they relate to an assumed cooperative and promoting function for spermatogenesis (24).

MATERIAL AND METHODS

RNA synthetic acitvities during spermatogenesis have been studied in mouse and human testes. Adult male mice, ranging from 30 to 45 days old, were injected with [^{3}H]uridine ([5,6-^{3}H]uridine sp act 42.4 Ci/mmol, New England Nuclear, Boston, Mass.) directly into both testes under the albuginea at a dose of 10 µCi per testis in a volume of 0.05 ml of sterile aqueous solution. As indicated before (26,27), we chose this route of injection on the basis of Monesi's results (38), recognizing the advantages of introducing the labeled compound directly into the incorporation site in adequate and known testicular concentrations thus permitting evaluation of responses in very short labeling times. The same route was also used for prolonged labeling periods. Testes were removed at the following postinjection intervals: 5, 15, 30 and 60 min; 3 and 24 hrs; 7, 8, 10 and 12 days. A period of twelve days is considered necessary for completion of the whole meiotic prophase cycle in the mouse (44).

Biopsy samples from testes of normal, untreated patients attending infertility clinics were examined. Upon removal, a few seminiferous tubules were incubated in Basal Medium (Eagle) with Earle's balanced salt solution containing 50 µCi/ml of [^{3}H]uridine (sp. act 42.4 Ci/mmol). After 3 hs of incubation at 34°C, the samples were rinsed several times with non-radioactive medium containing 100 µg/ml of cold uridine (Sigma Chemical Co., St. Louis, Mo.) and fixed therafter in 2.5% glutaraldehyde in 0.1 M phosphate buffer (pH 6.9) for 2 hs. Some samples were incubated further in the non-radioactive medium for another 30 min period before fixation. This procedure was designed to wash out unbound [^{3}H]-uridine from the incubated samples. We tested this procedures in specimens from mouse testes and compared the results with previous autoradiographic data obtained by injecting [^{3}H]uridine intra-testicularly. Similar nucleolar and chromosomal labeling sites were obtained with both procedures.

After post-fixation in osmium tetroxide, samples were embedded in Maraglas according to routine procedures. The rationale for procedures for our methods of light and electron microscope auto radiography and of techniques for preparing whole-mounts of spread mouse meiotic chromosomes and visualization of transcription with the electron microscope have been described in detail elsewhere (25,26,27).

TRANSCRIPTION IN SPERMATOGONIA

As indicated by Monesi (38), mouse spermatogonia incorporate actively [^{3}H]uridine into nucleoli and nucleoplasm. We have examined different spermatogonia types in light and electron micro-scope autoradiographic preparations of mouse testes. 5 min after an intratesticular injection of [^{3}H]uridine, silver grains are readily displayed on spermatogonia nuclei (25). Nuclear silver grains increase progressively with longer labeling times. 3 hr after a [^{3}H]uridine pulse, there is complete nucleolar and nucleoplasmic labeling of all types of spermatogonia in interphase (Figs. 1, 2, 3). At the same labeling time, silver grains can also be detected over the cytoplasm (Figs. 2, 3). Metaphase spermatogonia display a few silver grains associated with some chromosomal regions, whereas cytoplasmic labeling is diffuse (Fig. 4)   In this respect, mitotic cells are known to display a reduced capacity for RNA synthesis (2) and a striking decrease of chromatin template activity (23).

Monesi pointed out that [^{3}H]uridine incorporation rates are much higher in spermatogonia of type A than in spermatogonia of type B as observed in autoradiographic squash preparations of mouse testes (38). This difference in RNA synthesis was correlated with a greater chromatin condensation in type B spermatogonia nuclei

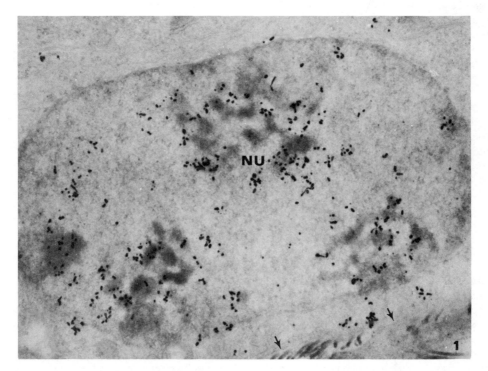

Figure 1. Mouse spermatogonia of type A. Several nucleolar masses
(NU) are labelled 3 h after a [^{3}H]uridine pulse. Arrows indicate
the position of the tubular wall. X 20,000

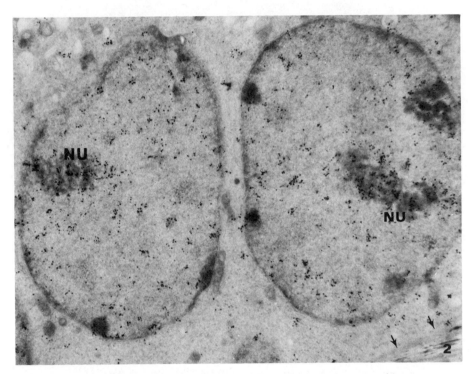

Figure 2. Mouse spermatogonia, presumably of intermediate type. Small clumps of chromatin are attached to the nuclear envelope. Nucleoli (NU) are well labeled with [^{3}H]uridine, after 3 hours. X 9,400

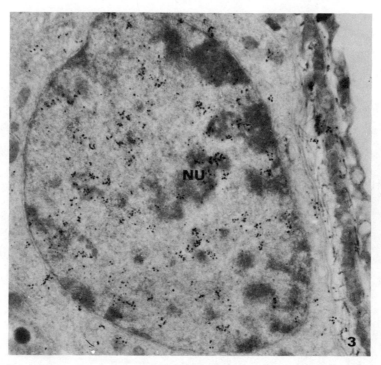

Figure 3. Mouse spermatogonia of type B. The larger chromatin
clumps are mainly associated with the nuclear envelope; small
chromatin clumps are scattered throughout the nucleus. (NU)
part of a centrally located nucleolus. X 18,600

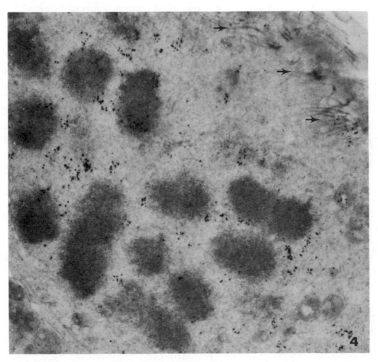

Figure 4. Mouse spermatogonia in metaphase. Arrows indicate collagen fibers of the tubular wall. X19,800

compared to a more dispersed chromatin pattern in type A
spermatogonia (38). However, since the maintenance of a constant
spermatogonial population involves several mitotic cycles (45)
giving rise to different types of spermatogonia type A which,
in turn, engender intermediate and type B spermatogonia, it is
possible to envisage fluctuations in transcription activity related to cell-cycle specific changes in chromatin template
capability as described in other somatic cells (40,42). Moreover, modifications in chromatin condensation have been described
by Oakberg (45) for the five classes of type A spermatogonia.
Therefore, it is reasonable to assume variations in RNA synthesis
within type A spermatogonia and as cells move from an early phase
(G_1,S) toward a late phase (S,G_2) in the cell cycle. Quantitative
analysis of autoradiographic changes occurring during transcription
in all spermatogonia types is difficult with the electron microscope
since the various types of spermatogonia type A are hard to
identify. Nevertheless, at the present time, it is clear that
all spermatogonia of the mouse testis are involved on a temporal
scale in both nucleolar and extranucleolar RNA synthesis.

TRANSCRIPTION DURING MEIOTIC PROPHASE

It has been thought that nucleolar RNA synthesis does not
occur during male gametogenesis (38,58) whereas ribosomal build up
during female gametogenesis has long been recognized. This has
posed an intriguing problem during the last ten years. Several
authors indicated the presence of an "inactive" nucleolus during
meiotic prophase of plants, insects and mammals (cf. in ref. 25).
Nevertheless, male meiotic cells are capable of nucleolar organization during early meiotic prophase stages. For instance,
Parchman and Lin (47) have provided evidence in lily microsporocytes
for nucleolar [3H]uridine labeling during leptotene stage. Moreover,
they indicated that this nucleolar labeling marks an RNA species
involved in the ribosomal pathway. They noted further that there
is a peak of ribosomal RNA labeling at leptotene, followed by a
decline in ribosomal maturation in further meiotic prophase stages.
Galdieri and Monesi (15), in a recent re-evaluation of ribosomal
RNA synthesis in mouse spermatocytes, suggested several hypotheses
which could account for the absence of ribosomal RNA synthesis in
mouse spermatocytes. Such hypotheses were based on an assumed lack
of [3H]uridine labeling of the nucleolus associated with the sex
chromosomes and the uncertain existence of autosomal nucleoli
(15). Yet autosomal nucleoli had been demonstrated previously in
light and electron microscope preparations of mouse (52), rat (57)
and human spermatocytes (13,53). Moreover, electron microscope
autoradiographic studies of nucleolar organization during meiotic
prophase in the mouse (25,26) using [3H]uridine as a precursor for
RNA, has revealed that nucleoli are indeed organized by autosomal

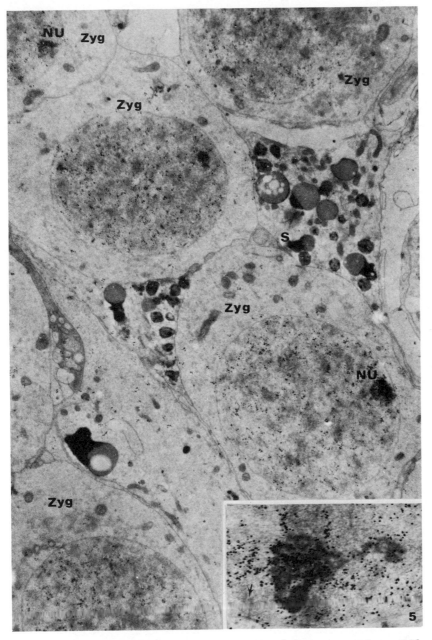

Figure 5. Zygotene (Zyg) spermatocytes of human testis. Silver grains are predominantly located over the nuclear structures. Nucleoli (NU), next to the nuclear envelope are labeled with [3H] uridine (incubation time: 3 hours). (S), portion of a Sertoli cell cytoplasm. X 6,600. Inset Detail of an autosomal nucleolus of an early pachytene human spermatocyte. The arrow indicates a section of a synaptonemal complex ending against the nuclear envelope. X 12,500.

bivalents in proximity to a chromosomal region designed as terminal or basal knob. This region, also identified as a paracentromeric heterochromatic region, presumably contains ribosomal DNA cistrons (25). Furthermore, [^{3}H]uridine labeled nucleoli have recently been described in light microscope autoradiographic preparations of rat spermatocytes and with electron microscope autoradiography in human spermatocytes (Fig. 5), thus confirming our original observation of nucleolar RNA synthesis by autosomal bivalents during early meiotic prophase stages (25). The condensed sex chromosomes display little or no RNA synthesis.

Autosomal bivalents are also involved in transcription of non-nucleolar species. Here, we review selected features of our recent studies on the molecular organization of spermatocyte genomes and their transcriptive activity.

Nucleolar RNA Synthesis During Meiotic Prophase

Our data in mouse (25,26) and human spermatocytes indicate a sequence of [^{3}H]uridine labeling associated with structural changes during nucleolar development. Fibrillar nucleolar components (identified from leptotene-early zygotene on) are followed by granular nucleolar components visible at late zygotene-early pachytene. Such a structural sequence, constantly observed in the nucleolar organization of different cells (16), is detected only in nucleoli associated with terminal knobs of some autosomal bivalents but not in the nucleolus which becomes associated with the sex chromosomes from middle pachytene on (26). Autoradiographic experiments in mouse testes have also shown (26) that nucleolar masses, once detached from their primary nucleolar site at middle pachytene, migrate toward the sex chromosomal pair, rearrange their nucleolar components and form a typical natural segregated nucleolus clearly evident at late pachytene. These segregated nucleoli associated with the sex chromosomes do not incorporate [^{3}H]uridine. This assumed migration of nucleolar structures and their later relationship with sex chromosomes appears to explain a puzzling fact described by several authors (28,50), namely that nucleoli, especially those associated with the sex chromosomes, do not incorporate labeled precursors for RNA.

In human spermatocytes this migrating behavior is usually not observed and autosomal nucleoli segregate at their primary autosomal origin after a decrease in [^{3}H]uridine uptake and upon completion of a full chromatin condensation at the terminal knob region (Tres, submitted for publication). In this respect, the fact that a progressive condensation of terminal knob regions correlates with a gradual decrease in [^{3}H]uridine labeling and the onset of a rearrangement of nucleolar components (nucleolar segregation) in human spermatocytes suggests that the template capability of ribosomal DNA cistrons, located in the proximity of the terminal knob region, is largely associated with a dispersed state of chromatin at the knob region.   Thus autosomal basal knobs are not conspicuous at leptotene-zygotene when [^{3}H]uridine-nucleolar labeling rises sharply to maximal levels.   They become evident throughout all pachytene stages in correlation with a lessened nucleolar RNA transcription.   As shown in Figure 5, zygotene human spermatocyte nuclei are evenly labeled with [^{3}H]uridine.   Peripheral autosomal nucleoli display a marked concentration of silver grains (inset, Fig 5).

Finally, results from in situ ribosomal RNA-DNA hybridization experiments in mouse and human somatic cells (19,20) do not support the idea of a nucleolar organizing function in sex chromosomes. These studies have indicated that several acrocentric autosomes (but not X and Y chromosomes) contain ribosomal DNA cistrons.

Chromosomal RNA Synthesis During Meiotic Prophase

A fuzzy appearance of pachytene autosomal bivalents due to lateral projections of chromatin fibers was recognized since several years ago.   This feature has been interpreted as an indication of template regions of meiotic chromosomes activated for transcription.   In fact, autoradiographic experiments indicate that [^{3}H]uridine is distributed along the bivalent margins (Figure 6). However, the identification of active sites of perichormosomal labeling has been difficult due to inadequate electron microscope resolution and poorly defined boundaries of meiotic chromosomes.   The use of whole-mount preparations of mouse pachytene spermatocytes obtained after dispersing cellular suspension in an air-liquid interface or by microcentrifugation techniques (26,27), has permitted a satisfactory display in the electron microscope of transcription complexes related to loosely extended chromatin loops along autosomal bivalents (Figs. 7 and 8).   Moreover, the use of autoradiographic procedures combined with whole-mount electron microscope techniques reveals "hot" [^{3}H]uridine-labeled spots corresponding to nucleolar masses attached to the terminal condensed region of some autosomal bivalents (25,26).   [^{3}H]uridine labeled regions extending along the sides of the paired autosomes (26) coincide with the presence of ribonucleoprotein fibrils (RNP) presumably representing primary products of the loops (heterogeneous nuclear RNA (hnRNA) complexed with proteins)   (Fig. 8).   RNP fibrils have a considerable length and are composed of granules ranging from 13 to 20 nm in diameter linked by thinner segments (inset Figure 8).   These fibrils readily disappear after RNAse treatment (26).   Accordingly, nuclear RNP particles isolated and purified from nuclei of different species have been identified as carrying hnRNA molecules complexed with proteins (33,51).   These RNP particles are rapidly labeled with [^{3}H]uridine and show varying sensitivity to RNAse on a RNAse-concentration dependent basis (51).

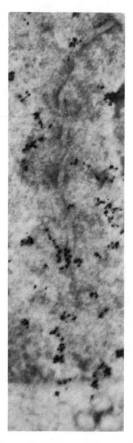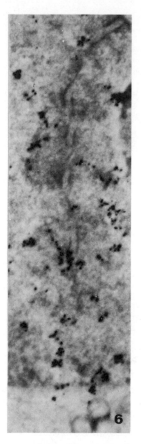

Figure 6. Stereo pairs of electron micrographs of an autosomal
bivalent of a mouse middle pachytene spermatocyte. [^{3}H]uridine
labeling: 3 hours . The perichromosomal location of silver grains
is apparent with this procedure. A three-dimensional stereo effect
can be achieved by direct observation of the micrograph pair in a
magnifying stereo-viewer. $\pm$ 5° tilting. X 12,000.

     One of the most interesting features of our autoradiographic
experiments is that nucleolar and chromosomal transcription during
meiotic prophase in mouse and human spermatocytes displays stage-
dependent variations. We have suggested that these variations may
be the consequence of a control mechanism acting on various genome
segments so that activation of ribosomal and non-ribosomal DNA
cistrons occurs at appropriate stages of meiosis (25,26). For
example, nucleolar RNA synthesis takes place during leptotene-
zygotene preceding chromosomal RNA synthesis at middle pachytene
during which no nucleolar RNA forms. Whether there is a direct
or indirect effect of androgen-protein complexes on transcription or
post-transcription processing in spermatocytes, as postulated for

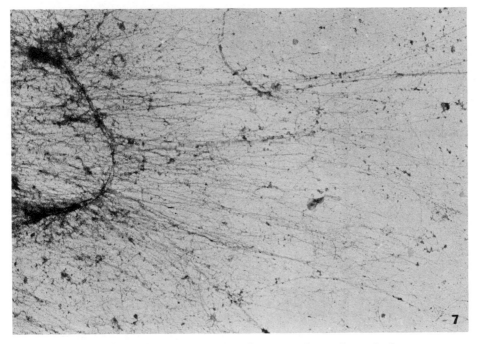

Figure 7. Electron micrograph of a portion of a whole-mount mouse autosomal bivalent with projecting and looping chromatin fibers ("lampbrush" chromosome). X 5,200.

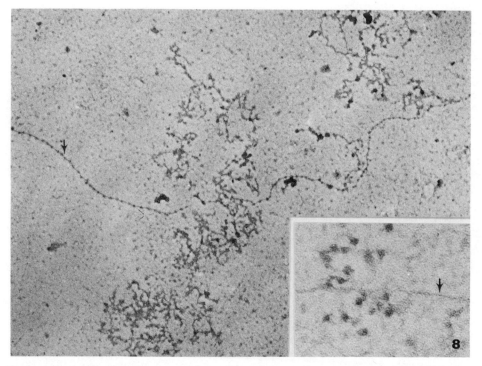

Figure 8.   Chromatin loop (arrow) of a pachytene mouse spermatocyte
displaying a beaded pattern.   The chromatin axis is related
to RNP fibrils of variable length presumably representing hnRNA-protein
molecules.   Microcentrifugation method (26,37).   X 45,900.   Inset:
Detail of similar RNP fibrils visualized with the spreading
method.   The particulate mature of the RNP chain is clearly observed.
The arrow indicates the chromatin fiber.   X 120,000.

other androgen-protein complexes in different target tissues (29), remains as an open question which merits further investigation. With regard to the biological significance of meiotic RNA synthesis, it may be suggested that different RNA species transcribed during well defined meiotic prophase stages, may provide specific trans- criptional and translational products necessary for intricate molecular events occurring during pairing and genetic exchange be- tween homologous chromosomes or for later stages of spermatogenesis.

TRANSCRIPTION DURING SPERMIOGENESIS

Autoradiographic data from the mouse testis obtained by localizing [^{3}H]uridine (38) and by an assay system for localization of endogenous RNA polymerase activity (39) indicate that post- meiotic transcription occurs in early steps of spermiogenesis. By way of illustration, Figure 9 depicts silver grains in nuclei of early spermatids (approximately step 3 of spermiogenesis) after a [^{3}H]uridine pulse of 3 hours. It is not possible to detect the presence or synthesis of RNA in late spermiogenic steps when rates of [^{3}H]arginine incorporation into arginine-rich sperm histone and other proteins containing arginine are increasing (27).

As RNA synthesis decreases in late spermatids, various morphological and biochemical changes take place. Spherical nuclei of early spermatids are transformed to a highly compact and elon- gated nuclear structures in late spermatids, while somatic histones are replaced by sperm histones (5). Whereas many details of acro- some and sperm tail formation in several species are well known from electron microscope studies of thin sections, it has been dif- ficult to recognize structural nuclear changes occurring during ter- minal stages of spermiogenesis because of the nuclear condensation. Appreciable information has been obtained from the application of the critical point method (64) and from electron microscope studies of whole-mount preparations of spermatids (31,64). Spermatid nuclei, can be opened at an air-liquid interface and then spread sufficiently so the nuclear content can be satisfactorily resolved by electron microscopy. We have used a procedure for visualization of spermatid genomes with the electron microscope based on a procedure first developed by Miller and Bakken (37) and adapted for the testis by Kierszenbaum and Tres (26,27). We have explored features of the molecular organization of genome segments during mouse spermiogenesis (27). In these studies, we have identified two distinct patterns of chromatin: a beaded type of chromatin associated with transcription complexes observed in early spermatids, and a smooth type of chroma- tin, not involved in transcription and evident in advanced spermatid genomes (27). The smooth type of chromatin tends to associate with adjacent smooth threads and, less frequently, with the beaded type, probably due to a progressive decrease of this type of fiber as

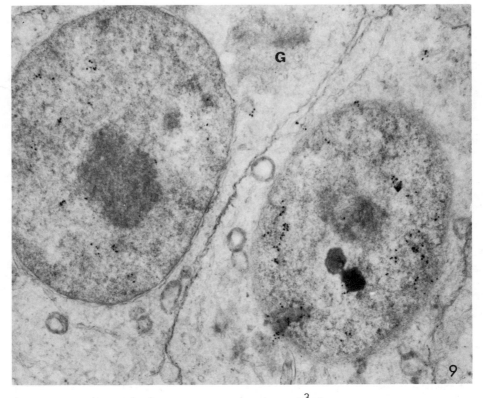

Figure 9. Mouse early spermatids. [³H]uridine labeling:
3 hours. X 3,000.

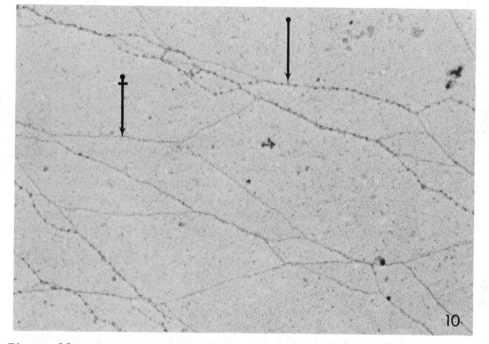

Figure 10. Two structural types of chromatin in a late spermatid genome (mouse). The plain arrow indicates a beaded type of chromatin. The crossed arrow points to a smooth type of chromatin. The associations of the two types of fibers (smooth-smooth; beaded-smooth) are well depicted. X 74,800.

sperminogenesis approaches completion (Figure 10). In eukaryotes,
chromatin is organized into globular subunit structures (DNA plus
somatic histones) adopting a typical array of beads on a string.
This subunit model has been supported by several biochemical and
physical studies (1,22,28,46,59,63).

Since a general hypothesis conceives that chemical modifications
of histones are involved in the control of chromatin structure and
function (56), one can assume that the replacement of somatic
histones by sperm histones in advanced spermiogenesis modifies
significantly the chromatin pattern, and accounts for the smooth
type of chromatin observed.

TRANSCRIPTION IN SERTOLI CELLS

Recent studies have attributed a key role to Sertoli cells
in the control of spermatogenesis. Several lines of evidence
indicate that Sertoli cells are able to secrete an androgen-binding
protein with high affinity for testosterone and DHT (17,19) after
stimulation by FSH (cf. in ref. #17,60). These findings,
together with the fact that these cells, comprising a unique
stable cell population in the seminiferous tubule, are closely
associated with spermatogonia, spermatocytes, and spermatids,
have led to the assumption that Sertoli cells may exercise some
kind of control favoring completion of spermatogenesis (55).

When RNA synthesis by Sertoli cells in adult mice is studied
by autoradiographic procedures, 5 min after a labeling pulse with
[^{3}H]uridine, nearly all radioactivity is localized in the nucleoplasm of Sertoli cells and in some types of spermatogonia (25).
After 15 minutes, silver grains appear on the nucleoplasm and nucleoli of Sertoli cells and spermatogonia. Between 60 min and 3 h
after [^{3}H]uridine administration, nuclear RNA synthesis in Sertoli
cells reaches a peak (Figure 11). A remarkable finding arises from
comparing the labeling patterns of spermatocytes with those of
Sertoli cells (Fig. 11). For instance, in spermatocytes, chromosomal labeling persists for longer times (7-10 days), when almost
all radioactivity has been lost from Sertoli cells. The persistance
of long-lived [^{3}H]uridine labeled species in pachytene spermatocytes
indicates that functional Sertoli cells and spermatocytes differ
from each other in post-transcriptional behavior. Since a significant amount of the heterogeneous nuclear RNA with rapid turnover is
metabolized in the nucleoplasm (61), we have assumed that the
remaining silver grains in spermatocytes probably correspond to
disintegrating products (25).

Furthermore, it has been reported (24) that mouse Sertoli cells
differ from each other in cytoplasmic patterns. One type shows even

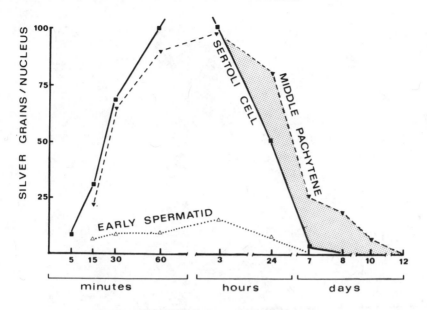

Figure 11. Comparative profiles of transcription of Sertoli cells, middle pachytene spermatocytes and early spermatids of the mouse testis after intratesticular administration of a [3H]uridine pulse, followed by different labeling times (5 min to 12 days). The gray area indicates the difference in post-transcriptional behavior between Sertoli cells and spermatocytes.

dilatations of endoplasmic reticulum (Figure 12), whereas the other lacks this type of dilatation (Figure 13). Both types are observed in the same seminiferous tubule and differ from each other in the uptake of [3H]uridine with slightly higher values of silver grain density appearing in the vacuolated type of Sertoli cell. These findings suggest the possibility of cyclic transcriptive functions of Sertoli cells. Cyclic activity may be consistent with results indicating that FSH activates the template function of Sertoli cells (see Means, this volume). On the other hand, gene activation preceding a translational function (34) leading to provision of "promoting factor(s)" for spermatogeneis has been postulated (24). A possible relation, if any, of Sertoli cell transcription to specific cell types or cell associations is being explored in our laboratory.

Aggregates of interchromatin granules are very conspicuous in Sertoli cells. Available data indicate that interchromatin granules contain RNA, presumably surrounded by a protein coat protecting them from RNAse degradation (cf. in ref. 25). Interchromatin granules in Sertoli cells are weakly labeled with [3H]uridine after a pulse

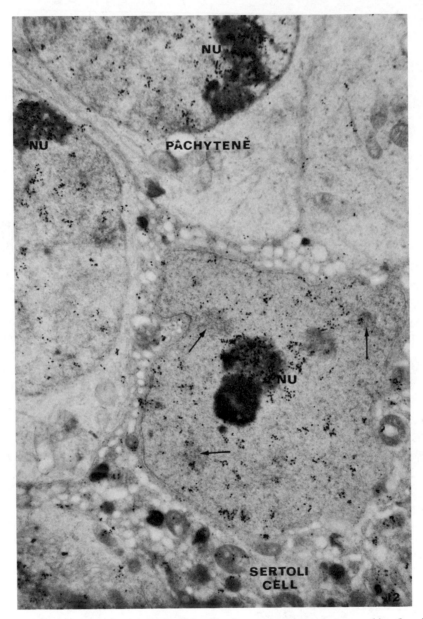

Figure 12.   Mouse Sertoli cell of the vacuolated type displaying
silver grains in the cytoplasm 3 hours after [³H]uridine-labeling
pulse.   The nucleus is well labeled, particularly the nucleoli
(NU).   Aggregates of interchromatin granules (arrows) and a
condensed chromatin structure next to the nucleolus are unlabeled.
Two closely related spermatocytes (middle pachytene) show
labeled autosomal nucleoli (NU).   Few silver grains are observed
in the cytoplasm of the spermatocytes.   X 11,220.

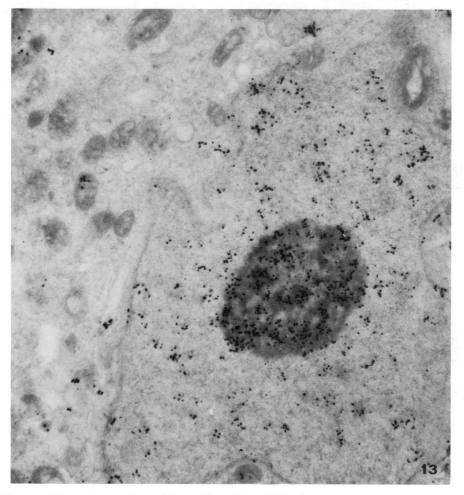

Figure 13. Mouse Sertoli cell. The cytoplasm is less vacuolated than in Figure 12. Silver grains predominate over the nucleus, especially on the nucleolus. X16,400.

of 3 h., in agreement with in vitro studies in other somatic cells, (Figure 12) and are completely unlabeled when sampled 8-12 days after isotope administration (24).

Nuclear RNP particles have been identified as subunit components of hnRNA-protein complexes on the basis of a rapid incorporation rate of [^{3}H]uridine and a high RNA complementary base ratio to DNA (33). A high endogenous protein kinase activity in RNP particles was recently reported. This activity was pronase sensitive and RNAse resistant. At this point, a systematic biochemical investigation aimed at characterizing RNP particles seems to be desirable since hnRNA-protein complexes and interchromatin granules differ from each other in their [3H]uridine uptake and RNAse sensitivity. This distinction appears necessary since, as has been suggested (30), steroid-receptor complexes can associate with RNP particles of target cells (50-80S), and hormonal binding can be abolished by protease and RNAse treatment (30).

REFERENCES

1. Baldwin, J.P., Boseley, P.G., Bradbury, .E.M., and Ibel, K., Nature 250: 2370, 1975.
2. Baserga, R., J. Cell Biol. 12: 633, 1962.
3. Beardsley, J.A., and Hilton, F.K., J. Reprod. Fert. 42: 361, 1975.
4. Blanchard, J.M., Ducamp, C., and Jeanteur, P., Nature New Biol. 253: 467, 1975.
5. Bloch, D.P. Genetics (Suppl.) 61: 93, 1969.
6. Braun, T., In Current Topics in Molecular Endocrinology, Dufau, M., and Means, A.R. (Eds.), Raven Press, N.Y., Vol. 1: 243-264, 1974.
7. Braun, T., and Sepsenwol, S., Endocrinology 94: 1028, 1974.
8. Bubenik, G.A., Brown, G.M., and Grota, L.J., Endocrinology 96: 63, 1975.
9. Cooke, B.A., De Jong, F.H., van der Molen, H.J., and Rommerts, F.F.G., Nature New Biol. 237: 255, 1972.
10. De Kretser, D.M., Catt, K.J., and Paulsen, C.A., Endocrinology 88: 332, 1971.
11. Desjardins, C., Zeleznik, A.J., Midgley, A.R., and Reichert, L.E., In Hormone Binding and Activation in the Testis, Dufau, M.L., and Means, A.R. (Eds.), Academic Press, N.Y., 1974.
12. Dorrington, H.J., and Fritz, I.B., Endocrinology 94: 395, 1974.
13. Ferguson-Smith, M.A., Cytogenetics 3: 124, 1964.
14. French, F.S., and Ritzen, E.M., Endocrinology 93: 88, 1973.
15. Galdieri, M., and Monesi, V., Exp. Cell Res. 80: 120, 1973.
16. Granboulan, N., and Granboulan, P., Exp. Cell Res. 38: 604, 1965.

17. Hansson, V., Trygstad, O., French, F.S., McLean, W.S., Smith, A.A., Tindall, D.J., Weddington, S.C., Petrusz, P., Nayfeh, S.N., and Ritzen, E.M., Nature 250: 387, 1974.

18. Heindel, J.J., Rothenberg, R., Robison, G.A., and Steinberger, A.J., Cyclic Nucleot. Res. 1: 69, 1975.

19. Henderson, A.S., Eicher, E.M., Yu, M.T., and Atwood, K.C., Chromosoma 49: 155, 1974.

20. Henderson, A.S., Warburton, D., and Atwood, K.C., Proc. Nat. Acad. Sci. (U.S.A.), 69: 3394, 1972.

21. Hildebrand, C.E., and Tobey, R.A., Biochem. Biophys. Res. Comm. 63: 134, 1975.

22. Hyde, J.E., and Walker, I.O., Nucleic Acid. Res. 2: 405, 1975.

23. Johnson, T.C., and Holland, J.J., J. Cell Biol. 27: 565, 1965.

24. Kierszenbaum, A.L., Biol. Reprod. 11: 365, 1974.

25. Kierszenbaum, A.L., and Tres, L.L., J. Cell Biol. 60: 39, 1974.

26. Kierszenbaum, A.L., and Tres, L.L., J. Cell Biol. 63: 923, 1974.

27. Kierszenbaum, A.L., and Tres, L.L., J. Cell Biol. 65: 258, 1975.

28. Kornberg, R.D., Science 184: 868, 1974.

29. Liao, S., Int. Rev. Cytol. 41: 87, 1975.

30. Liao, S., Liang, T., and Tymoczko, J.L., Nature New Biol. 241: 211, 1973.

31. Lung, B.J., J. Ultrastruct. Res. 22: 485, 1968.

32. Mancini, R.E., Castro, A., and Seiguer, A.C., J. Histochem. Cytochem. 15: 516, 1967.

33. Martin, T., Billings, P., Levey, A., Ozarslan, S., Quinlan, T., Swift, H., and Urbas, L., Cold Spring Harbor Symp. Quant. Biol. 38: 921, 1974.

34. Means, A.R., Endocrinology 89: 981, 1971.

35. Means, A.R., and Huckins, C., Endocrinology 94: Suppl., A-107, 1974.

36. Means, A.R., and Vaitukaitis, J., Endocrinology 90: 39, 1972.

37. Miller, O.L., and Bakken, A.H., Acta Endocrinol. 168(Suppl.): 155, 1972.

38. Monesi, V., Exp. Cell Res. 39: 197, 1965.

39. Moore, G.P.M., Exp. Cell Res. 68: 462, 1971.

40. Moser, G.C., Muller, H., and Robbins, E., Exp. Cell Res. 91: 73, 1975.

41. Mulder, E., Peters, M.J., De Vries, J., and van der Molen, H.J., Mol. Cell. Endocrinol. 2: 171, 1975.

42. Nicolino, C., Ajird, K., Borun, T.W., and Baserga, R., J. Biol. Chem. 250: 3381, 1975.

43. Noll, M., Nucleic Acid Res. 1: 1573, 1974.

44. Oakberg, E.F., Nature 180: 1137, 1957.

45. Oakberg, E.F., Anat. Rec. 169: 515, 1971.

46. Olins, A.L., Carlson, R.D., and Olins, D.E., J. Cell Biol. 64: 528, 1975.

47. Parchman, L.G., and Lin, K.C., Nature New Biol. 239: 235, 1972.

48. Pederson, T., Proc. Nat. Acad. Sci. (U.S.A.) 69: 2224, 1972.

49. Reddy, P.R.K., and Villee, C.A., Biochem. Biophys. Res.
     Comm. 63: 1063, 1975.
50. Ritzen, E.M., Nayfeh, S.N., French, F.S., and Dobbins, M.C.,
     Endocrinology 89: 143, 1971.
51. Sekeris, C.E., and Niessing, J., Biochem. Biophys. Res.
     Comm. 62: 642, 1975.
52. Solari, A.J., and Tres, L.L., Exp. Cell Res. 47: 86, 1967.
53. Solari, A.J., and Tres, L.L., J. Cell Biol., 45: 43, 1970.
54. Stefanini, M., De Martino, C., D'Agostino, A., Agrestini,
     A., and Monesi, V., Exp. Cell Res. 86: 166, 1974.
55. Steinberger, E., Physiol. Rev. 51: 1, 1971.
56. Sutton, W.D., Nature New Biol. 237: 70, 1972.
57. Urena, F., and Solari, A.J., Chromosoma 30: 258, 1970.
58. Utakoji, T. Exp. Cell Res. 42: 585, 1966.
59. Van Holde, K.E., Sahasrabuddhe, C.G., and Shaw, B.R.,
     Nucleic Acid Res. 1: 1579, 1974.
60. Vernon, R.G., Kopec, B., and Fritz, I.B., Mol. Cell. Endocrinol.,
     1: 167, 1974.
61. Weinberg, R.A., Ann. Rev. Biochem. 42: 329, 1973.
62. Woods, M.C., and Simpson, M.E., Endocrinology 69: 91, 1961.
63. Woodcock, C.L.F., J. Cell Biol. 59 (2, Pt. 2): 368A (abstract)
     1973.
64. Zirkin, B.R., J. Ultrastruct. Res. 36: 237, 1971.

HISTOCHEMICAL AND ULTRASTRUCTURAL OBSERVATIONS ON NORMAL AND FOLLICLE STIMULATING HORMONE-INJECTED PREPUBERAL RAT SERTOLI CELLS

Don F. Cameron and Roger R. Markwald

Department of Anatomy, Medical Univ. of South Carolina

80 Barre Street, Charleston, South Carolina 29401

Rat seminiferous tubules appear to be capable of limited steroid conversions. Christensen and Mason (1) and Hall, Irby and de Kretser (2) demonstrated the ability of isolated seminiferous tubules to convert labeled precursors to various C19-steroids. According to Bell, Vinson and Lacy (3), the seminiferous tubules have an equal or greater capacity than interstitial cells for converting progesterone to androgens. Of the intratubular cell types, both germinal cells (4) and Sertoli cells (5) have been hypothesized as participating in steroid anabolism. Of the gonadotropins, it appears that FSH stimulates the Sertoli cell (6,7) and that this cell is the primary target site of the hormone (8,9). By correlating ultrastructural observations of intratubular material with the results of histochemical demonstration of steroidogenic enzymes, this study offers evidence that during the period of prepuberal maturation the rat Sertoli cell (but not germinal cells) develops the potential to participate in steroid synthesis and that this potential is enhanced by FSH.

MATERIALS AND METHODS

Wistar rats (Albino Farms), maintained on a stock diet, were bred and the young weaned at three weeks of age. Of these newborn rats half of the males in each litter were used as controls (Group 1). The remaining males were assigned to one of three groups (Groups 2, 3, or 4) and received daily injections of FSH in 0.1 ml of saline. Two young female rats served as additional controls (Group 5).

Group 1 consisted of 52 rats sacrificed with sodium pento-

barbital at two weeks (3 rats), three weeks (13 rats), four weeks
(8 rats), five weeks (18 rats) or six weeks of age (10 rats).
Several rats were injected daily for 30 days with saline in an
amount identical with the experimental animals and sacrificed at
five and six weeks of age. These rats were used as sham controls.
Group 2 consisted of 14 rats injected daily for 30 days with 150 µg
FSH-Armour Standard (FSH-A) and sacrificed at five weeks (9 rats)
or six weeks of age (5 rats). Group 3 consisted of 15 rats injected
daily for 30 days with 1.66 mg FSH-A and sacrificed at five weeks
(11 rats) or six weeks of age (4 rats). Group 4 consisted of four
rats injected daily for 30 days with 150 µg FSH provided by the
National Institute of Arthritis and Metabolic Diseases (FSH-NIAMD-
B1, FSH activity 3.7 x NIH-FSH-S1 and LH activity 0.0045 x NIH-LH-
S1). They were sacrificed at five weeks (2 rats) or six weeks of
age (2 rats). These four rats were used as a control for the FSH-
A. Group 5 served as an additional quality control for the FSH.
One young female rat was injected with 150 µg FSH-A and another
with 150 µg FSH-NIAMD. Both were injected daily for seven days
and sacrificed at five weeks of age. Ovaries were collected and
processed for histologic observations (Table 1).

Testes were collected from all control and experimental male
rats (Groups 1-4). From each animal either the right or left gonad
(testis A) was divided in half and prepared for routine histologic
or ultrastructural examination. The remaining gonad (testis B)
was divided in half and prepared with silver for histologic examination or processed for histochemical observations.

Table 1
Distribution of control and experimental rats

Age Groups	Control	Experimental			Total
	Group 1	Group 2	Group 3	Group 4	
		FSH-Armour 150µg/day 30 days	FSH-Armour 1.66mg/day 30 days	FSH-NIAMD 150µg/day 30 days	
2 weeks old	3	0	0	0	3
3 weeks old	13	0	0	0	13
4 weeks old	8	0	0	0	8
5 weeks old	18	9	11	2	40
6 weeks old	10	5	4	2	21
TOTAL	52	14	15	4	85

For routine histology testis A was fixed 24 hours in Bouin's fluid, embedded in paraffin, sectioned, affixed to glass slides and stained with hematoxylin and eosin (H&E), Mallory's trichrome stain or Alcian Blue (pH 2.5)-Periodic Acid Schiff (PAS). For ultrastructural examination the remaining tissue of testis A was fixed in cold 6% glutaraldehyde-2% paraformaldehyde in 0.1M phosphate buffer (10). Fixed tissue was rinsed in phosphate-buffered sucrose, dehydrated in a graded series of cold alcohols and embedded in Epon 812. Ultrathin sections (silver-gold) were cut and double-stained in 1% uranyl acetate and 0.5% lead citrate.

For additional light microscopic study, tissue from testis B was prepared by silver impregnation to demonstrate the extent of Sertoli cell cytoplasm. Half of the gonad was fixed overnight in Bouin's fluid containing 2% silver nitrate (11) and subsequently reduced in freshly prepared Cajal's fluid for 22 hours (12). The remaining half of testis B was prepared for enzyme histochemical study. Fresh tissue was wrapped immediately in tin foil and flash frozen in liquid nitrogen. The frozen block was embedded in Ames O.C.T. compound, sectioned at 10μ at -17°C and affixed to glass slides. The slides were processed within 24 hours after sectioning in order to minimize possible enzymatic degeneration.

Enzyme Histochemical Incubation Media

Media were prepared immediately prior to staining for the histochemical demonstration of fluoride-sensitive (type B) esterase (B-Est.) and 3β-hydroxysteroid dehydrogenase (3βOLDH). Following exposure to medium for a specified period of time the slides were washed in distilled water, fixed in 10% phosphate-buffered formalin (pH 7.3 - 7.4) and mounted in water soluble glycerol jelly. Post-incubation procedure was the same for all slides. Esterase media were prepared according to Thompson's (12) modification of Gomori's original technique. Substrate medium for 3βOLDH was modified from Baillie *et al.* (13) and contained dehydroepiandrosterone or pregnenolone (0.6mM), NAD (0.6mM), sucrose (0.1M) and nitro-BT (NBT) (0.6mM) in 50.0 ml of 0.1M phosphate buffer (pH 7.4).

The reliability of the formazan reaction was tested by staining for NADH-diaphroase (14) and by frequently adding phenazine methosulfate (PMS) to the dehydrogenase media to insure transfer of hydrogen ions from the reduced coenzyme to the tetrazolium salt (15). Adult rat liver and adrenal gland served as positive control tissues for the histochemical reactions and these same tissues, heat inactivated for 15 minutes at 80°C, served as negative controls. Other controls included heat-inactivated testicular tissue (80°C water bath for 15 minutes) and omission of either substrate, coenzyme or capturing agent from the media.

RESULTS

The external genitalia appeared unaffected by the FSH treatment. In four experimental rats (three five week old rats and one
six week old rat) one testis contained a tumor-like growth and
weighed significantly more than the other gonad. These four rats
were excluded from the results. Testis weights, body weights, the
ratio of testis weight/body weight and tubule diameters of experimental animals (Groups 2, 3, and 4) were similar and not significantly different from comparable measurements taken from control
rats (Group 1) (Table 2).

The histologic, histochemical and ultrastructural observations
of the Sertoli cells in FSH-NIAMD injected rats (Group 4) were not
different from those Sertoli cell observations in the FSH-A injected
rat (Groups 2 and 3). Additionally, there appeared to be little
difference in results between rats from Groups 2 (5 weeks of age)
and 3 (6 weeks of age). Henceforth, "experimental rats" refers
collectively to rats from Groups 2, 3 and 4.

Sertoli Cells

Controls. At two weeks of age the Sertoli cell appeared undifferentiated. The cytoplasm was homogeneous and slightly eosinophilic and contained sparse deposition of silver. Its roughly
spherical nucleus contained granular chromatin and a prominent
nucleolus. The three week old Sertoli cell was similar in appearance to the two week old cell. By four weeks of age the cell was
more eosinophilic and argyophilic with increasing cytoplasmic
branching. By five and six weeks of age Sertoli cells of Group 1
rats were similar to adult Sertoli cells. The cytoplasm was eosinophilic, silver deposition was relatively high especially in the
distal periluminal cytoplasm. In some instances the Sertoli cell
cytoplasm of several tubules appeared in different early stages of
the Sertoli cell cycle as described by Elftman (16). However, the
proliferative stage of the Sertoli cell cycle was never seen in any
of the tubules of Group 1 animals.

Experimental. Following FSH injections germ cells were reduced in number while Sertoli cell cytoplasm of five and six week
old animals appeared more extensive. This resultant increase in
Sertoli cell cytoplasm reflected true hypertrophy as judged by
electron microscopy and not apparent hypertrophy due to the reduction in germ cells. The cytoplasmic ramifications of the cell
were extensive and there were many intercellular spaces toward the
luminal side. In many cases the nucleus of the Sertoli cell had
migrated away from its position near the base of the tubule and was
situated closer to the lumen. The cytoplasm was both more eosinophilic and argyophilic than the cytoplasm of control Sertoli cells.

Table 2

Average weights and tubule diameters of all control and experimental rats

Age	Control					Experimental	
	2 weeks	3 weeks	4 weeks	5 weeks	6 weeks	5 weeks	6 weeks
No. of Rats	3	13	8	18	10	22	11
Average* Body Weight (gms.)	37.0	45.3	55.6	90.3	131.6	91.2 (ns)	132.7 (ns)
Average** Testis Weight (gms.)	.0445	.0801	.1461	.4289	.6751	.3281 (ns)	.6174 (ns)
Testis Weight / Body Weight	.0012	.0017	.0025	.0047	.0051	.0042 (ns)	.0045 (ns)
Average*** Tubule Diameter (mm)	.00090	.00115	.00125	.00152	.00159	.00148 (ns)	.00140 (ns)

* Average of all the rats per age group

** Average of one testis per rat of all the rats in the age group

*** Average of eight tubules cut in cross section per testis of each rat in each age group

(ns) Average value not significantly different from control value $(p > .01)$

Enzyme Histochemical Observations

Relative staining intensities of all enzymes for Groups 1, 2, 3, and 4 are recorded in Table 3.

Diaphorase. All tubules from all animals observed contained diaphorase reaction product. Whereas staining in control tubules was generally diffuse, the deposition of reaction product within experimental rat tubules was intense and appeared to be more concentrated in that part of the tubule associated with Sertoli cell cytoplasm, the periluminal cytoplasm.

Type B Esterase (B-Est). In control tissue, intratubular negative staining of this steriodogenic enzyme was minimal at two weeks of age and increased slightly with age. Azo dye distribution through the tubules was diffuse in the two, three, and four week old animals. In the five and six week old control rats intratubular negative staining was slightly increased and was, generally, more concentrated in periluminal tissue. When compared with their controls, tubules of the five and six week old hormone-injected rats contained a greater amount of type B esterase as judged by the increase of negative staining. Much of the negative stained area was the periluminal cytoplasm suggesting that the increase of reaction product was in Sertoli cell cytoplasm.

3β-hydroxysteroid Dehydrogenase (3βOLDH). No enzyme activity was observed within the two and three week old control seminiferous tubules. Reaction product first appeared in the four week old rat, but only in a few tubules. Minimal staining in 5 week old control rats was generally limited to the basal area of the tubule but some reaction product was observed in the periluminal cytoplasm. At six weeks there was increased staining with control tubules. A detectable increase of the 3βOLDH formazan reaction product was observed in both the five and six week old experimental rat seminiferous tubules. The increase of formazan was notable in the periluminal cytoplasm and was deposited within the tubules similar to the characteristic trunk configuration of Sertoli cell cytoplasm as seen with silver staining.

Staining Controls. No tissue staining occurred when the specific substrate, the specific coenzyme or the capturing agent for each enzyme was deleted from the incubation medium. After protein deactivation all heat control tissue remained unstained and positive control tissue was always intensely stained. With the addition of phenazine methosulfate (PMS) to the 3βOLDH incubation medium, there was a slight increase of intratubular staining but it was more diffuse pink mono-formazan reaction product rather than the purple di-formazan.

Ultrastructural Observations

Control. The ultrastructure of the two and three week old
Sertoli cell was that of an undifferentiated cell which progressively took on the subcellular morphological characteristic of the
adult Sertoli cell. The two week old Sertoli cell contained few
organelles. There were mitochondria, an oval nucleus with a nucleolus and primitive cellular junctions (a narrowing of the distance
between cellular membranes) between adjacent Sertoli cells. By
four weeks of age the cell was larger and its nucleus was more
irregular in shape. There was an increase of smooth endoplasmic
reticulum (SER) and some mitochondria exhibited dilated cristae
similar to the cristae of mitochondria seen in steroid-producing
cells. By four weeks, limited interdigitation of adjacent Sertoli
cells was seen in the region closest to the basal lamina of the
seminiferous tubule and cellular junctions between adjacent Sertoli
cells were more numerous. Seminiferous tubules of the five week
old rats were in many respects characteristic of adult seminiferous
tubules. Sertoli cells were regularly spaced along the tubular
border and their nuclei, which were irregular in shape with occasional small nuclear clefts, contained an electron dense nucleolus.
At this time the SER, which was sometimes vesiculated, was prominent.
Generally, mitochondrial cristae were dilated (or tubular) in shape
although lamellar cristae were seen. Junctional specializations
between adjacent Sertoli cells, similar to the Sertoli cell junctions
described by Flickinger and Fawcett (17), were evident and were
flanked on either side by a flat cisternae of SER which was parallel
to the plasma membranes. On the cell side of the flanking reticulum
ribosomes were present in groups of about five or six. Occasionally,
an accumulation of electron dense filamentous material occurred
between the plasma membrane and the associated cisternae of SER.
Lipid droplets and a few electron dense, membrane bound bodies resembling lysosomes were found in the basal portion of the Sertoli
cytoplasm. Remaining cytoplasmic inclusions included free ribosomes,
Golgi apparati, and occasionally some microtubules. A number of
distended intercellular spaces were observed in the five week old
rat seminiferous tubule. Small cytoplasmic vesicles and infre-
quently caveolae were present in the basal cytoplasm.

Table 3

Histochemical reactions within the seminiferous tubules of all
control and experimental rats

	Control					Experimental	
Age	2 wks	3 wks	4 wks	5 wks	6 wks	5 wks	6 wks
Diaph.	++	+++	+++-	+++-	+++-	++++	++++
Est.	+	++	++	++-	+++	+++-	++++
Est.-Naf	+	+-	+	+	++	++-	++-
3 OLDH	0	0	+	+-	++-	+++	+++-

*Average intensity of intratubular reaction production; +, very
little reaction product; ++++, very heavy staining.

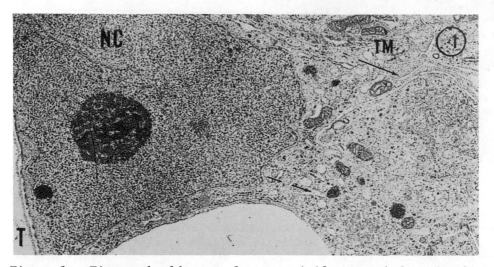

Figure 1.   Five week old control rat seminiferous tubule. At the
periphery of the tubule (T) a Sertoli cell nucleus contains a distinct nucleolus and a small nuclear cleft (NC).   SER (arrows) and
mitochondria with tubule-like cristae (TM) are evident. Although
the cell contains SER, it is underdeveloped and undilated.   The
cell is not highly characteristic of a steroid producing cell.
Uranyl acetate and lead citrate. 9,000X.

     The ultrastructure of six week old Sertoli cells looked similar
to adult rat Sertoli cells.   The major differences between the five
and the six week old cell was quantitative in nature rather than
qualitative.   Between five and six weeks there was more SER which
was often vesiculated.   Mitochondrial cristae were usually in a
tubular configuration and many mitochondria were crescent-shaped.
The nucleus was more irregular in shape than previously noted.
Interdigitations between adjacent Sertoli cells were more extensive
as were junctional specializations between Sertoli cells (Fig. 1).

     Experimental.   The changes seen in FSH-treated five and six
week old Sertoli cells (Groups 2, 3, and 4) were similar.

     The most conspicuous change after FSH injections was an in-
crease in and dilation of SER, which appeared highly stimulated,
filling most of the cytoplasm (Figs. 2, 3, 4).   Polysomes were
frequently seen.   One of the most noticeable observations was the
consistent appearance of an electron dense material resembling linear polyribosomes which sometimes ran the entire length of greatly
extended nuclear clefts (Figs. 2, 3, 6).   The Sertoli cell nucleus was highly irregular in shape and was often misplaced luminally.
Frequently it was encircled by microfilaments (Fig. 7).   The Sertoli

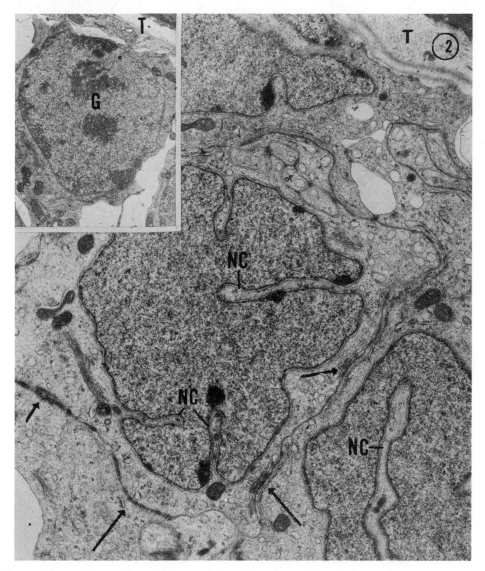

Figure 2. Six week old Sertoli cells from FSH-injected rat.
Sertoli cell nuclei are highly irregular in shape with numerous deep
nuclear clefts (NC). Often these clefts contain electron dense ma-
aterial. There is a large amount of vesiculated SER and an increased
number of junctional specializations (arrows). T=part of tubule
wall. Inset: Germinal cell nucleus of FSH-injected rat remains
oval in outline and there is very little SER. This ultrastructural
picture of germinal cells is consistent enough to serve as a subcellular landmark in distinguishing between SER-filled Sertoli cells
and germinal cells. Uranyl acetate and lead citrate. 9,500X.
Inset 5,600X.

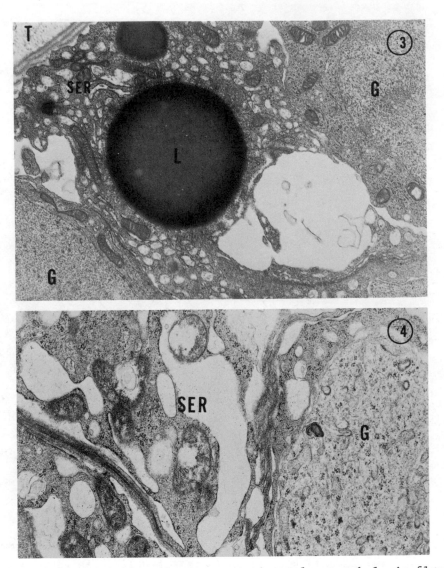

Figure 3.   The Sertoli cell of an experimental rat tubule is flanked
by germinal cells (G).   There is a large amount of SER in the Sertoli
cell cytoplasm filling the entire cell.   T=part of tubule wall.   L=
lipid.   Uranyl acetate and lead citrate.   8,500X.
Figure 4.   Higher power view of Sertoli cell cytoplasm and germinal
cell cytoplasm (G).   The SER is dilated, often being distended along
a Sertoli cell junction (SJ).   Uranyl acetate and lead citrate.
17,850X.

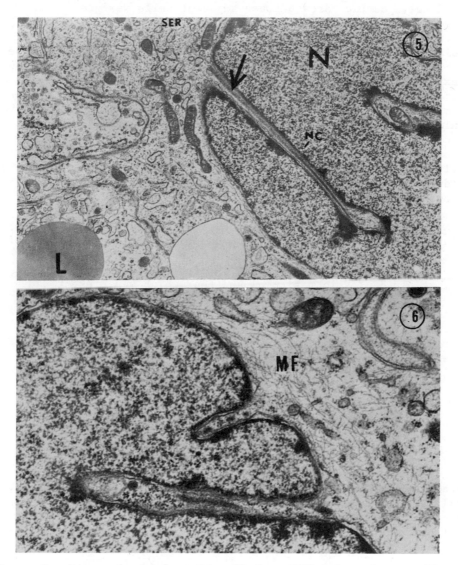

Figure 5. Six week old Sertoli cell from FSH injected rat. The Sertoli cell nucleus (N) contains an electron dense material (arrow) which is within a large nuclear cleft (NC). Uranyl acetate and lead citrate. 9,775X.

Figure 6. Microfilaments (MF) are often seen surrounding the nucleus of Sertoli cells in FSH-injected rats. Note the dense material within the nuclear clefts. Uranyl acetate and lead citrate. 24,875X.

cell-Sertoli cell interrelation was greatly affected in the FSH-treated rat. Surface area between adjacent cells was greatly increased due to extensive interdigitations particularly in basal regions of the cell. Accompanying this was an increased number of cellular junctions of the zonula adherens and zonula occludens type (Fig. 2). The specialized Sertoli cell junctions also were numerous and extended. The intercellular space between periluminal cytoplasm of adjacent Sertoli cells was quite extensive and numerous branches of Sertoli cytoplasm were distributed in the periluminal area of the seminiferous tubule. Included in the cytoplasm nearest the basal lamina of the tubule were numerous dense bodies resembling primary lysosomes. Their matrix varied in density with the smaller ones usually lighter than the larger ones. Most mitochondria were the tubular-vesicular type. There also appeared to be an increase in the number of microtubules within the Sertoli cell cytoplasm.

Germinal Cells. The fine structure of germinal cells was monitored only to establish orientation and to determine the extent of development of ultrastructural organelles associated with steroid synthesis. Control and FSH-treated rat germinal cells contained very little endoplasmic reticulum and that which was present was studded with ribosomes giving the appearance of rough endoplasmic reticulum (RER). These cells also contained mitochondria which were almost always in the condensed configuration (Fig. 3). Tubular cristae were never observed. These organelles and the lack of SER were sufficiently consistent to serve as landmarks for the identification of germinal cells at the electron microscopic level (Fig. 2 - inset).

DISCUSSION

The purpose of this investigation was to study the in vivo steroidogenic potential of the rat Sertoli cell and to see if FSH altered such a potential. The Sertoli cells of two to six week old normal rats were followed to determine if they developed morphologic characteristics associated with steroid anabolism. The same experimental parameters were used on a similar group of rats to determine if the steroidogenic profile of the cell was influenced by exogenously injected FSH. Specifically, this two part approach at clarifying the functional role of the Sertoli cell was carried out by staining for two enzymes involved in steroid synthesis and correlating these histochemical results with electron microscopic observations of the intratubular material, particularly the Sertoli cell.

The Sertoli cell developed from a relatively undifferentiated cell at two weeks of age to a well-differentiated adult cell at six weeks of age. The developmental observations corresponded closely to both the light and EM development of the cell as reviewed by Nagy

(18).   There was a period of rapid testicular development and Sertoli
cell differentiation between 21 and 35 days. This was comparable
to rapid Sertoli cell differentiation described in the mouse testis
between 7 and 14 days (19). During this period of rapid differentiation (21-35 days) in the rat there was a noticeable increase of
intratubular argentophilia which was accredited to an increased
amount of Sertoli cell cytoplasm, in which silver presumably was
bound to the smooth endoplasmic reticulum (SER) of the cell. This
staining technique showed five and six week old Sertoli cell cytoplasm to be truncated and periluminally distributed which is characteristic of adult Sertoli cells.

     After FSH was given to the prepuberal rats using an optimum
dosage of FSH for rats as defined by Lostroh (20), Sertoli cell
cytoplasm hypertrophied, became highly eosinophilic and argentophilic
and extended toward the lumen. Extensive periluminal cytoplasm and
trunk formations were evident. These light level observations of
both normal and hormone-treated Sertoli cells were supported by
the cells ultrastructure. In control rats between 21-35 days there
was a noticeable development of SER in Sertoli cells and many of
their mitochondria contained tubular-like cristae. The functional
presence of these organelles can be described as "being consistent
with the view that the cells are steroidogenic as judged by the presence of certain organelles found in other steroid-producing cells"
(5). After FSH-treatment the cell was packed with SER which often
appeared dilated (Figs. 1, 2, 3). Since the same fixative was
used for both control and experimental tissues, the dilation of SER
was believed to represent the functional state of the Sertoli cell and
not an artifact of fixation. Additionally, it appeared that all
of the Sertoli cell mitochondria were of the tubular-cristae type.
It is significant to note that in neither normal nor FSH-treated
rats the only other intratubular cell type, the germ cell, showed
no such ultrastructural evidence of steroid production (i.e.,
SER and tubular-cristae mitochondria).

     It would be difficult though to speculate on the steroidogenic
potential of the Sertoli cell based only on the presence of SER and
mitochondria. However, during the period of rapid differentiation
there was a concomitant accumulation of intratubular reaction products of 3β-hydroxysteroid dehydrogenase (3βOLDH) and type B esterase (B-Est.). Reaction products of these steroidogenic enzymes
were detected within the seminiferous tubule at three to four weeks
of age coinciding with the proliferative appearance of SER in the
Sertoli cell between 21-35 days. Also, the intratubular enzyme reaction products in normal rat tubules increased in amount between
four and six weeks as did the amount of Sertoli cell SER (see Table
3). In FSH-treated rats there was a marked increase of the intratubular 3βOLDH reaction product and a slight increase in B-Est. reaction product. Because of the distribution of reaction products

in intratubular trunks and periluminal cytoplasm it appeared that
the enzymes were most concentrated in Sertoli cells.

In order to evaluate these histochemical findings two questions
needed to be answered: Is the reaction product observed within the
seminiferous tubule a true representation of enzyme activity and in
which intratubular cell type are these enzymes located? Although
some investigators have stated that the intratubular 3βOLDH activity
is negligible (21,22,23), and other investigators have detected this
enzyme activity within seminiferous tubules (24,25,26). To deal with
possible enzyme diffusion during incubation and to maximize enzyme
viability all tissue sections were flash frozen in liquid nitrogen
(-70°C). Additionally, all incubation media were prepared with
sucrose and frequently with phenazine methosulfate (PMS) to insure
rapid hydrogen ion transfer and in situ reduction of the capturing
agent (14). The chromatogenic agent used in dehydrogenase media was
ditetrazolium salt nitro-BT which has the greatest substantive
properties of all tetrazoles (27). Finally the use of positive and
negative control tissue indicated that there was no non-enzymatic
reduction of the nitro-BT.

Since the above two enzymes are SER-bound (28), the cell containing them would necessarily have to have SER. Of the intratubular cell types it is only the Sertoli cell which contains conspicuous
amounts of this organelle. Its appearance and stimulation coincides
with the appearance and increased amounts of intratubular enzyme reaction products indicating enzyme localization in Sertoli cells.
Since it is evident that the Sertoli cell is the principle target
site for FSH (9) and that stimulation occurring in this cell is
affected by this hormone (8,29), it seems likely that the changes
observed in the experimental rat Sertoli cells were mediated via
FSH. Initial Sertoli cell stimulation (most likely due to FSH)
may occur between 21-35 days as suggested by the data presented
and supported by the fact that between 21-35 days there is a marked
elevation of rat serum FSH reaching a maximal level at 35 days (30).
While the presence of tubular-cristae mitochondria, SER and
steroidogenic enzymes does not prove that the Sertoli cell is involved in steroid synthesis, it does provide a strong indication
that this cell type has the potential to participate in some event(s)
of steroid modification. Additionally, since FSH stimulates a
corresponding increase of SER and the amount of some steroidogenic
enzymes it appears that this gonadotropin enhances (and possibly
initiates) the steroidogenic potential of Sertoli cells.

LITERATURE CITED

1.   Christensen, A.K., and Mason, N.R., Endocrinology 76: 911, 1956.
2.   Hall, P.E., Irby, D.C., and de Kretser, D.M., Endocrinology 84:
      488, 1969.

3. Bell, J.B.G., Vinson, G.P., and Lacy, D., Proc. Roy. Soc. Lond. B176: 433, 1971.
4. Yamada, M., Yasue, S., and Matsumoto, K., Endocrinology 93: 81, 1973.
5. Lacy, D., and Pettitt, A.J., Br. Med. Bull. 26:(1) 87, 1970.
6. Murphy, H.D., Proc. Soc. Exp. Biol. Med. 118: 1202, 1965.
7. Lostroh, A.J., Johnson, R., and Jordan, C.W., Jr., Acta Endocrin. 44: 536, 1963.
8. Dorrington, J.H., and Fritz, I.B., Endocrinology 94: 395, 1974.
9. Castro, A.E., and Seiguer, A.C., Proc. Soc. Exp. Biol. Med. 133: 582, 1970.
10. Karnovsky, M.J., J. Cell Biol. 27: 137A, 1965.
11. Elftman, H., Amer. J. Anat. 113: 25, 1963.
12. Thompson, S.W., In Selected Histochemical and Histopathological Methods. Charles C. Thomas Publ., Springfield, 1964, p. 1639.
13. Baillie, A.H., Ferguson, M.M., and Hart, D., Academic Press, 1966.
14. Pearse, A., In Histochemistry. Theoretical and Applied. Little, Brown and Co., Boston, 1960.
15. Van Wijhe, M., Blanchaer, M.C., and Jacyk, W.R., J. Histochem. Cytochem. 6: 225, 1958.
16. Elftman, H., Anat. Rec. 106: 31, 1950.
17. Flickinger, C., and Fawcett, D.W., Anat. Rec. 158: 207, 1967.
18. Nagy, F., Ph.D. Dissertation; Graduate School of the State University of New York, Upstate Medical Center in Syracuse, N.Y., 1969.
19. Flickinger, C., Z. Zellforsch. 78: 92, 1967.
20. Lostroh, A.J., Endocrinology 85: 438, 1969.
21. Maeir, D.M., Endocrinology 76: 463, 1965.
22. Levy, H., Deane, H.W., and Rubin, B.L., Endocrinology 65: 932, 1959.
23. Wattenberg, L.W., J. Histochem. Cytochem. 6: 225, 1958.
24. van Oordt, W.J., and Brands, F., J. Endocrin. 48: 1, 1970.
25. Gardner, P.J., and Shervey, C., Anat. Rec. 160: 351, 1968.
26. Woods, J.E., and Domm, L.V., Gen. Comp. Endocrin. 7: 559, 1966.
27. Pearse, A., and Hess, R., Experientia 17: 136, 1961.
28. Christensen, A.K., J. Cell Biol. 26: 911, 1956.
29. Braun, T., and Sepenwol, W., Endocrinology 94: 1028, 1974.
30. Swerdloff, R.S., Walsh, P.C., Jacobs, H.S., and Odell, W.D., Endocrinology 88: 120, 1971.

FOLLICLE STIMULATING HORMONE AND CYCLIC AMP DIRECTED CHANGES IN

ULTRASTRUCTURE AND PROPERTIES OF CULTURED SERTOLI CELL-ENRICHED

PREPARATIONS: COMPARISON WITH CULTURED TESTICULAR PERITUBULAR CELLS

Pierre S. Tung and Irving B. Fritz

Banting and Best Department of Medical Research,
University of Toronto, Toronto, Canada   M5G 1L6

INTRODUCTION

In a previous communication, we reported that addition of
follicle stimulating hormone (FSH) or dibutyryl cyclic AMP (dcAMP)
elicited pronounced structural changes in Sertoli cell-enriched preparations cultured in a serum-free defined medium (1).

We now provide additional information on the properties and
ultrastructure of these cells, and demonstrate several criteria
which strengthenoour conclusion that the cultured preparations consist
primarily of Sertoli cells. We shall also compare the structure
and properties of cultured testicular peritubular cells with those
of Sertoli cells.

MATERIALS AND METHODS

Cell Preparations

The Sertoli cells were isolated from testes of 20 day old
rats, and were cultured in a defined medium by methods described
in detail elsewhere (1,2). Peritubular cells were prepared from
comparable testes. Following the last of the previously described
sequential enzymatic treatments of the tubule segments with
collagenase (1), the supernatant fraction was freed of debris by
centrifugation at 60 g for 4 mins. Cells in the resulting supernatant fraction were collected by centrifugation at 60 g for 6 mins,
resuspended, washed with Hanks' buffer and then plated at a density
of 2-4 x 10^4 cells per dish. The identical treatment employed in
isolation of Sertoli cell-enriched preparations was used here, with

the exception that cells released into the supernatant fraction
were cultured.

Culture Conditions

Primary cultures of Sertoli cells were maintained as described
previously (2). Testicular peritubular cells were cultured in
supplemented minimal essential medium (MEM) with the addition of 10%
calf serum (1,2). The medium was changed every 2 days. After 6
days in culture, essentially all germ cells had detached. Subcultures were then prepared in the following manner. The cultures
were treated with 0.05% trypsin (Grand Island Biological) and
0.02% EDTA in Hanks' buffer, deprived of calcium and magnesium,
according to the procedure of Owens (3). Fibroblast-like cells were
detached during this treatment, while epithelial cells, if any, remained attached to the surface of the culture vessel. Material in
the suspending medium was centrifuged at 60 g for 4 min to sediment
debris. Fibroblast-like cells remaining in the supernatant fraction
were collected by further centrifugation at 360 g for 6 min, resuspended and washed in Hanks buffer. These cells were then plated
in the MEM, plus or minus 10% calf serum, at a density of 2-4 x 10^4
cells per dish for subculture.

Preparations of all cell types were incubated for varying
periods of time in the presence or absence of hormones or other
agents described in Results.

Morphological techniques used in this study were the same as
those described previously (1).

RESULTS AND DISCUSSION

Initial Partial Purification of Testicular Cell Preparations

Scanning and transmission electron micrographs of the
testicular preparations after different stages of sequential enzyme
treatment are shown in Figs. 1 and 2. After trypsin digestion, the
seminiferous tubule segments were free of interstitial elements
and blood vessels. After subsequent treatment with collagenase,
the washed tubules were essentially free of peritubular elements
(Figs. 1A-G and 2A-C). Finally, after agitation with a Pasteur
pipette, the tubular fragments were dispersed into aggregates
containing primarily Sertoli cells and germinal cells (Figs. 1H
and I and 2C). These Sertoli cell-enriched aggregates were plated
and cultured as described above.

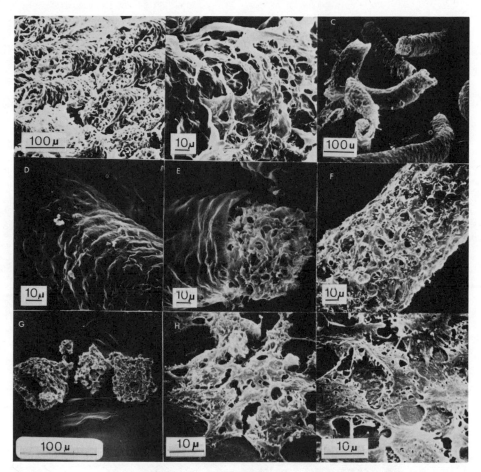

Figure 1.   Scanning electron micrographs of seminiferous tubule
fragments prior to and at different stages during sequential enzymatic
treatments.   (A) Crude testicular preparation after mincing (0.5mm),
illustrating segments of seminiferous tubules and masses of interstitial elements (x360).   (B) A higher magnification (x1,200) of a
seminiferous tubule segment, showing the external surface of the
lamina propria and attached endothelial cells.   (C) Testicular preparation after trypsin digestion and subsequent washing.   Note
complete removal of interstitial and supratubular material (x240).
(D & E) Segments of seminiferous tubule after trypsin digestion
(x1,200).   (F) A segment of seminiferous tubule after further
digestion with collagenase and subsequent washing, illustrating removal of peritubular elements (x1,200).   (G) Fragments of cell aggregates, ready for plating (x1,200).   (H) A colony of Sertoli cells
cultured 48 hours after plating.   The cavities depicted in this
picture represent space originally occupied by germinal cells (x3,000).
(I) Monolayer of Sertoli cells cultured 4 days after plating (x3,000).

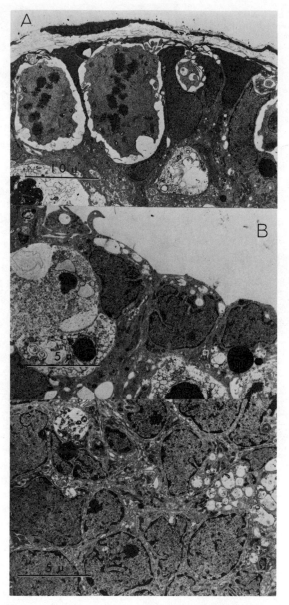

Figure 2.   Representative transmission electron micrographs of
seminiferous tubules at different stages during sequential
enzymatic treatment.   (A) Cross-section of seminiferous tubule
after treatment with trypsin (x1,925).   (B) Cross-section of
seminiferous tubule after collagenase treatment and subsequent
washing (x3,850).   Note removal of peritubular elements.   (C)   A
section of cell aggregate ready for plating (x3,850).

Structural Properties of Sertoli Cells and Peritubular Cells in Culture

With phase microscopy, the mosaic type of cell borders characteristic of epithelial cells was consistently observed in Sertoli cell-enriched cultures maintained in 10% calf serum (Fig. 3A). The cultured cells are not shaped as elongated columnar epithelium cells, characteristically seen in situ, but instead appear squamous. As the Sertoli cells migrated from the initially plated aggregates, they formed a relatively flat monolayer. Once the monolayer was established, the cells were never observed to form a criss-crossing or multilayered structure. The mitotic index during the first 6 days of culture was lower than 0.03% in MEM alone or in MEM containing calf serum, as measured in cells treated with colcemid (0.5 µg/ml) for 6 hrs (1).

Subcultures of testicular peritubular cells showed fibroblast-like characteristics. The peripheral cytoplasm of these cells was markedly extended into web-like structures, thus assuming a polyhedral form. Binucleated cells were occasionally encountered in cultures which were in exponential growth, and polynucleated up to hexanucleated cells have been noted in cells cultured for periods longer than 2 weeks. In contrast to the cultured Sertoli cell-enriched preparation, peritubular cells frequently criss-crossed and formed multilayers in culture (Fig. 3B). After reaching confluence, the cells in the multilayer continued to multiply along randomly arrayed axes. This resulted in the formation of ridges with diameters up to 200 µ (Fig. 3C). The mitotic index of subcultured cells in MEM containing 10% calf serum ranged from 0.8 to 1.8% during the first 6 days.

Ultrastructural Properties of Sertoli Cells and Peritubular Cells in Culture

Sertoli cells cultured in MEM containing 10% calf serum were observed to have many of the ultrastructural characteristics of Sertoli cells in situ described by Flickinger (4), Dym (5) and Fawcett (6). The unique tight junction with its associated cisterna between two Sertoli cells is illustrated in Fig. 4A. The characteristic Sertoli cell nucleolar structure, containing an electron dense well-delineated central element and more diffuse satellite structures (pars granularis, pars fibrilaris and pars amorpha), is shown in Fig. 4B. Other characteristic ultrastructural features were consistently observed in ultrathin sections of cultured Sertoli cells, including an elaborate Golgi apparatus (Fig. 4C), frequent lipid droplets, a perinuclear layer of microfilaments, an indented pleomorphic nucleus, a well-developed smooth endoplasmic reticulum and evidence of phagocytosis of foreign objects.

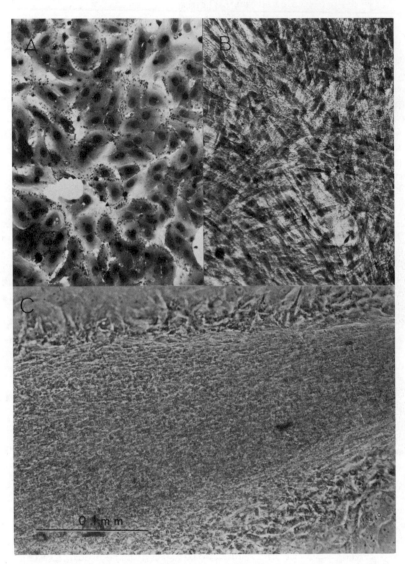

Figure 3.   Light photomicrographs of Sertoli cell-enriched preparations
(A) and peritubular cell preparations (B and C) cultured in MEM plus
10% calf serum (x300).   The mosaic-type cell borders and monolayer-
forming behavior of Sertoli cell-enriched preparations maintained
in culture for 6 days are depicted in "A"; "B" shows multi-layer-
forming behavior of peritubular cells cultured for 6 days; "C" shows
a representative large ridge-like structure, formed by subcultured
peritubular cells maintained for 10 days.

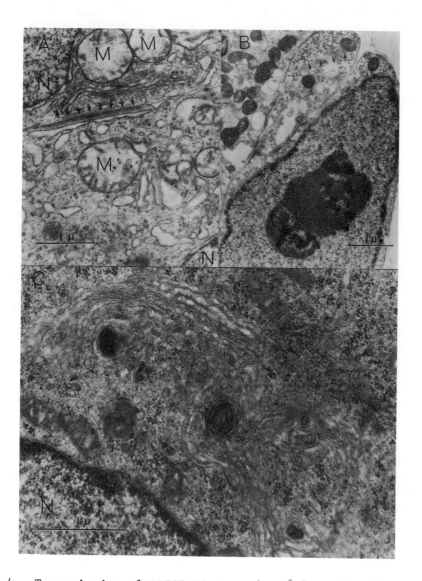

Fig. 4. Transmission electron micrographs of Sertoli cell-enriched preparations maintained for 6 days in MEM supplemented with 10% calf serum. A: Characteristic tight junctions are indicated by arrowheads, (N-nuclei, M-mitochondria) (x15,400); B: Detail of a nucleus showing the characteristic nucleolus and its 2 karyosomes (x12,070); arrowheads indicate cross sections of microtubules. C: Golgi complex in Sertoli cell (x24,200).

In contrast, peritubular cells maintained in culture under comparable condition had features similar to those described by Bressler and Ross (7) for fibroblasts and myoid cells from rat testis. The fine structures frequently observed in cultured peritubular cells included the dilated profiles of granular endo-plasmic reticulum and free ribosomes (Fig. 5B), along with membrane-bound electron dense bodies which occasionally give the appearance of autophagy (Fig. 5A). In addition, parallel arrays of fine filaments, similar to those reported in smooth muscle cells (8), were observed in the cultured peritubular cells. These filaments were oriented parallel to the long axis of the cell and were localized in the peripheral cytoplasm immediately below the plasma membrane (Fig. 5C). Interfilamentous dense bands similar to those present in smooth muscle cells (8) were associated with these filaments. The ultrastructural features described in these cultured peritubular cells in the polyhedral shape suggest their contractile nature, and indicate that they may be partially differ-entiated peritubular myoid cells.

Structural and Ultrastructural Responses of Cultured Cells to FSH or dcAMP

In our previous publication, data were presented showing the appearance of Sertoli cells cultured in the absence and presence of FSH in a defined medium (1). In FSH-treated preparations, cell nuclei appeared darker, in association with changes in cell shape, the surrounding cytoplasm appeared scant, and multiple cytoplasmic extensions were evident (1). Identical effects have been obtained when a 50X more highly purified preparation of FSH (contributed kindly by Dr. H. Papkoff) was used at concentrations of 0.05 to 0.2 µg/ml (data not shown). Even more striking effects of the same qualitative sort were observed in cells cultured in the presence of 0.1 mM dcAMP. Moreover, these morphological responses could be reverted to normal form in standard culture medium supple-mented with 10% calf serum. The morphological changes induced by FSH were not duplicated in cells cultured in the presence of luteinizing hormone (LH) (NIH S-18 ovine LH) at concentrations up to 10 µg/ml, or in the presence of 1 mM 5'-AMP or 0.1 mM sodium butyrate (1). Parallel experiments have now been performed with testicular peri-tubular cells, prepared as described in Methods. Fibroblasts from other sources are known to respond to dcAMP with striking mor-phological changes (9,10). Similar effects were obtained with our preparations of testicular peritubular cells. In contrast, there was no detectable effect of FSH, under all culture conditions employed, on the structure of any of the testicular peritubular preparations cultured. FSH-treated cells looked exactly like those of untreated cells shown in Fig. 3B. From these studies, we conclude that structural changes elicited in cultured Sertoli cells by FSH (1) cannot be induced in peritubular cells under all conditions employed thus far.

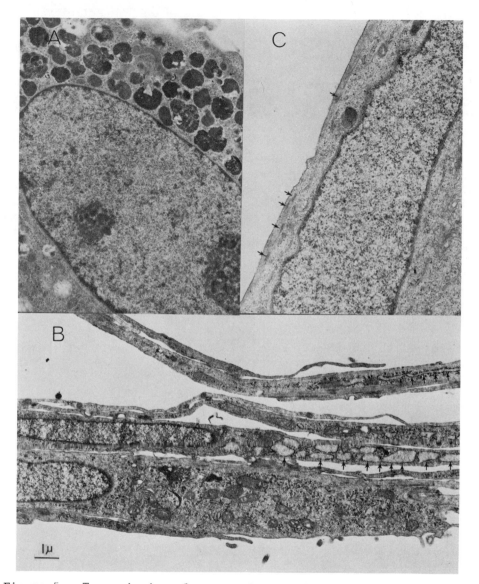

Figure 5.   Transmission electron micrographs of peritubular cells
grown for 6 days in MEM supplemented with 10% calf serum (x10,800).
A: A horizontal section showing membrane-bound electron dense bodies
in the cytoplasm.   B: A vertical section showing arrays of
filaments near the upper plasma membrane and the interfilamentous
dense bands (arrows).   C: Vertical sections of scraped cells showing
dilated profiles of granular endoplasmic reticulum in the cytoplasm immediately below the plasma membrane (arrows) and free ribosomes (x52,800).

Transmission electron microscopic studies of FSH-stimulated Sertoli cells revealed arrays of microtubules which are oriented parallel to the long axis of the cytoplasmic extensions (Fig. 6). A marked increase in free ribosomes was also evident throughout the cytoplasm of stimulated cells (Fig. 6 inset). Investigations are in progress to clarify whether such structural alterations are related in an obligatory fashion to biochemical functions stimulated in these cells, such as the synthesis and secretion of androgen binding protein (11,12).

The biochemical properties of Sertoli cell-enriched cultures, prepared in a manner similar to that described here, have been described elsewhere. The influences of FSH and dcAMP on androgen binding protein formation (11,12), incorporation of amino acids into protein (2) and steroid metabolism (13,14) have been investigated. All biochemical and morphological effects thus far elicited in these cells by FSH have been duplicated by addition of cAMP or dcAMP. These data are consistent with the hypothesis that FSH biological actions on Sertoli cells may be mediated by cAMP, since it is established that FSH addition to enriched Sertoli cell preparations from several sources results in increased cAMP formation (2,15,16).

Kodani and Kodani (17) reported that Sertoli cells were able to migrate from segments of seminiferous tubules maintained in organ culture, and could become attached as a monolayer to the incubation vessel. Their claim that populations of Sertoli cells could be maintained in culture indefinitely (17) was challenged by Steinberger et al. (18). The criticisms were based on the absence of an un-equivocal ultrastructural identification of the cell type being cultured, and the occurrence of frequent mitosis. Sertoli cells in rat testis in vivo cease mitosis by the 14th day of life (18-20). Steinberger et al. (18) suggested that the cell being cultured by Kodani and Kodani (17) may have been derived from other testicular elements, perhaps from fibroblasts or peritubular cells.

It is unlikely however, that peritubular cells or fibroblasts are present in Sertoli cell cultures described in the present communication, since they were stripped from the tubule following trypsin and collagenase digestion and dispersal (Fig. 1F). If an appreciable number of these cells were present, a markedly higher mitotic index should have been obtained. Testicular peritubular cell-preparations cultured in MEM containing serum were in fact shown to have a high mitotic rate. Germinal cells were present in the initial Sertoli cell aggregates, comprising up to 30% of the total cells at the time of preparation. Isolated germinal cells did not adhere to the surface of the vessels, in agreement with earlier observations by Kodani and Kodani (17). Those germinal cells which were trapped within the aggregates in culture were largely removed

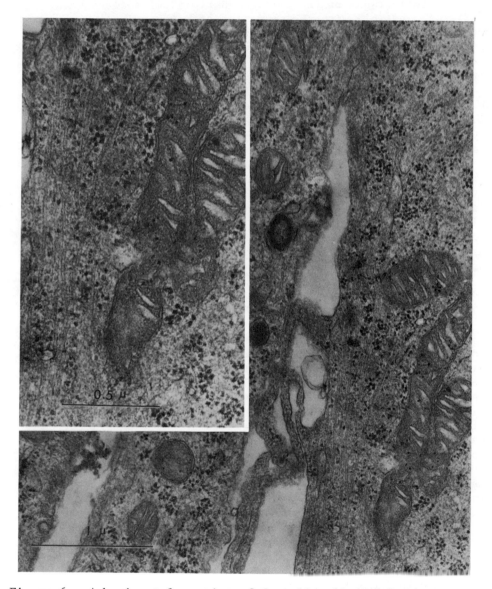

Figure 6. A horizontal section of Sertoli cell-enriched preparations maintained for 6 days in MEM and treated with 5 µg/ml
NIH S-10 ovine FSH during the last 24 hrs (x32,676); Inset: Higher
magnification of portion of the same section showing abundant
microtubules oriented parallel to the long axis of the cytoplasmic
extension, and free ribosomes (x52,800).

by washing the preparations which had been in culture for 48 hrs. The low mitotic index of the cultured Sertoli cells (less than 0.03%) is compatible with the cessation of mitosis in vivo of Sertoli cells by the 14th day of life in rats (18-20). From our differential cell counts, combined with other observations reported, we conclude that about 90% of cells in the Sertoli cell-enriched cultures are Sertoli cells (12). Further, they respond to FSH in ways consistent with the response of Sertoli cells in vivo to FSH. The increased rate of formation of ABP by isolated cells stimulated with FSH (11,12) supports the previous deductions from in vivo data that FSH increases ABP production in testis via stimulation of Sertoli cells (11,21-23).

Recently, Welsh and Wiebe (24) reported observations on "Rat Sertoli cells: A rapid method for obtaining viable cells", in which alternate procedures were employed to isolate Sertoli cell-enriched preparations for culture. These authors, working independently, employed sequential treatment of testes with collagenase and pancreatin, followed by sedimentation of cells through a sucrose density gradient.

SUMMARY AND CONCLUSIONS

Sertoli cell-enriched preparations, isolated from testes of 20 day old rats and maintained in primary culture in a defined medium, have been shown to respond to follicle stimulating hormone (FSH), cyclic AMP or dibutyryl cyclic AMP with characteristic morphological changes. The preparations form a monolayer of cells having a relatively uniform structure in which approximately 90% of the cells appear similar when cultured for 4 days or more. They have been identified as Sertoli cells by recognition of unique ultrastructural features, including the presence of tight junctions, in electron micrographs of the preparations. The structures of these cells have been examined with phase-contrast microscopy, scanning electron microscopy and transmission electron microscopy. With all these techniques employed, the appearance and properties of the Sertoli cell-enriched preparations have been shown to differ from those of cultured testicular peritubular cells. The Sertoli cell-enriched preparations, cultured in 10% calf serum in MEM, have a low mitotic index (less than 0.03%), whereas the peritubular cells have a mitotic index ranging from 0.8 to 2.2% when cultured under similar conditions. Peritubular cells frequently formed multilayers in culture, and criss-crossed each other. This behavior was not observed in Sertoli cell-enriched cultures. The fine structures observed in the cultured peritubular cells are reported, and are shown to differ from those in cultured Sertoli cell-enriched preparations. Peritubular cell structures were not altered following addition of FSH to the medium, under all conditions employed.

Thus, we conclude that these cultured cells are Sertoli cells which clearly differ from testicular peritubular cells cultured in parallel experiments.

Some of this information was presented at a poster session at the 1974 Cell Biology meetings (25).

LIST OF ABBREVIATIONS

FSH - follicle stimulating hormone; LH - luteinizing hormone; cAMP - 3'5-cyclic adenosine monophosphate; dcAMP - dibutyryl cAMP; MEM - supplemented Eagle's minimal essential medium (2); ABP - androgen binding protein.

ACKNOWLEDGEMENTS

We are indebted to Ms. Krystyna Burdzy and Ms. Edna Cartwright for excellent technical assistance, to Ernest Whitter for transmission electron micrographs and to Eric Lin for scanning electron micrographs. We also wish to thank Dr. Martin Dym for useful discussions on the structural characteristics of Sertoli cells, and for his many suggestions. The considerable importance of continuing dialogues with our colleagues, especially Dr. J.H. Dorrington, is gratefully acknowledged. We thank Mrs. Erene Stanley for typing the manuscript.

REFERENCES

1. Tung, P.S., Dorrington, J.H., and Fritz, I.B., Proc. Nat. Acad. Sci. (US), 1975 (in press).
2. Dorrington, J.H., Roller, N.F. and Fritz, I.B., Molec. Cell Endocrinol., 1975 (in press).
3. Owens, R.B., J. Nat. Cancer Inst., 52:1375, 1974.
4. Flickinger, C.J., Z. Zellforsch. Mikroskop. Anat., 78:92, 1967.
5. Dym, M., Anat. Rec., 175:639, 1973.
6. Fawcett, D.F., The ultrastructure and functions of the Sertoli cell. In: Handbook of Physiology on Male Reproduction, R.O. Greep and D.W. Hamilton (Eds.), Amer. Physiol. Soc., Washington, D.C., 1975, p. 21.
7. Bressler, R.S., and Ross, M.H., Exper. Cell Res., 78:295, 1973.
8. Campbell, G.R., Vehara, Y., Mark, G., and Burnstock, G., J. Cell Biol., 49:21, 1971.
9. Hsie, A.W., and Puck, T.T., PNAS 68:358, 1970.
10. Wahrman, J.P., Winand, R., and Luzzati, D., Nature New Biol., 245:112, 1973.

11. Fritz, I.B., Fommerts, F.G., Louis, B.G., and Dorrington, J.H.,
     J. Reprod. Fertil., 1975 (in press).
12. Fritz, I.B., Louis, B.G., Tung, P.S., Griswold, M., Rommerts,
     F.G., and Dorrington, J.H., this volume, 1975, p.
13. Dorrington, J.H., and Fritz, I.B., Endocrinology, 96: 1975,
     (in press).
14. Armstrong, D., Dorrington, J.H., and Fritz, I.B., This volume,
     1975, p.
15. Dorrington, J.H., and Fritz, I.B., Endocrinology, 94:395, 1974.
16. Means, A.R., Life Sci. 15:371, 1974.
17. Kodani, M., and Kodani, K., Proc. Nat. Acad. Sci., U.S., 56:
     1200, 1966.
18. Steinberger, E., Steinberger, A., and Ficher, M. Rec. Prog.
     Hormone Res., 26:547, 1970.
19. Nagy, F., J. Reprod. Fertil., 28:389, 1972.
20. Clermont, Y., and Perey, B., Am. J. Anat., 100:241, 1957.
21. Vernon, R.G., Kopec, B., and Fritz, I.B., Molec. and Cell.
     Endocrinol., 1:167, 1974.
22. Hansson, V., Trygstad, O., French, F.S., McLean, W.S., Smith,
     A.A., Tindall, D.J., Weddington, S.C., Petrusz, P., Nayfeh, S.M.,
     and Ritzen, E.M., Nature 250:387, 1974.
23. Tindall, D.J., Schrader, W.T., and Means, A.R., The pro-
     duction of androgen binding protein by Sertoli cells. In:
     Hormone Binding and Target Cell Activation in the Testis,
     M.L. Dufau and A.R. Means (Eds.), New York: Plenum Press,
     1974, p. 167.
24. Welsh, M.J., and Wiebe, J.P., Endocrinology, 96:618, 1975.
25. Tung, P.S., Dorrington, J., Rommerts, F., and Fritz, I.B.,
     J. Cell Biol., 63:353a, 1974.

POSSIBLE BOUNDARY TISSUE FUNCTION IN ISOLATED SEMINIFEROUS TUBULES

Robert S. Bressler

Department of Anatomy

Mount Sinai School of Medicine of the City University
of New York, Fifth Avenue & 100th Street, New York, N.Y.
10029

In view of the expanding use of isolated tubule preparations
since their introduction by Christensen and Mason (1), it may be
appropriate to consider the composition of such preparations. It
is frequently implied that the only functional components in tubules devoid of Leydig cells are the Sertoli cells and germinal
elements. It is the purpose of these remarks to focus attention
on the boundary tissue of the seminiferous tubules and the possibility that peritubular elements may be important participants of
tubular metabolism and physiology.

Several of the papers included in this book have indicated that
the younger the testis, the more difficult it is to separate the
tubules from the interstitial tissue. This is not surprising if
one considers the architecture of the interstitial compartment in
the early postnatal rat and mouse testis. Instead of a well defined double layer of cells such as that found in the adult, the
seminiferous cords of the newborn are surrounded by a homogeneous
population of polyhedral cells which grade to more flattened forms
further into the interstitium. (Fig. 1) Thus, there is no distinct
boundary between the peritubular cells and the interstitial elements
such as that provided by the lymphatic vessels described in the adult
(2) and along which a plane of separation is easily established.
It is probable that seminiferous tubules isolated from young
animals carry along a significant number of adjacent fibroblast-
like cells, some of which may be precursors of the Leydig cells
which ultimately populate the interstitium.

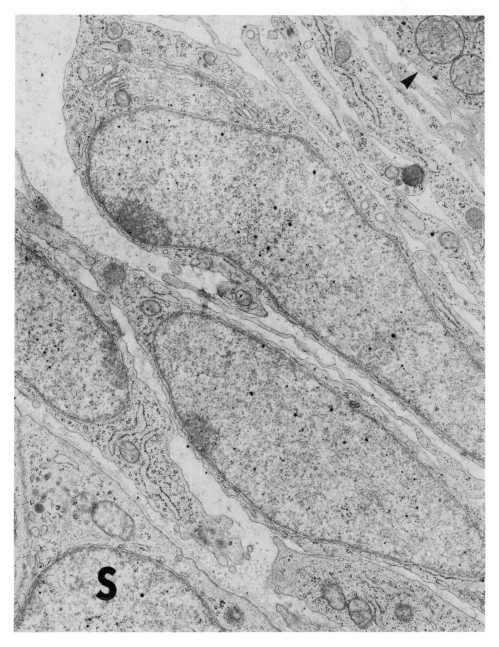

Figure 1. The edge of a seminiferous cord of a newborn mouse is
seen at the lower left hand corner (S) and part of a Leydig cell
at the upper right (arrowhead). Several layers of fibroblast-like
cells lie between them. x 15,100.

In the adult it is possible to achieve an apparently clean separation of seminiferous tubules. However, the possible existence of steroid metabolizing cells within the boundary tissue cannot be ignored. In studies of rabbit testicular tissue transplanted to ear chambers, Williams (3) described the appearance of new Leydig cells from fibroblast-like cells on the surface of some tubules. Subsequently, Fawcett and Burgos (4) reported electron microscopic observations consistent with the hypothesis that new Leydig cells arise from spindle shaped precursors associated with, and not readily distinguishable from cells in the lamina propria. The boundary tissue of seminiferous tubules in culture readily give rise to monolayers of cells (5,6), some of which have been shown to metabolize steroid (6).

These observations emphasize the danger of neglecting the possible activity of boundary tissue cells when drawing conclusions based on isolated seminiferous tubules. They also indicate the need for additional studies of preparations of isolated boundary tissue to determine its possible roles in tubular function.

REFERENCES

1. Christiansen, A.K. and Mason, N.R., Endocr. 76: 646, 1965.

2. Fawcett, D.W., heidger P.M. and Leah, L.V., J. Reprod. Fert. 19: 109, 1969.

3. Williams, R.G., Am. J. Anat. 86: 343, 1950.

4. Fawcett, D.W. and Burgos, M.H., Am. J. Anat. 107: 245, 1960.

5. Bressler, R.S. and Ross, M.H., Exp. Cell Res. 78: 295, 1973.

6. Dufau, M.L., de Kretser, D.M. and Hudson, B., Endocr. 88: 825, 1971.

CONFERENCE SUMMARY

H. J. van der Molen

Department of Biochemistry (Chemical Endocrinology)
Medical Faculty, Erasmus University Rotterdam,
The Netherlands

The second annual workshop on the testis was intended to
discuss the most recent information on steroid production and
metabolism in the seminiferous tubules and on the hormonal regulation of seminiferous tubular function. In this short summary,
I have arbitrarily selected several aspects that have emerged
from the discussions and which concern:

- some analytical/technical aspects
- the production of steroids by various cell types of the testis
- factors influencing testicular steroid production
- established characteristics of Sertoli cells
- steroids and the regulation of spermatogenesis

The main guideline for this selection has been a conviction that
correct answers to questions regarding biological problems cannot
be established without detailed information regarding the significance of experimental results, particularly when different technical
approaches tend to result in seemingly conflicting information.

Proper appreciation of the limitation of techniques is required
to prevent the implications that different data are unreconcilable.
A good case in point are the results that were presented on the
occurrence and distribution of 5α-reductase activity and 5α-reduced
steroids in testis. The seemingly conflicting results reported by
Rivarola, Dorrington and van der Molen can only be compared if
proper consideration is given to the different conditions that were
employed, i.e., the use of dissected tissue preparations without
any additions incubated with small amounts of substrate (Rivarola),
versus cultured intact Sertoli cells incubated with approximately

513

1×10^{-6}M testosterone (Dorrington), versus homogenized tissue preparations in the presence of added cofactors incubated with enzyme
saturating amounts of substrate (Van der Molen).

Another example that experimental conditions may influence the
results obtained was presented by Tamaoki, who after solubilization
of the microsomal 17β-hydroxysteroid dehydrogenase observed inhibition of the purified enzyme by testosterone rather than stimulation
which occurs with the microsomal enzyme preparation. It may also
help the comparison of results from different laboratories by ex-
pressing results of enzyme activities in enzyme units (μmol/min/per
mg protein). Although such activities for intact cells or unpurified
enzymes have no real biochemical meaning such standardization would
at least provide a basis for comparing differences in activity between different preparations.

A final technical comment concerning the interpretation of biochemical results may re-emphasize the discussion during the meeting
that the demonstration of steroid metabolizing enzyme activities
in testis tissues does not always imply a significant steroid production. In this respect observations presented by Armstrong
et al. on oestradiol-17β formation from added testosterone by
cultured Sertoli cells clearly demonstrate the potential for aromatization of testosterone in Sertoli cells. These results also show
that without added testosterone, and FSH or cyclic AMP little oestradiol was produced in cultured Sertoli cells. These observations
will certainly stimulate further work on the possible origin of
testicular oestrogens including measurement of both enzyme
activities and pool sizes of the steroids involved. Similar studies
will also be stimulated by Rivarola's observations on the distribution and the development with age of 5α-reductase activity and
5α-reduced androstane steroids in testis.

Possibilities were discussed for establishing morphological
criteria which might support the purity of a cell culture, the
purity of a subcellular fraction and changes in the morphology as
a result of experimental treatment. Although several electron
microscopic techniques are presently available (including standard
and scanning EM-cytochemistry involving capture reactions, autoradiography and labeling with antibodies - freeze cleaving - mor-
phometry), there was general agreement that light microscopy with
whole field observations, and low power pictures in general, are
also most revealing for evaluation of the morphologic quality of
cell preparations.

STEROIDS PRODUCED BY THE VARIOUS CELL TYPES OF THE TESTIS

One of the most interesting observations was the finding reported by Armstrong et al. of aromatization of testosterone in

Sertoli cells, which appears to be influenced by FSH and cyclic AMP.
Ewing showed that in the rabbit 5α-reduced steroid secretion clearly
originates from testicular testosterone and does not involve de
novo steroid production in the epididymis. Although the presence
of several steroid metabolizing enzyme activities (5α-reductase, 3α/
3β-dehydrogenases) in seminiferous tubules and Sertoli cells was
reported, it was also discussed that enzyme activities required
for de novo testicular testosterone production are mainly present
in the interstitium (Van der Molen, Purvis, Menard, Dorrington).
Christensen pointed at the possibility that macrophages occurring
in the interstitium and which are occasionally difficult to distinguish from Leydig cells, might also metabolize steroids.

There was general agreement that in the rat (Setchell, Bartke)
the profile and concentrations of steroids in rete testis fluid
were similar to those in testicular venous blood. It is also of
interest (Bartke) that the maintenance of spermatogenesis in hypophysectomized rats correlates well with steroid levels in rete
testis fluid and that FSH in this respect might possibly potentiate
the effect of LH on testosterone production which would result in
increased levels of testosterone in rete testis fluid rather than
in blood. Ritzen et al. have shown a good correlation of the concentrations of testosterone and dihydrotestosterone with the
concentration of ABP in rabbit rete testis fluid, indicating a
possible role of ABP in the seminiferous tubular accumulation of
androgen as well as the transport of androgen to the epididymis.

FACTORS INFLUENCING TESTICULAR STEROID PRODUCTION

Setchell emphasized the importance of a "blood-testis
barrier" and demonstrated from elegant analyses of steroids in
rete testis fluid, blood and testicular lymph that different steroids
do penetrate tubular tissue at different rates. Whereas testosterone and dehydroepiandrosterone show a rapid transfer into
rete testis fluid, dihydrotestosterone, oestradiol-17β and cortisol
show a much slower entry, and cholesterol does not enter at all.

In addition to the "blood-testis barrier", several other
barriers which might affect free diffusion of steroids through
the testis were also discussed.

Free showed some provocative data of a counter current
mechanism in steroid transfer from the venous effluent through
the pampiniform plexis into the testicular arterial blood. The
increase of steroid concentrations in testicular arterial blood
makes it theoretically unattractive to use peripheral plasma
levels of steroids rather than testicular arterial levels when
calculating steroid production rates from venous arterial
differences. This counter current steroid transfer may not be

ubiquitous among all species, but these differences do not appear to
relate to the presence of testosterone binding globulin (TeBG).

Some new effects of LH and FSH on steroid production and
metabolism were presented. Addition of FSH to cultured Sertoli cell
preparations increased the formation of cAMP, ABP (Dorrington and
Fritz), and stimulated the aromatization of testosterone (Armstrong
et al.). The rate of conversion of testosterone to oestradiol in
Sertoli cells appeared to be stimulated only by FSH or cAMP and not
by LH. A combination of a stimulating effect of LH on the conversion
of cholesterol to testosterone in the Leydig cell and of FSH on the
Sertoli cells might suggest a synergistic effect of LH and FSH on
testicular oestradiol-17β production in situations when testosterone
production would be rate limiting.

Some of the effects of trophic stimulation on 5α-reductase as
discussed by Nayfeh again emphasized the importance in considering
the proper conditions of animals used and the quality, duration and
mode of administration of LH and FSH. Depending on the time after
hypophysectomy Nayfeh reported an unexpected stimulatory effect of
LH on 5α-reduction in whole testis homogenates and of FSH on this
enzyme activity in isolated interstitial tissue from immature rats.
In experiments reported by Dorrington 5α-reductase in isolated seminiferous tubules and Sertoli cells from mature rats appeared not to
be affected by gonadotrophins. This might indicate an age difference
in response or a mediating function of other testis cell types for
the effects of FSH and LH on 5α-reductase as reported by Nayfeh.

A possible role of prolactin in regulating steroid production,
was not discussed during the workshop and the possible role of
ABP in this regard was only speculated upon but not tested.

BINDING PROTEINS AND RECEPTORS

There is now evidence that the androgen binding protein (ABP)
and an androgen receptor are both present, and probably produced,
in Sertoli cells (French, Fritz, Mulder). The best supporting
evidence since the 1974 meeting in Houston was presented by Fritz
et al. for ABP production in cultures of isolated Sertoli cells.
The different characteristics of testicular androgen binding
protein (ABP) and the testicular androgen receptor were discussed
by French and coworkers. Means showed for the prenatally irradiated
male rat a close correlation between the effect of FSH on
testicular ABP and effects of FSH on parameters that are now
generally believed to be involved in the action of trophic
hormones such as cAMP, protein kinase, RNA polymerase and protein
synthesis. Apart from such correlations nothing is known about
the precise interrelationships between these parameters and ABP
production. Other studies (French, Mulder) also reported on androgen
receptors in testes of prenatally irradiated rats. In this respect

the gradually developing custom to call the prenatally irradiated
male rat a "Sertoli Cell Only" (SCO) rat might be discouraged.
Germ cells are clearly reduced or absent in the testes of such
irradiated rats, and there is a relative preponderance of
Sertoli cells. However, all other cells including Leydig cells and
peritubular elements are still present, so that the indication
"Sertoli Cell Only" is clearly a misnomer.

A comparison of the effects of FSH on the production of ABP
in different experimental in vivo or in vitro models shows
interesting differences which require further explanation.
Whereas Means for prenatally irradiated rats observed a maximal
stimulation of i.v. administered FSH on ABP already after 2 h, the
effects of FSH reported by Hansson in hypophysectomized rats,
Ritzen in cultured tissue and Fritz in Sertoli cell cultures were
much slower. Also the lack of a clear effect of testicular
testosterone on ABP production by some groups in contrast with the
clear stimulation of epididymal ABP observed after testosterone
treatment by Hansson et al. indicates that a proper comparison
of the turnover of ABP in different systems and/or under different
conditions is required. This appears particularly important
in selecting a proper system for the study of the possible
biological action(s) of ABP.

If many details of the physiology of testicular ABP remain
to be resolved, even less is known about the significance of the
testicular androgen receptor, which is present in the seminiferous
tubules, probably in Sertoli cells (Mulder, French). The presence
of an androgen receptor also in testis interstitial tissue cannot
be ruled out on basis of the presently available information
(French , Mulder). Sar and coworkers showed autoradiographic
evidence that after administration of labeled testosterone
and dihydrotestosterone radioactivity was clearly localized over
nuclei of interstitial tissue. The need to consider in addition
to the mere presence of steroid receptors also the possible
function of such receptors in steroid action was emphasized by
Bardin. Apart from the occurrence of this receptor there is,
however, no experimentally verified evidence for its possible
function.

ESTABLISHED CHARACTERISTICS OF SERTOLI CELLS

Steroid metabolism and regulation of the function of the
seminiferous tubules were main topics of the workshop, but most of
the discussion in this respect was concentrated around one single
cell type of the seminiferous tubules, i.e., the Sertoli cells.
Although possible functions of Sertoli cells have been inferred
for many years from microscopic observations, it is only in the last

few years that several biochemical parameters have been studied in
Sertoli cells. The role and function of Sertoli cells as discussed during the workshop include: nutrition and other interactions with germ cells, phagocytosis, secretion of ABP and other
proteins, several enzyme activities for steroid metabolism, androgen
receptors, cAMP production, protein kinase, RNA polymerase,
thymidine incorporation into DNA, protein synthesis and the effects
of trophic hormones (mainly FSH) on these parameters. The incorporation of thymidine into nuclei of Sertoli cells of 20 and 30
day old rats without cell division and the increase of this incorporation under the influence of FSH and dibutyryl cAMP as
reported by Fritz et al. requires further investigation. It is
important to determine the mechanisms involved since the absence
of cell division is considered (A. Steinberger) an important
criterion in establishing the purity of Sertoli cells from rats
older than 15 days.

REGULATION OF SPERMATOGENESIS

    Despite the wealth of morphologic and biochemical parameters
of testis function, no significant breakthrough has yet emerged
concerning the biochemical mechanism of hormonal regulation of
spermatogenesis. This may be due partly to the lack of information
about the detailed biochemistry of the different cell types during
development of spermatogenesis. In this respect it would be
surprising if any of the relatively rapid effects of hormones which
were discussed during the workshop can ultimately explain the cell
differentiation during spermatogenesis. It appears more likely
that initiation as well as maintenance of spermatogenesis could
depend on the continuous presence or absence of hormonal stimuli
rather than on rapid fluctuations. Huckin's observation, that
the formation of tight junctions between Sertoli cells is not
dependent on the presence of germ cells may be significant. This
observation may offer a simpler model for the biochemical evaluation
of the formation of such tight junctions which have often been
inferred as important for development of spermatogenesis. This
model might offer an opportunity to study the now well-known correlation between the arrest of spermatogenesis and Sertoli cell
production of ABP following hypophysectomy.

    Steroid involvement in the regulation of spermatogenesis has
become more complicated now that it is known that androgen
production occurs mainly in the interstitial compartment but
androgen receptors are present mainly in the seminiferous tubules,
wheras Sertoli cells may have the capacity for oestradiol-17β
production while a receptor for oestradiol-17β has only been
demonstrated in interstitial tissue.

The wealth of new information presented at the workshop provoked many hours of fruitful discussion, resulting not only in the formulation of new questions, but also in an evaluation of the priority and meaning of "established" facts. The object of <u>Dr. Sherins</u> and the planning committee in providing a forum for the exchange of the most recent observations on testis function, particularly of the seminiferous tubules was most certainly achieved. One of the other valuable aspects of the workshop was the opportunity to discuss both scientific and other problems during the excellent social program which was extremely well organized by <u>Drs. French, Nayfeh</u> and colleagues. The success of both the planning committee and the local committee left the participants in no doubt about the desirability of continuing this annual testis workshop next year and the years to come.

ACKNOWLEDGEMENTS

The responsibility for the (arbitrary) selection of topics for this summary rests completely with the author, who is, however, most grateful to Drs. Frank French, Irving Fritz and Dick Sherins for their comments and corroboration of the factual information.

INDEX

(Listed by Chapter Numbers)

A

B